Early Brain Damage

Volume 2
Neurobiology and Behavior

BEHAVIORAL BIOLOGY

AN INTERNATIONAL SERIES

Series editors

James L. McGaugh

Department of Psychobiology
University of California
Irvine, California

John C. Fentress

Department of Psychology
Dalhousie University
Halifax, Canada

Joseph P. Hegmann

Department of Zoology
The University of Iowa
Iowa City, Iowa

Holger Ursin, Eivind Baade, and Seymour Levine (Editors), Psychobiology of Stress: A Study of Coping Men

William W. Grings and Michael E. Dawson, Emotions and Bodily Responses: A Psychophysiological Approach

Enoch Callaway, Patricia Tueting, and Stephen H. Koslow (Editors), Event Related Brain Potentials in Man

Larry L. Butcher (Editor), Cholinergic–Monoaminergic Interactions in the Brain

Aryeh Routtenberg (Editor), Biology of Reinforcement: Facets of Brain-Stimulation Reward

Richard N. Aslin, Jeffrey R. Alberts, and Michael R. Petersen (Editors), Development of Perception: Psychobiological Perspectives. Vol. 1: Audition, Somatic Perception, and the Chemical Senses; Vol. 2: The Visual System

Joe L. Martinez, Jr., Robert A. Jensen, Rita B. Messing, Henk Rigter, and James L. McGaugh (Editors), Endogenous Peptides and Learning and Memory Processes

James W. Maas (Editor), MHPG: Basic Mechanisms and Psychopathology

Harman V. S. Peeke and Lewis Petrinovich (Editors), Habituation, Sensitization, and Behavior

C. Robert Almli and Stanley Finger (Editors), Early Brain Damage, Volume 1: Research Orientations and Clinical Observations

Stanley Finger and C. Robert Almli (Editors), Early Brain Damage, Volume 2: Neurobiology and Behavior

In preparation

Martin Reite and Tiffany Field (Editors), The Psychobiology of Attachment
Stanley D. Glick (Editor), Cerebral Lateralization in Nonhuman Species

Early Brain Damage

Volume 2
Neurobiology and Behavior

EDITED BY

STANLEY FINGER
Department of Psychology and Neurobiology Program
Washington University
St. Louis, Missouri

C. ROBERT ALMLI
Programs in Occupational Therapy and Neural Sciences
Departments of Anatomy and Neurobiology,
  Preventive Medicine, and Psychology
Washington University School of Medicine
St. Louis, Missouri

1984

ACADEMIC PRESS, INC.
(Harcourt Brace Jovanovich, Publishers)
Orlando   San Diego   San Francisco   New York   London
Toronto   Montreal   Sydney   Tokyo

To our families:
Wendy, Robbie, and Brad
Sheila, Todd, and Lynn

ACADEMIC PRESS, INC.
Orlando, Florida 32887

United Kingdom Edition published by
ACADEMIC PRESS, INC. (LONDON) LTD.
24/28 Oval Road, London NW1 7DX

Library of Congress Cataloging in Publication Data

Main entry under title.

Early brain damage.

(Behavioral biology)
Order of editors' names reversed on v. 2.
Includes bibliographical references and index.
Contents: v. 1. Research orientations and clinical
observations -- v. 2. Neurobiology and behavior.
1. Brain damaged children. 2. Developmental
neurobiology. 3. Developmental psychobiology.
I. Almli, C. Robert. II. Finger, Stanley. III. Series:
Behavioral biology (New York, N.Y. : 1978) [DNLM:
1. Brain damage, Chronic--In infancy and childhood.
2. Brain injuries--In infancy and childhood. WS 340 E12]
RJ496.B7E27 1984   618.92'8   83-25833
ISBN 0-12-052901-7 (v. 1 : alk. paper)
ISBN 0-12-052902-5 (v. 2 : alk. paper)
PRINTED IN THE UNITED STATES OF AMERICA

84 85 86 87   9 8 7 6 5 4 3 2 1

Contents

I. Anatomy and Physiology

3. **Lesion-Induced Sprouting in the Red Nucleus at the Early Developmental Stage**

   Yutaka Fujito, Shuji Watanabe, Hisashi Kobayashi, and Nakaakira Tsukahara

4. **Multiple Effects of Lesions on Brain Structure in Young Rats**

   Mark R. Rosenzweig, Edward L. Bennett, and Marie Alberti

II. Behavioral Biology

5. **A New Perspective for the Interpretation of Early Brain Damage**

   Robert L. Isaacson and Linda Patia Spear

6. **Early Brain Damage and Time Course of Behavioral Dysfunction: Parallels with Neural Maturation**

   C. Robert Almli

7. **Behavioral and Anatomical Studies of Rats with Complete
or Partial Decortication in Infancy**

Ian Q. Whishaw and Bryan Kolb

8. **Functional Development of the Prefrontal System**

*Arthur J. Nonneman, James V. Corwin, Christie L. Sahley,
and John P. Vicedomini*

9. **The Effects of Early Cerebellar Hemispherectomy in the Rat:
Behavioral, Neuroanatomical, and Electrophysiological Sequelae**

Albert Gramsbergen and Jos IJkema-Paassen

10. **Neonatal Cerebral Hemispherectomy: A Model for Postlesion
Reorganization of the Brain**

Jaime R. Villablanca, J. Wesley Burgess, and Bobby Jo Sonnier

III. Variables Interacting with Early Brain Damage

Contributors

Numbers in parentheses indicate the pages on which the authors' contributions begin.

Marie Alberti (49), Melvin Calvin Laboratory, University of California, Berkeley, California 94720

C. Robert Almli (99), Programs in Occupational Therapy and Neural Sciences, Departments of Anatomy and Neurobiology, Preventive Medicine, and Psychology, Washington University School of Medicine, St. Louis, Missouri 63110

Larry L. Bellinger[1] (269), Department of Physiology, Baylor College of Dentistry, Dallas, Texas 75246

Edward L. Bennett (49), Melvin Calvin Laboratory, University of California, Berkeley, California 94720

Lee L. Bernardis (269), Department of Medicine, State University of New York at Buffalo, Buffalo, New York 14215

J. Wesley Burgess (179), Mental Retardation Research Center, UCLA School of Medicine, Los Angeles, California 90024

[1]Present address: Department of Animal Physiology, University of California, Davis, California 95616.

Richard G. Burright (291), Department of Psychology, and Center for Neurobehavioral Sciences, State University of New York at Binghamton, Binghamton, New York 13901

James V. Corwin (138), Department of Neurology, J. Hillis Miller Health Center, University of Florida College of Medicine, Gainesville, Florida 32610

Peter J. Donovick (291), Department of Psychology and Center for Neurobehavioral Sciences, State University of New York at Binghamton, Binghamton, New York 13901

Francoise Eclancher (349), Laboratoire de Neurobiologie des Comportements, Universite Louis Pasteur, 67000 Strasbourg, France

Stanley Finger (327), Department of Psychology and Neurobiology Program, Washington University, St. Louis, Missouri 63130

Yutaka Fujito[2] (35), Department of Biophysical Engineering, Faculty of Engineering Science, Osaka University, Toyonaka, Osaka 560, Japan

Albert Gramsbergen (155), Department of Developmental Neurology, University Hospital Groningen, 9713 EZ Groningen, The Netherlands

Alfred Heller (17), Department of Pharmacological and Physiological Sciences, University of Chicago, Chicago, Illinois 60637

Philip C. Hoffmann (17), Department of Pharmacological and Physiological Sciences, University of Chicago, Chicago, Illinois 60637

Jos IJkema-Paassen (155), Department of Developmental Neurology, University Hospital Groningen, 9713 EZ Groningen, The Netherlands

Robert L. Isaacson (73), Department of Psychology, State University of New York at Binghamton, Binghamton, New York 13901

Hisashi Kobayashi (35), Division of Biochemistry, Institute of Biological Sciences, Mitsui Pharmaceuticals, Mobara, Chiba 297, Japan

Bryan Kolb (117), Department of Psychology, University of Lethbridge, Lethbridge, Alberta, Canada T1K 3M4

Arthur LaVelle (3), Department of Anatomy, University of Illinois College of Medicine, Chicago, Illinois 60612

Faith W. LaVelle (3), Department of Anatomy, Loyola University, Stritch School of Medicine, Maywood, Illinois 60153

Augustus R. Lumia (253), Department of Psychology, Skidmore College, Saratoga Springs, New York 12866

Robert L. Meisel (253), Department of Neurobiology and Behavior, The Rockefeller University, New York, New York 10021

[2]Present address: Department of Physiology, Sapporo Medical College, S. 1, W. 17, Sapporo 060, Japan.

Donald R. Meyer (211), Laboratory of Comparative and Physiological Psychology, Ohio State University, Columbus, Ohio 43212

Patricia Morgan Meyer (211), Laboratory of Comparative and Physiological Psychology, Ohio State University, Columbus, Ohio 43212

Dwight M. Nance (313), Department of Anatomy, Dalhousie University, Halifax, Nova Scotia, Canada B3H 4H7

Arthur J. Nonneman (138), Department of Psychology, Kastle Hall, University of Kentucky, Lexington, Kentucky 40506

Mark R. Rosenzweig (49), Department of Psychology, University of California, Berkeley, California 94720

Benjamin D. Sachs (253), Department of Psychology, The University of Connecticut, Storrs, Connecticut 06268

Christie L. Sahley (138), Department of Psychology, Yale University, New Haven, Connecticut 06520

Daniel Simons (327), Department of Physiology, University of Pittsburgh Medical School, Pittsburgh, Pennsylvania 15261

Bobby Jo Sonnier (179), Mental Retardation Research Center, UCLA School of Medicine, Los Angeles, California 90024

Linda Patia Spear (73), Department of Psychology and Center for Neurobehavioral Sciences, State University of New York at Binghamton, Binghamton, New York 13901

Peter D. Spear (229), Department of Psychology, The University of Wisconsin—Madison, Madison, Wisconsin 53706

Nakaakira Tsukahara (35), Department of Biophysical Engineering, Faculty of Engineering Science, Osaka University, Toyonaka, Osaka 560, Japan

John P. Vicedomini (138), Department of Psychology, University of Kentucky, Lexington, Kentucky 40506

Jaime R. Villablanca (179), Departments of Psychiatry and Anatomy, Mental Retardation Research Center and Brain Research Institute, UCLA School of Medicine, Los Angeles, California 90024

Shuji Watanabe (35), Division of Biochemistry, Institute of Biological Sciences, Mitsui Pharmaceuticals, Mobara, Chiba 297, Japan

Ian Q. Whishaw (117), Department of Psychology, The University of Lethbridge, Lethbridge, Alberta, Canada T1K 3M4

Bruno Will (349), Laboratoire de Neurobiologie des Comportements, Universite Louis Pasteur, 67000 Strasbourg, France

Preface

The first volume of *Early Brain Damage* represented an attempt to bring together recent findings and thoughts about brain lesions early in life as they pertain directly to clinical populations. In this context, pathological states both in children and in animal models of early brain insult were described. Among the topics addressed were the effects of early brain damage on the functional asymmetry of the human brain, findings pertaining to the cognitive development of the brain-damaged child, and functional differences between focal and diffuse early injuries. Research strategies and broad theoretical issues also were examined by some of the contributors to the first volume.

Volume 2 deals more with controlled experimentation on laboratory animals such as monkeys and rats. In addition, this volume emphasizes the anatomical and physiological correlates of early brain-insult as much as it does the behavioral changes that may follow central nervous system damage early in life. Thus, although the orientation is different from Volume 1, one should not consider this collection in isolation, but rather as a continuation of the first book placed under separate cover. The neurobiological and behavioral findings described here often stem from clinical observations and questions, and can be related to issues and problems in the clinical fields.

This volume is divided into three sections. The first examines recent advances in anatomy and physiology and covers such topics as axonal sprouting and changes in brain areas somewhat removed from the actual site of damage. The second section is the longest and emphasizes what is known about the behavioral effects of specific lesions, such as those of the frontal or posterior cortical areas. The anatomical correlates of these effects are also examined in these highly integrative chapters. The final section examines some factors that can affect the response to early brain damage—factors such as genetics, environmental conditions after early injury, and the differential effects resulting from sparing small fragments of a brain area. This third section is based on the observation that, even with lesions that look the same, the human behavioral response to early brain damage is rarely uniform. Animal research on factors such as those just described may help to explain this variability, which is a known characteristic of clinical populations.

As with Volume 1, the contributors to the second volume are individuals who are well known in their areas and who have been working for some time studying the effects of early brain damage. Hence, each chapter was designed to describe many studies on a particular phenomenon rather than a single experiment in great detail. Contributors were asked to emphasize important new findings and to integrate their results and ideas with those reported by other experimenters working on similar or closely related projects. The studies themselves use a wide variety of experimental techniques and laboratory approaches, and in this regard can be viewed as representative of the efforts that characterize the present thrust to learn more about the effects of early brain damage. It can be said that this volume indirectly looks at the issues of where experimentation on early brain damage has come from, where it is now, and where it may be going in the near future.

It is our hope that this collection will lead to a greater appreciation of the effects of early brain-damage, and will show why we believe that brain lesion phenomena should be evaluated in a developmental context. We hope these chapters will stimulate both further experimentation on brain damage early in life and new approaches to some of the problems outlined here. Most importantly, we hope the chapters presented here will eventually lead to improved methods for preventing early brain damage and for dealing with those children who suffer brain injuries.

Contents of Volume 1

Research Orientations and Clinical Observations

Early Brain Damage

Volume 2
Neurobiology and Behavior

I

Anatomy and Physiology

1

Neuronal Reaction to Injury during Development

*Arthur LaVelle
and Faith W. LaVelle*

Introduction to the Field

Most of the descriptions of cytological changes resulting from axon severance pertain to the neurons of adult animals and typically include cell swelling, nuclear eccentricity of position, and chromatolysis ("destaining") of cytoplasmic Nissl substance. It is known from electron microscopy that Nissl substance consists of stacks of rough endoplasmic reticulum (RER) in the cytoplasm and that chromatolysis results from fragmentation and dispersal of this RER, reflecting an underlying metabolic adaptation that is essentially geared toward protein synthesis for axon regeneration. For extensive appraisals of the retrograde reaction in mature neurons, see Grafstein and McQuarrie (1978) or Lieberman (1971, 1974).

It is clear that immature neurons react differently to axon severance, depending on their developmental state (see LaVelle, 1973, for a historical review). Very young motor neurons die within several days after severance from their peripheral field, but, in both central and peripheral neurons of different vertebrate species, this sensitivity decreases with developmental age.

Why neuronal survival varies directly with age is not yet fully understood. It has been postulated that early motor neuroblasts, after establishing connections with peripheral myoblasts, become dependent on the uptake and storage of trophic substances supplied by the target field, and that death from axotomy is not due directly to trauma but to the loss of these substances. Longer survival after injury at later ages would result from a greater storage of these substances (Prestige, 1967). This viewpoint has been strongly advocated by Hamburger and Oppenheim in their review (1982), and it receives impetus from the work of experimental embryologists who have shown neuroblasts "competing" for available target connections in order to survive.

In another review of the field, Cunningham (1982) forcefully argues that, in itself, the concept of competition for target connections is inadequate to explain the causes for neuronal cell death and survival. He hypothesizes that a proper balance of input from both afferent (presynaptic) and target cells defines the level of survival as well as the mode of degeneration for a particular type of neuroblast.

The idea of competition implies the idea of competence. Considering the inevitability of biological variability, it is likely that at this early stage some neuroblasts do not measure up in their ability to respond to complex conditions. During the critical period of establishing target connections, the many unknown stresses or variations in the microenvironment, coupled with the necessary cell responses induced by target contacts, may exceed the adaptive capacity of the cells.

We believe that an analysis of factors related to survival and competence must include consideration of the cell's inherent metabolic capabilities. It seems certain that during normal development, neuroblasts that achieve their target connections receive some signal that triggers a genetically directed program for a new level of morphological differentiation and synthetic integration. This involves intense protein synthesis and rapid, phenomenal cell growth (Hydén, 1943). At the very early stages of migration and presynaptic outgrowth, the genomically driven complement for protein synthesis, represented within the neuroblast by nucleoli, ribosomes, endoplasmic reticulum, and mitochondria, is minimally developed (LaVelle & LaVelle, 1970; Tennyson, 1970). Subsequent cell growth is accompanied by a striking elaboration of the nuclear and cytoplasmic structures underlying protein synthesis. The most visible organelles involved in this synthesis in the neuron are the nucleolar apparatus and the cytoplasmic components organized as Nissl substance.

The nucleolus has a special significance in protein synthesis and cell survival. Its evolving structure during development and its alterations during cell injury reflect essential, immediately adjacent, transcriptive activities being performed by the genome (Busch & Smetana, 1970; Radouco-Thomas, Nosal, & Radouco-Thomas, 1971). It should be pointed out that in the large motor neurons of mammals the typically single, predominant nucleolus is preceded in an earlier stage by multiple nucleoli (Figure 1). Furthermore, the nucleolar apparatus itself undergoes a prolonged sequence of cytological and functional development that includes both fetal and postnatal periods. The position of the birth time of the animal in relation to this sequence can be deceptive. In the guinea pig, for example, which has a gestation period of 68 days, neuronal nucleolar development is largely completed before birth (LaVelle, 1956). In the hamster, with a gestation period of 16 days, the multiple nucleoli of early development are still the rule during the first postnatal week, and nucleolar maturation is not completed in facial motor and neocortical pyramidal cells until about 20–25 days after birth (Buschmann & LaVelle, 1981; Kinderman & LaVelle, 1977; LaVelle & LaVelle, 1958a; McLoon & LaVelle, 1981b). In facial motor neurons of the rat, with a gestation period of 22 days, multiple nucleoli are seen at birth (Søreide, 1981), but subsequent maturational steps have not been timed. We emphasize that progression from multiple to single nucleoli is a discrete developmental event, as is increase in nucleolar size or attainment of central dominance in nucleolar position, and that all of these involve changes at both the intranucleolar and genomic levels.

Developmental stages of the nucleolus are closely associated with stages in Nissl body formation (LaVelle, 1956). As nucleolar numbers decline and RNA-rich nucleolar substance gradually builds up into a dominant, frequently single nucleolar apparatus (consisting of nucleolar substance and associated chromatin; see Figure 1), increased numbers of free polysomes become attached to cisternae to form RER. The greatest aggregates of stacked arrays of RER (Nissl bodies) appear contemporaneously with the mature nucleolar apparatus (Buschmann & LaVelle, 1981; LaVelle & LaVelle, 1970; Tennyson, 1970).

After studying the development of hamster facial neurons in some detail, we have hypothesized that the increasing ability with age of the neurons to survive axon severance can be closely correlated in time with the cytological maturation of the cell's organelle system for protein synthesis, and, therefore, with the cell's competence to maintain itself both structurally and functionally. Although the direction of neuronal differentiation and growth results from an interplay between the cell's genome, specific cytoplasmic effects, and important

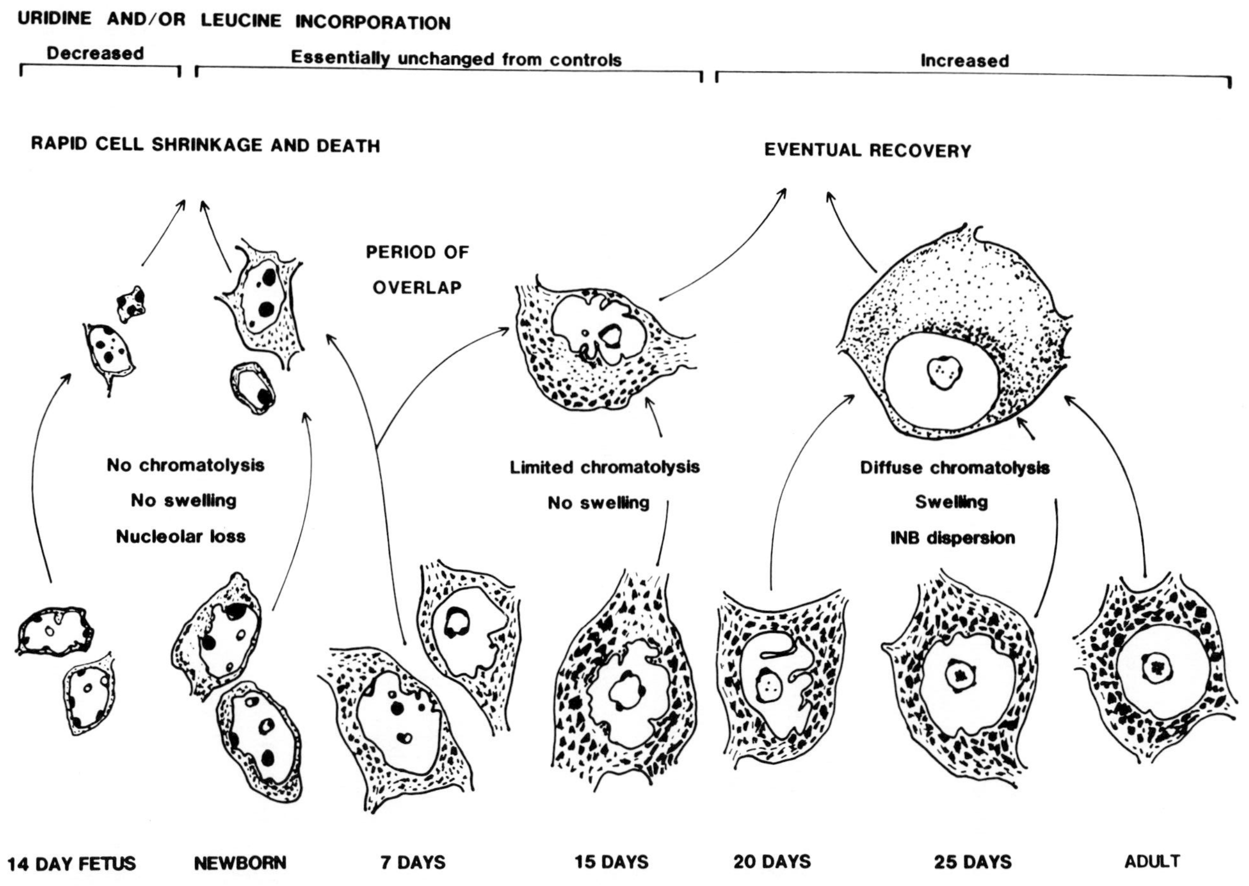

URIDINE AND/OR LEUCINE INCORPORATION

Decreased   Essentially unchanged from controls   Increased

RAPID CELL SHRINKAGE AND DEATH   EVENTUAL RECOVERY

PERIOD OF OVERLAP

No chromatolysis
No swelling
Nucleolar loss

Limited chromatolysis
No swelling

Diffuse chromatolysis
Swelling
INB dispersion

14 DAY FETUS   NEWBORN   7 DAYS   15 DAYS   20 DAYS   25 DAYS   ADULT

ancillary influences derived from the microenvironment (Jacobson, 1978; Spratt, 1964), the enactment of this direction is made via the neuron's capacity to synthesize proteins.

Most of the following account of the cytological effects of axotomy is based on our work with hamster facial motor neurons because it provides the most complete picture, in a single species, of the cytological and metabolic patterns of reaction to direct injury at successive developmental stages. Like most studies of axon severance, ours deals with neurons that have already progressed through the early stages of cell division, migration, and process outgrowth and have made their axonal connection with peripheral targets. Altogether, in this whole field of study, very little has been done on the cytological effects of axon severance *before* the establishment of connections. As is noted in this description, the early period of graded sensitivity to the lethal effects of axotomy corresponds temporally to the period of initial nucleolar formation. Later, when cell survival is high, the more subtle, differentiative nucleolar alterations that occur suggest that stage-specific changes in nucleolar function are still actively involved.

Cytological Maturation Related to Nature of Response to Injury

Effects of Injury during Early Stages after Peripheral Connection

NORMAL FETAL DEVELOPMENT

In the hamster, facial nerve outgrowth into the hyoid arch begins during the 9th fetal day; by Day 11, the fibers have attained their adult pattern of distribution (Boyer, 1953). By Day 14, column formation is evident in stained, transverse sections through the facial nuclear group (LaVelle & LaVelle, 1959). Little is known about the timing of the arrival of afferents to the nuclear group, although the late entrance of pyramidal tract fibers into the field occurs at about 4 days after birth (Rey & Kalil, 1981). During the last quarter of gestation (Days

Figure 1. Summary of reactions of hamster facial motor neurons to axotomy at different developmental stages. Cytoplasmic Nissl substance is shown as stained with thionin. Nucleolar substance is shown as light areas surrounded by dark clumps of chromatin. In the 25-day cell and in the adult cell, the intranucleolar body (INB) is shown as a dark aggregation of ribonucleoprotein (RNP) granules within the nucleolus. Note that the degree of normal nuclear invagination is greatest at 15 and 20 days. Changes in labeled isotope incorporation are indicated at top of figure.

12–16), RNA-rich nucleolar substance forms within the neuronal nuclear chromatin bodies as areas that lightly stain with basic dye but are achromatic with the Feulgen technique for DNA. Cytoplasm-containing fine basophilic particles form a thin layer around nuclei, except where it is concentrated on one side or at opposite poles of the cell.

FETAL OPERATIONS

With severance in utero of the facial nerve by electrocautery at 14 days, and after a postoperative time of 17 hours, enough cells have reacted so that a sequence of degenerative stages can be observed (LaVelle & LaVelle, 1959). The apparent initial effect involves the regression of nucleolar material resulting in a dark-staining, Feulgen-positive chromatin body; this is seen in certain cells that otherwise show no apparent thinning of cytoplasmic basophilia (see Figure 1, fetal cells). Subsequent degenerative steps involve progressive cell shrinkage and darkening, with eventual disappearance of the cells within 48 hours. The now-familiar pattern of rapid cell loss with relatively few really degenerated stages being visible at any given time is a characteristic of the reaction.

To our knowledge, severance of a single peripheral nerve in utero has not been reported by anyone else. Amputation of fetal limbs and sectioning of fetal spinal cords, however, have resulted variably in chromatolysis, cell degeneration, and cell loss (see review by Hess, 1957).

An autoradiographic study in our laboratory shows that the 14-day fetal neurons, 17 hours after electrocautery, are able to incorporate [³H]uridine injected into the mother, but that this incorporation is depressed relative to the unoperated side (Clark & LaVelle, 1983), indicating a decreased synthesis of RNA. We emphasize that the sequelae of synthetic events, stemming from the nucleolus and relayed through to the cytoplasm, are associated at this time with an incompletely formed cytology. With further development of this cytological basis, the effects of axotomy become less severe.

EFFECTS OF INJURY DURING THE PERIOD OF RAPID NEURONAL GROWTH

NORMAL EARLY POSTNATAL DEVELOPMENT

At birth, after 16 days' gestation, the typical hamster facial neuron contains four or five nucleoli in various stages of development (Figure

1). Usually one nucleolus is larger than the others. After birth there is a gradual, normal decrease in nucleolar number, resulting by postnatal Day 7 in a large, centrally placed nucleolar apparatus that either is alone or predominates over one or two smaller ones in the same nucleus. By 15 days, nucleolar, nuclear, and somal size are nearly indistinguishable from that of adult neurons. The configuration of the nucleolar apparatus, usually one in number and centrally positioned within the nucleus, is now essentially mature and consists of nucleolar substance proper that is surrounded by small particles of nucleolus-associated chromatin. Along with nucleolar growth and maturation, there also occurs a concomitant increase in cytoplasmic Nissl substance (LaVelle & LaVelle, 1958a, 1970). This period of rapid somal growth is also associated with a high quantity of invaginated nuclear envelope (LaVelle & Buschmann, 1983), suggestive of a very active nuclear–cytoplasmic exchange (Hydén, 1943).

EARLY POSTNATAL OPERATIONS

When the facial nerve is transected in the hamster at birth, initial nucleolar loss occurs and is inevitably followed by neuronal death. Axotomy performed at 7 and 15 days postnatal ages, when the neurons are structurally more mature, results in chromatolysis (dispersal of Nissl substance), without any pronounced nucleolar alteration in the cells that survive. A limited, central type of chromatolysis thus becomes the paramount reaction as the nucleolar apparatus attains its segregated, more mature configuration and, presumably, its greater synthetic capability. During this period, survival time also increases, from complete degeneration of the whole facial neuronal group within 6 days after axotomy at birth, to nearly 90% survival 30 days after axotomy at 15 days postnatal age (LaVelle & LaVelle, 1958a, 1958b) (see Figure 1, newborn to 15-day cells).

As detailed elsewhere (LaVelle, 1973), a few investigators, using limb ablation and axon section of other nerves in other animals, have described sequences that very much parallel our own. Although none of these studies focused primarily on steps in nucleolar development, they nevertheless demonstrated age-dependent reactions that might have been related to differentially labile phases of nucleolar development and hence of protein production. Søreide (1981) has severed facial neurons of rats at various postnatal stages. At birth, when there were multiple nucleoli (see Figure 1a, Søreide, 1981), neuronal chromatolysis and eventual cell death occurred. Axon injury at successively later ages, as single nucleoli became predominant (see Figures 2–5, Søreide, 1981), resulted in more cell survival and lessened

chromatolysis. Although species differences in the direction of chromatolysis with age were apparent when compared with the hamster,
Søreide's results appear to us to indicate that cell survival was associated with continued nucleolar maturation and increasing associated synthetic competence.

As work in our laboratory shows, axotomy at birth, 7, 9, and 15
days postnatal ages results in no significant differences in uridine
incorporation between control and operated sides (Clark & LaVelle,
1983; Jones & LaVelle, 1983; Kinderman & LaVelle, 1977). This is
also generally observed with [³H]leucine, an amino acid precursor,
after axon section at 15 days (Griffith & LaVelle, 1971; McLoon &
LaVelle, 1981a, 1981c). An exception does occur, however, if observation is delayed until 30 days after an operation performed at 15 days
postnatal age (McLoon & LaVelle, 1981c). At this later postoperative
time, when these animals have reached 45 days of age, there is a
small but significant rise in incorporation on the operated side over
that of the control, a trend that foreshadows the typical reaction of
axotomized adult neurons. Thus, despite the stress of trauma, the
young neurons have reached a stage of development that enables
them to incorporate at a more mature level. This fits well with our
speculation (LaVelle & LaVelle, 1975; McLoon & LaVelle, 1981a,
1981c) that during the accelerated somal growth period, beginning at
birth and culminating at 15 days, axotomy cannot stimulate the surviving cells beyond what is already maximal synthetic output. Following the end of the growth period, however, a leveling of synthetic
activity normally occurs, and trauma can elicit incorporative levels
over that of normal cells, as cells seek to repair the damage done and
replace the cytoplasm lost.

Effects of Injury during the Period of Final Cytological Maturation

NORMAL FINAL MATURATIONAL CHANGES

The final stage of nucleolar maturation in hamster facial neurons
occurs between 20 and 25 days postnatal ages (Figure 1). In the majority of nucleoli, during this time, ribonucleoprotein (RNP) granules
aggregate into a large, centrally located cluster, which we have
termed the *intranucleolar body* (INB) (LaVelle & LaVelle, 1975). The
segregation of components such as the RNP granules has been in-

terpreted to indicate a reduction in RNA synthesis (Busch & Smetana, 1970; Miller & Gonzales, 1976). We have suggested, therefore, that during the period of earlier rapid somal growth, the associated lack of INBs indicates a phase of high nucleolar metabolism in which reserve quantities of RNP granules cannot be accumulated for INB formation. At the end of the growth period, however, when the normal requirements for utilization appear to be less, the formation of the INB indicates that a more than sufficient supply of ribosomal precursors has now been synthesized (Kinderman & LaVelle, 1976; LaVelle & LaVelle, 1975; McLoon & LaVelle, 1981b). In this regard it is of interest that there is normally a significant, sharp decline in the quantity of invaginated nuclear envelope between 20 and 25 days (LaVelle & Buschmann, 1983), indicating again a more restricted metabolic rate of protein synthesis.

THE SWELLING REACTION

In hamsters, the retrograde reaction already described for 15 days postnatal age, although different in character from the reaction at earlier ages, is still not the mature one. When, however, the facial nerve is severed at 20 days, a distinctly different sort of response occurs (see Figure 1, 20-day to adult cells). This is characterized by a significant swelling of the nucleolar apparatus, nucleus, soma, and mitochondria, accompanied by a diffuse type of chromatolysis not seen in animals operated on at 15 days of age. The increased somal size persists throughout the reaction period and is associated with regenerative activity within the cell (LaVelle, 1973). According to Lieberman (1971), both somal and mitochrondrial swelling in axotomized adult neurons seem to be well-established phenomena.

DISPERSION OF INTRANUCLEOLAR BODIES

What appears to be the final cytological component of the retrograde reaction resides in changes of the intranucleolar body (INB). With axotomy of adult facial neurons, the INB disperses within 3 days and does not begin to reappear until about 25 days postoperative, long after Nissl bodies have been reconstituted in the cytoplasm (LaVelle & LaVelle, 1975) (see Figure 1, 25-day to adult). Further experiments have shown, after combined ligature and axotomy at different ages before, during, and after INB formation, that the more immature the nucleolar apparatus is, the longer it takes for

reconstitution of the INB (McLoon & LaVelle, 1981b; Smith & La-
Velle, 1976).

Incorporation studies on axotomized hamster facial neurons support the cytological evidence that the 15–25-day age period involves
a critical change in the maturation of the protein-synthesis system in
these neurons, as reflected by the structure of the nucleolus. Unlike
the younger postnatal cells, which showed no significant differences
between operated and control sides, facial neurons severed at 20 and
25 days, as well as those severed in the adult, incorporated tritiated
leucine and uridine at significantly higher levels than did control
cells at all postoperative ages, with the differences being greater in
the older operative series (Griffith & LaVelle, 1971; Kinderman &
LaVelle, 1977; McLoon & LaVelle, 1981a, 1981c).

Considerations in Comparing Results
and Drawing Conclusions

As summarized by Geist (1933), the cell-body reaction to injury is
conditioned by such variables as elapsed time after injury, distance
of the injury from the cell body, neuronal type, and animal species
and age. In addition, the regenerative action by the neuron may be
influenced by the presence of remaining collaterals (Lieberman,
1974), by surrounding glial cells (Jacob & Durica, 1983), or by substances derived from peripheral connections (Kristensson & Sjöstrand, 1972; Prestige, 1967). Despite general awareness of the multiple influences affecting the neuron, investigators in this field
nevertheless can still not explain the extremes of reaction that may
occur following nerve section. Particularly perplexing examples are
the highly differential results between severance of central and peripheral processes of sensory ganglion cells (Grafstein & McQuarrie,
1978; Lieberman, 1971, 1974), or the marked disintegration of facial
motor neurons after axotomy in the adult mouse (Torvik & Skjørten,
1971) compared to the nearly complete survival of facial neurons
after axotomy in the adult hamster (Jacob & Durica, 1983; LaVelle &
LaVelle, 1958a, 1975).

The exact signal responsible for inducing the somal reaction to
injury is also uncertain (Cragg, 1970), although evidence indicates
that retrograde transport, possibly of a substance liberated at the site
of injury, may be involved (Singer, Mehler, & Fernandez, 1982). Trauma itself probably initially induces a reaction, whatever the inter-

mediary signal may be, as is indicated by Watson's results (1968) with mature neurons in which ribosomal synthesis was again increased by a second cutting of axons that had not yet reestablished peripheral connections. In cultured neurons, which also lack terminal connections, compression injury to their axons resulted in retrograde responses that were less severe the older the cells were (Levi & Meyer, 1945).

In their study on the microchemical analysis of axotomized single neurons, Brattgård, Edström, and Hydén (1957, p. 323) stated a basic perspective that cannot be overemphasized: "The primary problem is at the level of gene action on the cytoplasm and action of external or cell milieu factors back on the genes of the nucleus." We would stress, additionally, that the whole spectrum of regulatory and trophic influences achieves its effects through the capacity of the neuron's synthetic mechanism to produce protein for repair and regeneration.

Under certain conditions the capacity of this mechanism can be limiting. Lieberman (1974) has argued, on the basis of Watson's data (1968), that when axotomy is close to the cell body, cell death many ensue if nucleolar response in metabolic output is too small or too short to support the required axonal growth. Because the degree of nucleolar structural advancement or complexity is highly variable, even among different adult neuronal types (LaVelle, 1956; LaVelle & LaVelle, 1983), it follows that reactive competence among these types might also be expected to differ and could be related to their nucleolar structure and associated synthetic activity. However, there are insufficient data available to relate variations in nucleolar structure and competence with specific degrees of reactive or regenerative capacity in most of the neuronal types in which the retrograde reaction has been observed, because the cytological status of their nucleolar structure has rarely been determined and described. In the studies on the effects of injury on developing neurons, particularly, it is our view that assessments of (1) nucleolar structure at the time of application of the injurious agent or insult, as well as of (2) the length of postoperative period allowed for appearance of the reaction, are crucial in any interpretation of results. This is especially so when results from different cell types and from different species are compared.

We suggest, therefore, that comparative studies on the effects of injury on both developing and mature neurons should include accurate descriptions of nucleolar cytology, number, and size. It seems clear that an understanding of the differential reactions of developing and mature neurons to trauma depends on a knowledge of a multiplicity of conditions, including pre- and postsynaptic connections, the surrounding micromilieu, and the intrinsic cytology underlying synthetic competence. Not all of these categories have been adequately documented for any given neuronal type. When they are, we can perhaps better approach the fundamental problem of genetic control of neuronal function and reactivity to injury.

Summary Statements

Following the attainment of terminal axon connections, neuronal maturation is accompanied by a changing pattern of cytological and metabolic reaction to injury inflicted at successive stages. Intrinsic to this pattern is the increasing tendency of developing neurons to survive injury. As observed with the hamster facial motor neurons, this changing reaction pattern is closely associated with the maturation of the organelle system for protein synthesis, as particularly exemplified by the nucleolar apparatus. Thus, the capacity for heightened survival with age can be associated with the increasing capacity of the developing neuron to maintain itself.

We interpret our own findings to indicate that as the neuronal synthetic mechanism matures, the neuron becomes less dependent on peripheral connections for its maintenance. To carry this premise further, we would suggest that should all things, in terms of trophic input and microenvironment, be equal, then the state of cellular synthetic competence could be the deciding factor in enabling a particular neuron or neuronal group to survive the stresses of disease or trauma.

References

Boyer, C. C. (1953). Chronology of development for the golden hamster. *Journal of Morphology, 92,* 1–37.

Brattgård, S.-O., Edström, J.-E., & Hydén, H. (1957). The chemical changes in regenerating neurons. *Journal of Neurochemistry, 1,* 316–323.

Busch, H., & Smetana, K. (1970). *The nucleolus.* New York: Academic Press.

Buschmann, MB. T., & LaVelle, A. (1981). Morphological changes of the pyramidal cell nucleolus and nucleus in hamster frontal cortex during development and aging. *Mechanisms of Ageing and Development, 15,* 385–397.

Clark, P., & LaVelle, A. (1983). ³H-uridine incorporation in normal and axotomized immature hamster facial motor neurons. *Society for Neuroscience Abstracts, 9,* 46.

Cragg, B. G. (1970). What is the signal for chromatolysis? *Brain Research, 23,* 1–21.

Cunningham, T. J. (1982). Naturally occurring neuron death and its regulation by developing neural pathways. *International Review of Cytology, 74,* 163–186.

Geist, F. D. (1933). Chromatolysis of efferent neurons. *Archives of Neurology and Psychiatry, 29,* 88–103.

Grafstein, B., & McQuarrie, I. G. (1978). Role of the nerve cell body in axonal regeneration. In C. W. Cotman (Ed.), *Neuronal plasticity* (pp. 155–195). New York: Raven.

Griffith, A., & LaVelle, A. (1971). Developmental protein changes in normal and chromatolytic facial nerve nuclear regions. *Experimental Neurology, 33,* 360–371.

Hamburger, V., & Oppenheim, R. W. (1982). Naturally occurring neuronal death in vertebrates. *Neuroscience Commentaries, 1,* 39–55.

Hess, A. (1957). The experimental embryology of the foetal nervous system. *Biological Reviews, 32,* 231–260.

Hydén, H. (1943). Protein metabolism in the nerve cell during growth and function. *Acta Physiologica Scandinavica, 6*(Suppl. XVII), 1–136.

Jacob, S. K., & Durica, T. E. (1983). Variations in the glial response following axotomy of different cranial nerves of the hamster. *Anatomical Record, 205,* 90A.

Jacobson, M. (1978). *Developmental neurobiology* (2nd ed.). New York: Plenum.

Jones, K. J., & LaVelle, A. (1983). A time course study of axotomy-induced changes in RNA synthesis and nucleolar morphology in immature and mature hamster facial neurons. *Society for Neuroscience Abstracts, 9,* 46.

Kinderman, N. B., & LaVelle, A. (1976). Ultrastructural changes in the developing nucleolus following axotomy. *Brain Research, 108,* 237–247.

Kinderman, N. B., & LaVelle, A. (1977). Uridine incorporation by axotomized facial neurons. *Anatomical Record, 187,* 624.

Kristensson, K., & Sjöstrand, J. (1972). Retrograde transport of protein tracer in the rabbit hypoglossal nerve during regeneration. *Brain Research, 45,* 175–181.

LaVelle, A. (1956). Nucleolar and Nissl substance development in nerve cells. *Journal of Comparative Neurology, 104,* 175–205.

LaVelle, A. (1973). Levels of maturation and reactions to injury during neuronal development. *Progress in Brain Research, 40,* 161–166.

LaVelle, A., & Buschmann, MB. T. (1983). Nuclear envelope invaginations in hamster facial motor neurons during development and aging. *Developmental Brain Research, 10,* 171–175.

LaVelle, A., & LaVelle, F. W. (1958a). The nucleolar apparatus and neuronal reactivity to injury during development. *Journal of Experimental Zoology, 137,* 285–315.

LaVelle, A., & LaVelle, F. W. (1958b). Neuronal swelling and chromatolysis as influenced by the state of cell development. *American Journal of Anatomy, 102,* 219–241.

LaVelle, A., & LaVelle, F. W. (1959). Neuronal reaction to injury during development: Severance of the facial nerve *in utero. Experimental Neurology, 1,* 82–95.

LaVelle, A., & LaVelle, F. W. (1970). Cytodifferentiation in the neuron. In W. A. Himwich (Ed.), *Developmental neurobiology* (pp. 117–164). Springfield, IL: Thomas.

LaVelle, A., & LaVelle, F. W. (1975). Changes in an intranucleolar body in hamster facial neurons following axotomy. *Experimental Neurology, 49,* 569–579.

LaVelle, F. W., & LaVelle, A. (1983). A difference in the nucleoli of Purkinje cells of the nodular lobe of the hamster cerebellum. *Brain Research, 265,* 119–124.

Levi, G., & Meyer, H. (1945). Reactive, regressive and regenerative processes of neurons cultivated *in vitro* and injured with the micromanipulator. *Journal of Experimental Zoology, 99,* 141–181.

Lieberman, A. R. (1971). The axon reaction: A review of the principal features of perikaryal responses to axon injury. *International Review of Neurobiology, 14,* 49–124.

Lieberman, A. R. (1974). Some factors affecting retrograde neuronal responses to axonal lesions. In R. Bellairs & E. G. Gray (Eds.), *Essays on the nervous system* (pp. 71–105). London: Clarendon.

McLoon, L. K., & LaVelle, A. (1981a). Tritiated leucine incorporation in the developing hamster facial nucleus with injury: A liquid scintillation study. *Developmental Brain Research, 1,* 237–248.

McLoon, L. K., & LaVelle, A. (1981b). Long-term effects of regeneration and prevention of regeneration on nucleolar morphology after facial nerve injury during development. *Experimental Neurology, 73,* 762–774.

McLoon, L. K., & LaVelle, A. (1981c). Tritiated leucine incorporation in the developing hamster facial neurons with injury: An autoradiographic study. *Experimental Neurology, 74,* 573–586.

Miller, L., & Gonzales, F. (1976). The relationship of ribosomal RNA synthesis to the formation of segregated nucleoli and nucleolus-like bodies. *Journal of Cell Biology, 71,* 939–949.

Prestige, M. C. (1967). The control of cell number in the lumbar ventral horns during the development of *Xenopus laevis* tadpoles. *Journal of Embryology and Experimental Morphology, 18,* 359–387.

Radouco-Thomas, C., Nosal, Gl., & Radouco-Thomas, S. (1971). The nuclear-ribosomal system during neuronal differentiation and development. In R. Paoletti & A. N. Davison (Eds.), *Chemistry and brain development* (pp. 291–307). New York: Plenum.

Reh, T., & Kalil, K. (1981). Development of the pyramidal tract in the hamster. I. A light microscopic study. *Journal of Comparative Neurology, 200,* 55–67.

Singer, P. A., Mehler, S., & Fernandez, H. L. (1982). Blockade of retrograde axonal transport delays the onset of metabolic and morphologic changes induced by axotomy. *Journal of Neuroscience, 2,* 1299–1306.

Smith, G., & LaVelle, A. (1976). Differential changes involving an intranucleolar body after either nerve crush or combined ligature/axotomy. *Anatomical Record, 184,* 533–534.

Søreide, A. J. (1981). Variations in the axon reaction in animals of different ages. *Acta Anatomica, 110,* 40–47.

Spratt, N. T., Jr. (1964). *Introduction to cell differentiation.* New York: Reinhold.

Tennyson, V. M. (1970). The fine structure of the developing nervous system. In W. A. Himwich (Ed.), *Developmental neurobiology* (pp. 47–116). Springfield, IL: Thomas.

Torvik, A., & Skjørten, F. (1971). Electron microscopic observations of nerve cell regeneration and degeneration after axon lesions. I. Changes in the nerve cell cytoplasm. *Acta Neuropathologica, 17,* 248–264.

Watson, W. E. (1968). Observations on the nucleolar and total cell body nucleic acid of injured nerve cells. *Journal of Physiology, 196,* 655–676.

2

Embryonic Dopaminergic Neurons in Culture and as Transplants

Philip C. Hoffmann
and Alfred Heller

Introduction

Dopaminergic neurons with cell bodies located within the mesencephalon innervate a number of important telencephalic structures including the frontal cortex, the nucleus accumbens, and the corpus striatum. Abundant evidence has been collected implicating these neurons in locomotor, ingestive, and emotional behaviors (Seiden & Dykstra, 1977). Important classes of pharmacological agents, notably the neuroleptic drugs, are believed to exert many of their therapeutic as well as their adverse effects through interactions with these neurons and neurons to which they project. Most important from the point of view of brain damage, the loss of these neurons is most assuredly responsible for Parkinson's disease, and pharmacotherapy using the precursor of dopamine, L-dopa, has proved to be an effective, albeit limited, therapy for this extrapyramidal disorder.

Studies on the development of these neurons in the intact animal have shown that they are born over a 3-day time span, beginning with embryonic Day 13 and extending to embryonic Day 15, with the vast majority being born on gestational Day 14. Both the older histofluorescent (Olson & Seiger, 1972) and the newer immunocytochemical techniques (Specht, Pickel, Joh, & Reis, 1981) have demonstrated the formation of axonal processes that extend into the developing striatum as early as embryonic Day 15. However, the extensive collateralization and arborization of the axonal field within the striatum is a postnatal event and extends for up to 60 days after birth. This has been demonstrated with both histochemical and biochemical techniques (Coyle & Henry, 1973; Porcher & Heller, 1972; Tennyson, Barrett, Cohen, Cote, Heikela, & Mytilineou, 1972).

Early experiments using unilateral lesions of the medial forebrain bundle, through which the axons of the dopaminergic neurons pass on their way to the corpus striatum and the frontal cortex, demonstrated the feasibility of selectively damaging these fibers, although nondopaminergic neurons whose axons pass through the same region no doubt are also destroyed by the lesion (Moore, Bhatnagar, & Heller, 1971; Ungerstedt, 1971). Subsequently, 6-hydroxydopamine has been used by several investigators as a selective agent for destroying dopaminergic axons and cell bodies (Jonsson, 1980). With the proper dosage regimen, and using desipramine to protect noradrenergic neurons, it is possible to obtain a selective and virtually complete denervation of target structures that are normally innervated by dopaminergic neurons (Miller, Heffner, Kotake, & Seiden, 1981). Interestingly, in contrast to the norepinephrine-containing neurons of the locus coereleus, which exhibit extensive axonal sprouting after axotomy (Moore, Björklund, & Stenevi, 1971), there is no evidence that a similar phenomenon occurs with dopaminergic neurons. However, as is discussed in the following, it has been possible to partially "reinnervate" denervated target structures of these dopaminergic neurons by using transplants containing embryonic dopaminergic neurons.

A wide variety of functional and behavioral effects result from destruction of dopaminergic neurons either in the adult (Ungerstedt, 1971; Zigmond & Stricker, 1974) or in the neonatal animal (Erinoff, MacPhail, Heller, & Seiden, 1979; Shaywitz, Yager, & Klopper, 1976). For example, as is discussed more extensively in Chapter 5, Volume 1, during the development of the rat, a wave of locomotor hyperactivity begins on Day 10 of postnatal life, peaks at Day 15, and is suppressed by Day 21. Bilateral destruction of dopaminergic neurons prior to 10 days of postnatal age results in a locomotor hyperactivity syndrome in which the normal suppression does not occur. Destruction of the same neuronal systems after the normal suppression of the wave of hyperactivity produces no increase in spontaneous locomotor activity. Thus in this particular instance there appears to be an age-dependent sensitivity of the brain to the presence of these dopaminergic neurons, and the functional consequences of their loss can differ as a function of age.

Results such as these suggesting a role for dopaminergic neurons in the development of behaviors have led investigators to study in some detail the development, differentiation, and maturation of dopaminergic neurons. However, the neuronal organization in the intact developing embryonic brain is complex, and it is difficult to control many experimental variables during the time of this development. Therefore a characterization of the mechanisms responsible for the normal differentiation of these catecholamine-containing neurons has not been achieved.

Embryonic Dopaminergic Neurons in Primary Monolayer Cultures

In vitro methods using tissue culture have been applied to the problems of the development of central dopaminergic neurons. Primary monolayer cultures of dissociated embryonic tissue of the rostral mesencephalic tegmentum have been studied in considerable detail with the use of mechanically dissociated cells from 13-day-old embryos plated onto collagen- and polyornithine-coated glass coverslips (Prochiantz, di Porzio, Kato, Berger, & Glowinski, 1979). With the appropriate culture conditions, the neurons were found to survive for several weeks. Moreover, the dopaminergic neurons could be identified histochemically as well as by the specific uptake of [^{3}H]dopamine. The cultured neurons were capable of synthesizing [^{3}H]dopamine from [^{3}H]tyrosine. On the basis of both histochemical observations and changes in biochemical indices, the dopaminergic neurons were found to differentiate, whether or not striatal target cells were present. However, the simultaneous presence of striatal cells in the monolayer cultures was found to stimulate the development of the dopaminergic neurons: There was an increase in the maximal velocity for specific uptake of [^{3}H]dopamine. This increase was at least twofold, regardless of the age of the cocultures. Additional evidence suggesting enhanced development due to the simultaneous presence of striatal target cells was found in the twofold enhancement of synthesis of [^{3}H]dopamine from [^{3}H]tyrosine observed in older cultures of 12 to 15 days of age.

Additional studies of such cultures revealed that they responded to depolarizing agents with release of [^{3}H]dopamine (Daguet, di Porzio, Prochiantz, Kato, & Glowinski, 1980). For example, a 5-minute pulse of 60 mM potassium resulted in a marked efflux of radioactivity with at least 75% of the radioactivity being associated with dopamine. Veratridine was also shown to stimulate the release of dopamine through a calcium-dependent mechanism, and tetrodotoxin prevented such veratridine-evoked release of transmitter. These studies suggest that the dopaminergic neurons grown in primary culture develop and retain their functional integrity.

In order to assess the role of glial cells in the maturation of the dopaminergic neurons and on the effects of striatal cells upon such maturation, the experiments were repeated with serum-free media, which allows for the generation of a virtually pure neuronal population (di Porzio, Daguet, Glowinski, & Prochiantz, 1980). The resulting decrease in the number of glia in the primary monolayer cultures was found to affect neither the maturation of the dopaminergic cells nor the stimulatory effect on their development by simultaneous addition of striatal cells. On the basis of autoradiographic analysis of the number of dopaminergic cells, the authors suggested that the stimulatory effect of the target cells was directly related to increased capacities for [³H]dopamine uptake and synthesis per dopaminergic neuron.

In order to determine whether diffusable or membrane-bound factors were involved in the stimulatory effect of striatal target cells, the in vitro development of embryonic mesencephalic dopamine neurons was studied in primary monolayer cultures exposed to striatal membranes that had been isolated from postnatal mice of various ages (Prochiantz, Daguet, Herbet, & Glowinski, 1981). The magnitude of [³H]dopamine uptake was used as an index of maturation. It was found that striatal membranes from 2- and 3-week-old animals were capable of stimulating the maturation of dopaminergic neurons, but that membranes prepared from 1-week-old or adult animals was ineffective. This result was interpreted as implying that a developmentally regulated membrane-bound "factor" was involved in the stimulatory effect of striatal target cells on dopaminergic neuron development. The factor seemed to be specific to the dopaminergic neurons, for striatal membranes had no effect on hippocampal cell development.

It has been reported that the addition of GM_1 monosialoganglioside ($10^{-8}–10^{-6}M$) produces an increased rate of neurite outgrowth associated with increased development of dopaminergic parameters ([³H]dopamine uptake, [³H]dopamine synthesis, and tyrosine hydroxylase-like immunoreactivity) in such cocultures of primary monolayers of dopaminergic cells with their striatal target cells (Leon, Dal toso, di Porzio, Facci, Mazzari, & Toffano, 1982). This effect of GM_1 monosialoganglioside may be related to its effects in apparently promoting reinnervation by dopaminergic neurons of the unilaterally denervated striatum in vivo (Toffano, Savoini, Moroni, Lombardi, & Agnati, 1982).

Further study of primary monolayer cultures of dopaminergic neurons has shown that the uptake of exogenous catecholamine can be detected within 24 hours after plating and precedes the appearance of tyrosine hydroxylase-like immunoreactivity, which is first demonstrable at 48 hours (Berger, di Porzio, Daguet, Gay, Vigny, Glowinski, & Prochiantz, 1982). The number of neurons appears to increase for up to 4 days if uptake of exogenous norepinephrine is used as an index, and for up to 10 days if determined by the appearance of tyrosine hydroxylase immunoreactivity. Endogenous stores of dopamine are seen only after 3 weeks in vitro using fluorescence histochemistry. At this culture age, the number of neurons present is independent of the assay technique used. In these experiments the presence of striatal target cells has no effect either on the sequential appearance of the markers or on the number of dopaminergic neurons (Berger *et al.*, 1982).

Embryonic Dopaminergic Neurons
in Three-Dimensional Aggregate Cultures

It is apparent from the studies just described that embryonic dopaminergic neurons can survive and differentiate in an essentially normal manner in primary monolayer cultures. Moreover, they appear to interact with striatal target cells in a manner that promotes maturation of the dopaminergic neurons. However, in such monolayer cultures, the neurons are restricted to developing in essentially two dimensions. This constraint can be avoided by the use of the dissociated cell-reaggregation system pioneered by Garber and Moscona (1972). In this system, areas of the embryonic brain containing dopaminergic neurons are dissected and dissociated into single-cell suspensions using trypsin and mechanical shearing forces. When the cell suspensions are placed with culture media in flasks in a rotatory incubator shaker, three-dimensional aggregates are formed. As described by Monroy and Moscona (1979, p. 170):

> Immediately following their dissociation, the separated cells begin to project from their surfaces numerous elongated processes referred to as filopodia, which often exceed in length the diameter of the cell. By means of these probe-

like projections, cells make initial point-contacts, often across large distances. The aggregates continue to increase in size by further recruitment of single cells and of smaller cell clumps which merge into the larger aggregates. Within the aggregates, cells move about and take up preferred positions depending upon cell type; that is they sort out, thereby progressively reconstructing the histologic pattern of their tissue of origin. Thereupon, cell movements largely cease, intercellular contacts become stabilized in part by means of specialized cell junctions, and the reconstituted tissue resumes its differentiation. This sequence in most cases takes 12–24 hours.

Early studies showed that aggregates formed from dissociated *whole* embryonic rat or mouse brains developed levels of specific activity of neuron-specific enzymes comparable to adult levels in vivo (Honegger & Richelson, 1977). In addition, [^{3}H]dopamine was synthesized from [^{3}H]tyrosine; it could be depleted by reserpine, and the rate of dopamine synthesis was decreased by tetrodotoxin and increased by veratridine, suggesting that the rate of dopamine synthesis in such aggregates is directly related to the electrical activity of certain neuronal cells contained within the aggregates (Honegger & Richelson, 1979).

Levitt, Garber, and Moore (1976) first applied the reaggregation technique to embryonic mesencephalic tissue containing the dopaminergic neurons, after dissection from the remainder of the embryonic mouse brain. In these experiments the tissue was dissociated and reaggregated for short periods of time (24–72 hours), and the resulting aggregates were treated by the Falck–Hillarp histofluorescence method to visualize the dopamine cells. Fluorescent cells were found to be distributed evenly in both the initial cell suspension and in 24-hour aggregates; by 48 hours, fluorescent cells were observed to be clustered in small groups, but by 72 hours, a band of closely associated fluorescent cells was described.

This result was interpreted as suggesting the sorting out of dopaminergic neurons and their association with one another subsequent to aggregate formation, an event qualitatively similar to the formation of a nuclear group in vivo. These visual impressions were subsequently confirmed by quantitative morphometric analysis, which demonstrated a nonhomogeneous distribution of dopaminergic neurons within the aggregates at 3, 7, and 12 days in culture (Hemmendinger, Garber, Hoffmann, & Heller, 1981a). Furthermore, the coculture of dopaminergic neurons with dissociated cells from both target and nontarget areas did not affect the ability of the dopaminergic neurons to sort out in this manner. These results show clearly that embryonic dopaminergic neurons retain one of the most important properties of developing neurons in situ; namely, the ability to selectively associate with one another to produce nuclear groups of neurons within the brain.

It has also been shown that another important property of developing neurons, the ability to form neuronal processes, both dendrites and axons, is retained by dissociated cells following reaggregation (Hemmendinger, Garber, Hoffmann, & Heller, 1981b). It was found that the formation and/or maintenance of axons or dendrites by these neurons is critically dependent on the nature of the cells with which they interact within the aggregates. Thus, dopaminergic neurons that are allowed to reaggregate with their nearest neighbors of the rostral mesencephalon form extensive dendritic arborizations but no discernible axons after 7 days in culture. In marked contrast, dopaminergic neurons form and maintain axons when cocultured for 7 days with dissociated cells of target areas such as the corpus striatum or the frontal cortex. In addition, the axonal patterns formed in association with such target cells are target-area specific: Dense axonal plexi are formed in coaggregates of dopamine neurons of the rostral mesencephalic tegmentum with cells of the corpus striatum (RMT–CS), whereas less dense patterns, in which single axons with beaded varicosities can be seen coursing through the neuropil, are formed in association with dissociated cells of the frontal cortex (RMT–FCx). These patterns mimic those found in these target areas in vivo. Other studies using the more sensitive aluminum sulfate adaptation of the Falck–Hillarp procedure (Loren, Björklund, Falck, & Lindvall, 1980) also show the individual dopaminergic axons with beaded varicosities in the RMT–CS coaggregates, although the number of such fibers is much greater than is the case with RMT-FCx, and the fluorescent fibers are very often pericellular in nature. An interesting contrast is provided by the development of dopaminergic neurons when cocultured for 7 days in the presence of dissociated telecephalic cells that are not part of their normal target area, for example, the occipital cortex (RMT–OCx). Under these circumstances dopaminergic cell bodies are found to be present in the coaggregates, but very few dendritic and axonal processes are formed and/or maintained (Hemmendinger et al., 1981b).

These experiments in the dissociated cell reaggregate system demonstrate that there is target-cell-dependent proliferation and/or maintenance of axonal processes by dissociated embryonic dopaminergic neurons. This result strongly supports the idea that the cells themselves possess the requisite information for these interactions. Moreover, these morphologically demonstrable effects of target cells may be related to the enhanced maturation of dopaminergic neurons seen in the earlier discussed primary monolayer studies.

In contrast to the studies in primary monolayer culture, which showed no difference in dopamine cell number as a function of the presence or absence of target cells, there is a clear-cut enhancement of dopamine cell survival in the reaggregate system in the presence of target cells (Hoffmann, Hemmendinger, Kotake, & Heller, 1983). After 7 days in culture, approximately 4 times as many dopaminergic neurons are found in RMT–CS coaggregates and $1\frac{1}{2}$ times as many in RMT–FCx coaggregates as are found in aggregates of RMT alone or in RMT–OCx or RMT–tectal coaggregates. The enhanced survival probably depends on the ability of the dopaminergic neurons to make contacts with their normal target cells, although an enhanced "capture" of dopaminergic neurons by target cells during the early stages of the formation of the aggregates has not been ruled out.

Reaggregates are formed from dissociated single-cell suspensions. Therefore, the information necessary for target-cell-dependent enhanced dopamine cell survival, as well as axonal proliferation and/or maintenance, must reside in the neurons themselves. Initial attempts to identify factors involved in these phenomena have involved the preparation of membrane fractions from a target area, corpus striatum (CS), and from a nontarget area, tectum (T) (Heller, Hoffmann, & Wainer, 1983). These membranes were then added to a mixture of single dissociated cells from the RMT and the T. Tectal cells were used to maintain equivalent numbers of cells in the various coaggregates. After 8 days in culture, the resulting aggregates were harvested, sectioned and examined under the fluorescence microscope, and the number of dopamine neurons present in randomly selected sections were counted. Compared to RMT–T–CS coaggregates constituted from *intact* cells, RMT–T coaggregates to which tectal membranes had been added yielded only 26% as many dopamine neurons. In contrast, in RMT–T coaggregates to which CS membranes had been added, 69% as many dopamine neurons were found as were present in RMT–T–CS coaggregates produced from *intact* cell populations. Dopaminergic axons (assessed independently by three investigators observing randomized color photomicrographs) in RMT–T–CS coaggregates constituted from intact cells were present in 87% of the sections, whereas only 7% of the sections from coaggregates to which tectal membranes had been added exhibited axons. However, 64% of the sections to which CS membranes had been added had axonal processes. Neither dopamine cell survival nor axonal development was influenced by the supernatant fractions resulting from the membrane preparation. It therefore seems likely that membrane-bound macromolecules are involved in target-cell-dependent enhancement of embryonic dopamine neuron survival as well as in axonal development and/or maintenance (Heller, Hoffmann, & Wainer, 1983).

The time course of the differentiation of dopamine neurons in coculture with their CS target cells over a period of 3 weeks has been examined (Kotake, Hoffmann, & Heller, 1982). Fluorescent cell bodies and patches of punctate pericellular fluorescence representing axonal plexi and containing sufficient *endogenous* dopamine to allow for their visualization were only obtained in the coaggregates after 2 and 3 weeks in culture. Punctate pericellular fluorescence could also be detected in 3- and 7-day coaggregates if following the harvest of the coaggregates they were exposed to $10^{-6}M$ dopamine for 10 minutes in order to load the dopaminergic neuronal processes with dopamine. Biochemical analysis showed that 7-day cultures contained approximately 1 ng dopamine/mg protein, whereas 14-day cultures contained 4.6 ng dopamine/mg protein and 21-day cultures contained 22.6 dopamine ng/mg protein. This increasing dopamine content undoubtedly explains the appearance of endogenous histofluorescence in the 14- and 21-day cultures. The density of the pericellular fluorescence increased with time in culture, as was to be expected given the increasing dopamine content.

In addition, the ability of the dopaminergic neurons to accumulate and retain exogenous dopamine increased with increasing time in culture, reaching a maximum of 82 ng dopamine/mg protein/10 minutes after 3 weeks. This value was 12 times greater than that achieved with 3-day cultures. Three- and 7-day cocultures were much less sensitive to the depleting effects of either reserpine or 6-hydroxydopamine than were 14-and 21-day cocultures. Taken together, these results demonstrate the development in vitro of uptake and storage mechanisms for the accumulated amine. Thus, as in the primary monolayer system, the development of a number of biochemical parameters for the dopaminergic neurons appears to take place in the aggregates in culture in a manner that is to a large extent indistinguishable from that seen in the intact brain.

To further assess the functional integrity of dopaminergic neurons contained within RMT–CS coaggregates, the capacity of the dopaminergic neurons to release [³H]dopamine in response to a number of chemical stimuli was assessed (Shalaby, Kotake, Hoffmann, & Heller, 1983a). Following 17 to 22 days in culture, the coaggregates were incubated in $5.6 \times 10^{-6}M$[³H]dopamine, washed, and then superfused for a period of 2 hours at the rate of 100 μl/minute. Two-minute fractions of the superfusate were collected and counted for radioactivity. [^{3}H]dopamine was spontaneously released at the rate of approximately 1% of the tissue stores every 2 minutes. Depolarization of the neurons with 70 mM potassium over an 8-minute period increased the release of radioactivity by a factor of six, whereas a smaller depolarization produced by 50 mM potassium increased release by a factor of two. This depolarization-induced release of [^{3}H]dopamine was found to be dependent on the presence of extracellular calcium. In addition, a dose-dependent release of [^{3}H]dopamine occurred with superfusion of the indirectly acting sympathomimetic amine d-amphetamine. A peak release of 8.9% of the tissue stores of ^{3}H was induced by $10^{-4}M$ d-amphetamine; $10^{-5}M$ induced 4.4%, $10^{-6}M$ induced 1.9%. A neuropeptide, substance P, also caused a twofold increase in release of [^{3}H]dopamine, although a high concentration ($10^{-4}M$) was required to produce a statistically significant effect. This result presumably reflects the fact that there are substance P neuronal inputs from the corpus striatum to the dopaminergic neurons of the substantia nigra in situ.

Tetrodotoxin ($2.5 \times 10^{-6}M$), which blocks voltage-dependent sodium channels in excitable tissues, caused a 40% decrease in the spontaneous release of radioactivity, suggesting the presence of spontaneous electrical activity within the dopaminergic neurons contained within the coaggregates. The fact that tetrodotoxin also blocks substance P-induced release strongly implies that substance P activates the dopaminergic neurons, which in turn release their transmitter substance. The fraction of the spontaneous release of radioactivity that is tetrodotoxin-sensitive was twice as large in aggregates composed of RMT neurons alone as it was in RMT–CS coaggregates (Shalaby, Kotake, Hoffmann, & Heller, 1983b). It appears that the presence of striatal cells within the coaggregate suppresses the spontaneous neuronal activity that is revealed by the tetrodotoxin sensitivity. In this regard, there appears to be an inhibitory γ-aminobutyric acid-containing pathway from the striatum to the substantia nigra in vivo (Fonnum, Grofova, Rinvik, Storm-Mathison, & Wallberg, 1974; Swift, Hoffmann, & Heller, 1978). It is interesting to speculate that the suppression of neuronal activity in the presence of striatal cells could be due to the establishment in the coaggregates in vitro of such an inhibitory input.

The potential involvement of dopaminergic mechanisms in the target-cell-dependent proliferation and maintenance of dopaminergic axonal processes has also been examined by determining the effect of pharmacological agents that interfere with dopaminergic function in a number of different ways (Kotake, Shalaby, Hoffmann, & Heller,

1983). Since the accumulation and retention of dopamine appears to parallel the morphologically observed proliferation of axonal networks within RMT–CS coaggregates, dopamine retention and accumulation was used as a quantitative index of such proliferation. Chronic exposure of RMT–CS coaggregates to the dopamine antagonists spiroperidol and d-butaclamol ($10^{-7}M$) from 1 through 14 days following reaggregation resulted in a reduction of approximately 40% in the capacity of these coaggregates to accumulate and retain endogenous dopamine. The finding that the isomer l-butaclamol, which is inactive as a dopamine antagonist at an equivalent concentration, did not reduce dopamine accumulation in coaggregates that had been exposed in an identical manner suggests that the drugs' effects on development may be mediated through dopamine receptors. Interference with process formation and/or maintenance can also occur with drugs that interact with dopaminergic neurons in other ways, as shown by the fact that treatment with α-methylparatyrosine ($10^{-4}M$), an inhibitor of tyrosine hydroxylase, or with tetrodotoxin ($10^{-6}M$) also resulted in a 40–50% reduction in the ability of the neurons to accumulate and retain dopamine. These experiments suggest that the activity of dopaminergic neurons and the integrity of dopamine receptors are involved in the normal development of the dopaminergic neurons in vitro.

Transplantation of Embryonic Dopaminergic Neurons into Adult Rodent Brains

The robustness of embryonic dopamine neurons in culture, as reflected in either primary monolayer culture or in the three-dimensional aggregate system, is mirrored by the ability of embryonic dopamine-containing neurons to partially reinnervate the striatum of adult animals in which the nigrostriatal dopaminergic projection has been destroyed. Following unilateral destruction of the substantia nigra with 6-hydroxydopamine, such lesioned animals exhibit pronounced rotational behavior after systemic administration of the dopamine receptor agonist apomorphine (Perlow, Freed, Hoffer, Seiger, Olson, & Wyatt, 1979) or of metamphetamine (Björkland & Stenevi, 1979). Denervated rats that had stable patterns of rotation were subjected to grafting with pieces of embryonic ventral mesencephalon containing the substantia nigra into the lateral ventricle adjacent to the striatum (Perlow al., 1979), or into a cavity created through the parietal cortex and corpus collosum just over the dorsal surface of the striatum (Björklund & Stenevi, 1979). Some weeks after the transplant, the animals were again tested for rotation in response to the same dose of apomorphine (Perlow et al., 1979) or of metamphetamine (Björlund & Stenevi, 1979). Animals that received the transplants containing embryonic dopamine neurons demonstrated a greater reduction in turning behavior than did control animals, suggesting at least a partial functional reinnervation by the dopaminergic neurons.

Histochemical procedures demonstrated that the transplanted embryonic neurons sent dopamine-containing fibers into the denervated striatum, where they formed terminal networks. There was a good correlation between the magnitude of the ingrowth of dopamine-containing fibers and the decrease in the turning response to dopaminergic agonists. These histochemical observations were supported by biochemical measurements that demonstrated increases in dopamine concentrations in areas of the striatum adjacent to the transplants (Freed, Perlow, Karoum, Seiger, Olson, Hoffer, & Wyatt, 1980).

Further studies with such transplanted animals have demonstrated less asymmetry in *spontaneous* rotational behavior than with control animals (Björklund, Dunnett, Stenevi, Lewis, & Iversen, 1980; Dunnett, Björklund, Stenevi, & Iversen, 1981a). Moreover, when tested for behavior that reflected spontaneous choice in a T maze, the rats with transplants often chose the side of the T maze (30–40%) that was contralateral to the lesion, whereas control-lesioned rats virtually always (97%) selected the arm of the T maze ipsilateral to the 6-hydroxydopamine lesion. However, animals receiving the transplant did not compensate for the sensory–motor deficits that resulted from the lesion.

In animals that were bilaterally lesioned and received bilateral transplants, the lesion-induced adipsia, aphagia, and akinesia were unaffected by the transplants (Björklund, Stenevi, Dunnett, & Iversen, 1981). From these observations the conclusion was drawn that the improved motor behavior was due to the reinnervation by the transplants of the dorsal aspect of the striatum, whereas the failure of the transplants to improve sensory–motor performance or to cause recovery from the consummatory deficits was due to the inability of the transplants to reinnervate the remaining neostriatum (Björklund et al., 1981).

This interpretation received strong support in the later demonstration that shifting the site of the transplant to a cavity in the lateral cortex led to a reinnervation of the ventral and lateral aspects of the striatum (Dunnett, Björklund, Stenevi, & Iversen, 1981b). In such transplanted animals, there was significant restoration of sensory–motor performance and, strikingly, no change in drug-induced rotational behavior. As noted earlier, drug-induced rotational behavior in unilaterally lesioned animals had been alleviated by transplants placed to reinnervate the dorsal aspect of the striatum. Additionally, animals receiving the lateral transplants showed a marked reduction in the akinesia produced by bilateral lesions. These experiments strongly suggest that dopaminergic innervation to the striatum is topographically organized with respect to particular kinds of behavior.

It has also been found that transplantation of murine embryonic mesencephalic dopamine neurons can result in a functional reinnervation of the denervated striatum in adult rats (Björklund, Stenevi, Dunnett, & Gage, 1982). Out of 18 animals, 10 had surviving dopamine neurons after 6 months. There was a good correlation between the degree of reinnervation and compensation in the turning behavior elicited by metamphetamine or apomorphine. The dopamine neurons that survived were found on the surface as well as in the depth of the recipient striatum. The remaining bulk of the transplant had been almost completely reabsorbed. On the basis of these observations the authors suggest that the migratory capacity of the embryonic neurons that are contained within the transplant may be of special importance in their ability to escape immunologically mediated rejection. These experiments demonstrated that transplantion of embryonic dopamine neurons, followed by functionally significant consequences, can be accomplished across immunological barriers, even in the absence of immunosuppressive treatment.

Other studies have demonstrated that adult adrenal medullary chromaffin cells can be substituted for the fetal mesencephalic grafts (Freed, Morihisa, Spoor, Hoffer, Olson, Seiger, & Wyatt, 1981). Such transplants produce a subsequent reduction of about 50% in the apomorphine-induced turning behavior that results from the unilateral denervation of the striatum. Histofluorescent observations showed that the catecholamine-containing chromaffin cells had developed polygonal morphology and had grouped themselves into one or two small clusters within the graft. Moreover, some of these cells had fine elongated processes, only a very few of which were seen entering the recipient brain. These results suggest that catecholamines or other substances produced in the graft can diffuse into the striatum in sufficient amounts to reduce the apomorphine-induced rotation in the lesioned animals. The incomplete transformation of the chromaffin cells toward the neuronal phenotype is explained by the authors on the basis of the absence of nerve growth factor (Freed *et al.*, 1981).

In an attempt to determine whether the transplanted embryonic dopamine neurons released dopamine from nerve terminals upon activation of the dopamine-containing cell bodies or if there was simple spontaneous release of dopamine into the striatum, the ability of transplants to maintain intracranial self-stimulation was examined (Fray, Dunnett, Iversen, Björklund, & Stenevi, 1983). Unilateral lesions were produced with 6-hydroxydopamine, and transplants either of embryonic substantia nigra or of embryonic isotopic cortex were placed into cortical cavities created above the dorsal surface of the striatum. After 4 months, bipolar stimulating electrodes were implanted into the surviving grafts. The animals were trained to perform intracranial self-stimulation 1 week after electrode placement. On the last 3 days, responses to a constant current intensity were determined. Of the 10 animals that had received the nigral embryonic transplant, 9 consistently responded at a greater rate than either rats that had received cortical transplants or rats in which the electrodes were implanted directly into the denervated striatum. Moreover, the nigra-transplant rats showed the typical increase in rate following administration of amphetamine, and this increment could be blocked by the neuroleptic drug α-flupenthixol. Fluoresence histochemistry showed that reinnervation by the grafts ranged from $\frac{1}{8}$ to $\frac{1}{3}$ of the dorsal aspect of the striatum. Histological examination revealed that in the animals with nigral transplants that had self-stimulated, the electrode tip was near dopamine neurons or their outgrowing fibers. The results of these experiments suggest that the transplanted dopamine neurons can be activated in such a way that the axons carry information to the striatum and thereby sustain intracranial self-stimulation. It is quite remarkable that these dopamine nerve cell bodies do not appear to require their normal location within the brain in order to sustain this behavior.

Within less than 4 years, it has been possible to exploit the remarkable viability of embryonic dopamine neurons to apparently reverse behavioral abnormalities associated with experimental destruction of these neurons in the adult animal. The results of such experiments clearly challenge previously held notions about the reversibility of the consequences of certain types of brain damage, and they may be applicable in certain clinical conditions.

Acknowledgments

That part of the research described here that was conducted in the authors' laboratories was supported by grants from the National Institute of Mental Health (MH 28942) and the Brain Research Foundation of Chicago. We thank E. Dimapalis, L. Hemmendinger, F. Karapas, C. Kotake, and I. Shalaby for their participation in various aspects of this work, and J. DeGroot for manuscript preparation.

References

Berger, B., di Porzio, U., Daguet, M.-C., Gay, M., Vigny, A., Glowinski, J., & Prochiantz, A. (1982). Long-term development of mesencephalic dopaminergic neurons of mouse embryos in dissociated primary cultures: Morphological and histochemical characteristics. *Neuroscience, 7,* 193–205.

Björklund, A., Dunnett, S. B., Stenevi, U., Lewis, M. E., & Iversen, S. D. (1980). Reinnervation of the denervated striatum by substantia nigra transplants: Functional consequences as revealed by pharmacological and sensorimotor testing. *Brain Research, 199,* 307–333.

Björklund, A., & Stenevi, U. (1979). Reconstruction of the nigrostriatal dopamine pathway by intracerebral transplants. *Brain Research, 177,* 555–560.

Björklund, A., Stenevi, U., Dunnett, S. B., & Gage, F. H. (1982). Cross-species neural grafting in a rat model of Parkinson's disease. *Nature, 298,* 652–654.

Björklund, A., Stenevi, U., Dunnett, S. B., & Iversen, S. D. (1981). Functional reactivation of deafferented neostriatum by nigral transplants. *Nature, 289,* 497–499.

Coyle, J. T., & Henry, D. (1973). Catecholamines in fetal and newborn rat brain. *Journal of Neurochemistry, 21,* 61–67.

Daguet, M.-C., di Porzio, U., Prochiantz, A., Kato, A., & Glowinki, J. (1980). Release of dopamine from mesencephalic dopaminergic neurons in primary cultures in absence or presence of striatal target cells. *Brain Research, 191,* 564–568.

di Porzio, U., Daguet, M.-C., Glowinski, J., & Prochiantz, A. (1980). Effect of striatal cells on *in vitro* maturation of mesencephalic dopaminergic neurons grown in serum-free conditions. *Nature, 288,* 370–373.

Dunnett, S. B., Björklund, A., Stenevi, U., & Iversen, S. D. (1981a). Behavioral recovery following transplantation of substantia nigra in rats subjected to 6-OHDA lesions of the nigrostriatal pathway. 1. Unilateral lesions. *Brain Research, 215,* 147–161.

Dunnett, S. B., Björklund, A., Stenevi, U., & Iversen, S. D. (1981b). Grafts of embryonic substantia nigra reinnervating the ventrolateral striatum ameliorate sensorimotor impairments and akinesia in rats with 6-OHDA lesions of the nigrostriatal pathway. *Brain Research, 229,* 209–217.

Erinoff, L., MacPhail, R. C., Heller, A., & Seiden, L. S. (1979). Age-dependent effects of 6-hydroxydopamine on locomotor activity in the rat. *Brain Research, 164,* 195–205.

Fonnum, F., Grofova, I., Rinvik, E., Storm-Mathison, J., & Wallberg, F. (1974). Origin and distribution of glutamate decarboxylase in substantia nigra of the cat. *Brain Research, 71*, 77–92.

Fray, P. J., Dunnett, S. B., Iversen, S. D., Björklund, A., & Stenevi, U. (1983). Nigral transplants reinnervating the dopamine-depleted neostriatum can sustain intracranial self-stimulation. *Science, 219*, 416–419.

Freed, W. J., Morihisa, J. M., Spoor, E., Hoffer, B. J., Olson, L., Seiger, A., & Wyatt, R. J. (1981). Transplanted adrenal chromaffin cells in rat brain reduce lesion-induced rotational behavior. *Nature, 292*, 351–352.

Freed, W. J., Perlow, M. J., Karoum, F., Seiger, A., Olson, L., Hoffer, B. J., & Wyatt, R. J. (1980). Restoration of dopaminergic function by grafting of fetal substantia nigra to the caudate nucleus: Long-term behavioral, biochemical, and histochemical studies. *Annals of Neurology, 8*, 510–519.

Garber, B. B., & Moscona, A. A. (1972). Reconstruction of brain tissue from cell suspensions. I. Aggregation patterns of cells dissociated from different regions of the developing brain. *Developmental Biology, 27*, 217–234.

Heller, A., Hoffmann, P. C. & Wainer, B. (1983). Enhancement of dopamine neuron survival and axonal proliferation by membranes from striatal target cells. *Abstracts of the Society for Neuroscience 9*, 10.

Hemmendinger, L. M., Garber, B. B., Hoffmann, P. C., & Heller, A. (1981a). Selective association of embryonic murine mesencephalic dopamine neurons *in vitro. Brain Research, 222*, 417–422.

Hemmendinger, L. M., Garber, B. B., Hoffmann, P. C., & Heller, A. (1981b). Target neuron-specific process formation by embryonic mesencephalic dopamine neurons *in vitro. Proceedings of the National Academy of Science, 78*, 1264–1268.

Hoffmann, P. C., Hemmendinger, L. M., Kotake, C., & Heller, A. (1983). Enhanced dopamine cell survival in reaggregates containing telencephalic target cells. *Brain Research, 274*, 275–281.

Honegger, P., & Richelson, E. (1977). Biochemical differentiation of aggregating cell cultures of different fetal rat brain regions. *Brain Research, 133*, 329–339.

Honegger, P., & Richelson, E. (1979). Neurotransmitter synthesis, storage and release by aggregating cell cultures of rat brain. *Brain Research, 162*, 89–107.

Jonsson, G. (1980). Chemical neurotoxins as denervation tools in neurobiology. *Annual Review of Neurosciences, 3*, 169–187.

Kotake, C., Hoffmann, P. C., & Heller, A. (1982). The biochemical and morphological development of differentiating dopamine neurons coaggregated with their target cells of the corpus striatum *in vitro. Journal of Neuroscience, 2*, 1307–1315.

Kotake, C., Shalaby, I., Hoffmann, P., & Heller, A. (1983). Effect of dopamine antagonists tetrodotoxin and alpha-methyl-p-tyrosine on development of dopamine neurons in reaggregating cocultures of midbrain and striatum. *Federation Proceedings, 42*, 880.

Leon, A., Dal toso, R., di Porzio, U., Facci, L., Mazzari, S., & Toffano, G. (1982). The effect of striatal target neurons on the maturation *in vitro* of mesencephalic dopaminergic neurons is potentiated by GM_1 ganglioside. *Abstracts of the Society for Neuroscience, 8*, 760.

Levitt, P., Moore, R. Y., & Garber, B. B. (1976). Selective cell association of catecholamine neurons in brain aggregates *in vitro. Brain Research, 111*, 311–320.

Loren, I., Björklund, A., Falck, B., & Lindvall, O. (1980). The aluminum-formaldehyde (ALSA) histofluorescence method for improved visualization of catecholamines and indoleamines. *Journal of Neuroscience Methods, 2*, 277–300.

Miller, F. E., Heffner, T. G., Kotake, C., & Seiden, L. S. (1981). Magnitude and duration and hyperactivity following neonatal 6-hydroxydopamine is related to the extent of brain dopamine depletion. *Brain Research, 229,* 123–132.

Monroy, A., & Moscona, A. A. (1979). *Introductory concepts in developmental biology* (170). Chicago: University of Chicago Press.

Moore, R. Y., Bhatnagar, R. K., & Heller, A. (1971). Anatomical and chemical studies of a nigro-neostriatal projection in the cat. *Brain Research, 30,* 119–135.

Moore, R. Y., Björklund, A., & Stenevi, U. (1971). Plastic changes in the adrenergic innervation of the rat septal area in response to denervation. *Brain Research, 33,* 13–35.

Olson, L., & Seiger, A. (1972). Early prenatal ontogeny of central monoamine neurons in the rat. Fluorescence histochemical observations. *Zeitschrift Anatomisches Entwicklungsgeschichte, 137,* 301–346.

Perlow, M. J., Freed, W. J., Hoffer, B. J., Seiger, A., Olson, L., & Wyatt, R. J. (1979). Brain grafts reduce motor abnormalities produced by destruction of nigrostriatal dopamine system. *Science 204,* 643–647.

Porcher, W., & Heller, A. (1972). Regional development of catecholamine biosynthesis in rat brain. *Journal of Neurochemistry, 19,* 1917–1930.

Prochiantz, A., di Porzio, U., Kato, A., Berger, B., & Glowinski, J. (1979). *In vitro* maturation of mesencephalic dopaminergic neurons from mouse embryos is enhanced in presence of their striatal target cells. *Proceedings of the National Academy of Science, 76,* 5387–5391.

Prochiantz, A., Daguet, M.-C., Herbet, A., & Glowinski, J. (1981). Specific stimulation of *in vitro* maturation of mesencephalic dopaminergic neurons by striatal membranes. *Nature, 293,* 570–572.

Seiden, L. S., & Dykstra, L. A. (1977). Dopamine, norepinephrine, and behavior. In *Psychopharmacology: A behavioral and biochemical approach* (pp. 117–171). New York: Van Nostrand-Reinhold.

Shalaby, I., Kotake, C., Hoffmann, P. C., & Heller, A. (1983a). Release of dopamine from coaggregate cultures of mesencephalic tegmentum and corpus striatum. *Journal of Neuroscience, 3,* 1565–1571.

Shalaby, I., Kotake, C., Hoffmann, P. C., & Heller, A. (1983b). Release of dopamine in aggregate cultures of midbrain neurons: Effect of striatal cells. *Federation Proceedings, 42,* 880.

Shaywitz, D. A., Yager, R. D., & Klopper, J. H. (1976). Selective brain dopamine depletion in developing brains: An experimental model of minimal brain dysfunction. *Science, 191,* 305–308.

Specht, L. A., Pickel, V. M., Joh, T. H., & Reis, D. J. (1981). Light microscopic immunocytochemical localization of tyrosine hydroxylase in prenatal rat brain. I. Early ontogeny. *Journal of Comparative Neurology, 199,* 233–253.

Swift, R. M., Hoffmann, P. C., & Heller, A. (1978). Activity-dependent changes in substantia nigra γ-aminobutyric acid. *Brain Research, 156,* 181–186.

Tennyson, V. M., Barrett, R. E., Cohen, G., Cote, L., Heikela, R., & Mytilineou, C. (1972). The developing neostriatum of the rabbit: Correlation of fluorescence histochemistry, electron microscopy, endogenous dopamine levels and (^{3}H) dopamine uptake. *Brain Research, 46,* 251–285.

Toffano, G., Savoini, G., Moroni, F., Lombardi, M. G., & Agnati, L. F. (1982). Lesioning and recovery of nigro-striatal dopaminergic neurons: Effect of GM_1 ganglioside treatment. *Abstracts of the Society for Neuroscience, 8,* 916.

Ungerstedt, U. (1971). Striatal dopamine release after amphetamine or nerve degeneration revealed by rotational behavior. *Acta Physiologica Scandinavica*, (Suppl. 367), 49–68.

Zigmond, M. J., & Stricker, E. M. (1974). Ingestive behavior following damage to central dopamine neurons: Implication for homeostasis and recovery of function. In E. Usdin (Ed.), *Neuropsychopharmacology of monoamines and their regulatory enzymes* (pp. 385–401). New York: Raven.

3

Lesion-Induced Sprouting in the Red Nucleus at the Early Developmental Stage

Yutaka Fujito, Shuji Watanabe,
Hisashi Kobayashi,
and Nakaakira Tsukahara

Introduction

Sprouting and the formation of new synapses is one of the possible mechanisms for recovery of function after brain damage and perhaps one of the neuronal bases for the adaptive properties, such as learning and memory, of the normal brain. It is generally agreed that the extent and degree of axonal sprouting and synaptogenesis is more remarkable after denervation in the early developmental stage than in the adult stage (see Cotman & Lynch, 1976; Lund, 1978; Tsukahara, 1981 for reviews). After unilateral enucleation in neonates, for example, axons from the intact retina invade an inappropriate lamina in the dorsal lateral geniculate nucleus (Guillery, 1972; Hickey, 1975), and an aberrant ipsilateral pathway from the remaining eye arises in the superior colliculus (Lund & Lund, 1971, 1976). After unilateral destruction of the cerebral cortex in neonatal rats, abnormal projections from the remaining cerebral cortex have been shown to appear in the red nucleus, pons, superior colliculus, dorsal column nuclei, medullary reticular formation, and spinal cord (Hicks & D'Amato, 1970; Leong, 1976; Leong & Lund, 1973; Nah & Leong, 1976a, 1976b). Neonatal hemicerebellectomy results in the appearance of uncrossed cerebello–thalamic and cerebello–rubral projections (Castro, 1978; Kawaguchi, Yamamoto, Samejima, Itoh, & Mizuno, 1979; Lim & Leong, 1975). In addition, it is well established that sprouting occurs in the adult central nervous system and also that the newly formed synapses are functional (Cotman & Lynch, 1976; More, Björklund, & Stenevi, 1971; Murakami, Katsumaru, Saito, & Tsukahara, 1982; Murakami, Tsukahara, & Fujito, 1977; Raisman, 1969; Steward, Cotman, & Lynch, 1973; Tsukahara, Hultborn, & Murakami, 1974; Tsukahara, Hultborn, Murakami, & Fujito, 1975a).

Red nucleus (RN) neurons of cats provide a good substrate for examining whether new, functional synapses are formed following partial denervation. RN neurons have two major synaptic inputs, one from the contralateral nucleus interpositus (IP) of the cerebellum onto the proximal portion of the soma–dendritic membrane of the cells and the other from the ipsilateral cerebral cortex onto the distal dendrites. The segregation of the two kinds of input on the RN cell membrane characterizes postsynaptic potentials (EPSPs) in RN cells. The EPSPs produced by the corticorubral dendritic synapses are characterized by a slow-rising time course due to the distortion of the waveform during the electrotonic propagation of EPSPs from dendrites to the soma, whereas the EPSPs produced by the IP-rubral somatic synapses are characterized by a fast-rising time course (Tsukahara & Kosaka, 1968; Tsukahara, Murakami, & Hultborn, 1975b). After destruction of the contralateral IP in adult cats, a new fast-rising component appeared in the corticorubral EPSPs and was interpreted as being produced by the newly formed synapses located on the proximal portion of the soma–dendritic membrane of RN cells (Tsukahara et al., 1974, 1975a). There is also evidence to suggest that sprouting and the formation of new synapses occurs in the intact RN of adult cats following cross-innervation of forelimb flexor and extensor nerves (Fujito, Tsukahara, Oda, & Yoshida, 1982; Tsukahara & Fujito, 1976; Tsukahara, Fujito, Oda, & Maeda, 1982). This evidence suggests that sprouting occurs without lesions and is likely to underlie the neuronal mechanism for the adaptive properties of the brain in response to the environmental changes.

In this chapter we show our physiological investigations on sprouting and the formation of synapses in the kitten RN after destruction of the ipsilateral cerebral cortex. Attention is focused on several kinds of specificity of organization of newly formed corticorubral projection from the contralateral cerebral cortex (Fujito, Tsukahara, & Yoshida, 1980; Tsukahara & Fujito, 1981; Tsukahara, Fujito, & Kubota, 1983). In addition, the effect of gangliosides, which are major lipid constituents of brain tissue and a possible neurite-elongation factor (Rapport & Gorio, 1981), on the formation of new projections in the RN from the contralateral cerebral cortex following lesions of the ipsilateral cerebral cortex is examined.

Sprouting and Formation of New Synapses in Red Nucleus Neurons following Ipsilateral Cerebral Cortex Lesions

SYNAPTIC ORGANIZATION OF THE NORMAL KITTEN
RED NUCLEUS

We examined synaptic organization of the RN of normal kittens 37–132 days old. Procedures for intracellular recording from neurons of left-side RN were essentially the same as those employed previously (Tsukahara et al., 1975a). However, the difference in size and shape between the young and the adult cat brain necessitated a recalibration of stereotaxic coordinates. C_1 and L_1 spinal segments were exposed and stimulated on the right surface to identify RN neurons by antidromic activation. RN cells activated from both C_1 and L_1 were designated L-cells; those activated only from C_1, C-cells (Tsukahara & Kosaka, 1968). Corticorubral fibers were stimulated at two levels, within the sensory–motor cortex (SM) and at the cerebral peduncle (CP).

Cerebrorubral and cerebellorubral projections were examined in normal kittens. Stimulation of the contralateral IP of the cerebellum produced fast-rising EPSPs (Figure 1[a]) with a mean latency of 1.0 msec and time to peak of 0.75 msec, as occurs in adult RN (Tsukahara & Kosaka, 1968). No detectable EPSPs were induced by stimulation of the ipsilateral IP, as is shown in Figure 1(b). Slow-rising dendritic EPSPs (Figure 1[c]) and, in some cases, succeeding IPSPs (not illustrated) were induced by stimulating the ipsilateral cerebral SM or its efferent fibers at the CP, as occurs in normal cats. The mean latency and time to peak of the EPSPs of the ipsilateral CP were 1.4 msec and 3.4 msec, respectively. Stimulation of the contralateral SM or CP did not produce any detectable EPSPs in the majority of RN cells, as is shown in Figure 1(d). These results indicate that the synaptic organization of the RN is virtually the same in kitten and adult (Figure 1[e]). Fibers from the contralateral IP terminate on the soma or the promixal dendrites of RN cells, where-

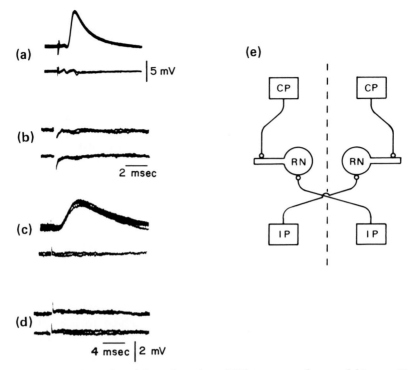

Figure 1. EPSPs induced in red nucleus (RN) neurons of normal kittens. Upper traces of (a–d) represent intracellular records. Lower traces of (a–d) are the corresponding extracellular records. (a) EPSPs produced in an RN neuron by stimulation of the contralateral nucleus interpositus (IP) of the cerebellum. (b) records induced by stimulation of the ipsilateral IP. (c) EPSPs elicited by stimulation of the ipsilateral cerebral peduncle (CP). (d) stimulation of the contralateral CP which produces no response. Voltage calibration in (d) also applies to (a–c). Time calibrations in (b) and (d) also apply to (a) and (c), respectively. (e) synaptic connections of the kitten RN. A dashed line represents the midline.

as fibers from the ipsilateral cerebral cortex make contact on the remote dendrites of RN neurons.

Newly Appearing Postsynaptic Potentials
in the Red Nucleus following Ablation
of the Ipsilateral Cerebral Cortex

The ipsilateral (left) frontal cerebral cortex, the sensory–motor cortex, the frontal portion of the parietal association cortex, and the surrounding cortex were ablated by aspiration under direct vision in kittens from 17to 149 days of age. These chronic kittens were reared for periods of time greater than 3 weeks, ranging from 20 to 247 days (mean = 105 days), after the cerebral destruction until the time of the acute experiments. In these chronic cats, three sprouting sources were found: (1) Stimulation of the contralateral SM or CP produced slow-rising EPSPs, as is exemplified in Figure 2(a); (2) Slow-rising EPSPs were produced in some cells by stimulation of the ipsilateral IP, as is shown in Figure 2(b); (3) Stimulation of the contralateral IP sometimes induced a slow-rising component that was superimposed on the normal fast-rising EPSPs, as is shown in Figure 2(c). The mean times to peak of the EPSPs of the contralateral CP, the ipsilateral IP, and the later component of the contralateral IP were 3.4 msec, 2.9 msec and 2.8 msec, respectively. The mean latency for the con-

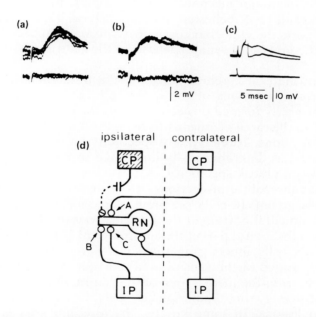

Figure 2. Newly appearing EPSPs in kitten RN cells following lesions of the ipsilateral cerebral cortex. (a) newly appearing EPSPs from stimulation of the contralateral cerebral penduncle (CP) (upper trace). Corresponding extracellular records are represented by the lower traces in (a–c). (b) newly appearing EPSPs produced by stimulation of the ipsilateral nucleus interpositus (IP). (c) slow-rising EPSPs superimposed on the normal fast-rising EPSPs by stimulation of the contralateral IP. Voltage calibration in (b) also applies to (a). Time calibration in (c) also applies to (a) and (b). (d) connections of newly formed synapses in the kitten RN following ablation of the ipsilateral cerebral cortex. Arrows indicate newly formed synapses. Dotted line represents the midline. Shade shows the lesion.

tralateral CP was 1.7 msec and that for the ipsilateral IP was 1.5 msec.

The newly appearing slow-rising EPSPs that were induced by stimulation of these three sprouting inputs, the contralateral CP and the ipsilateral and contralateral IP, were less sensitive to membrane potential displacement than were the fast-rising EPSPs of the contralateral IP. Therefore, these newly formed synapses, produced following unilateral cerebral cortex destruction, are located on the distal dendrites of RN cells.

Among these three sprouting inputs, there was an interesing tendency for only one source to produce new synapses in 50 (80%) of the 62 RN cells in which all three possible sources were tested. This evidence suggests some competitive interaction between the three sources of synaptogenesis. It has been shown that competitive interaction is the major mechanism in developing mammalian muscle (Betz, Caldwell, & Ribchester, 1980; Willshaw, 1981). The present result supports the view that competitive interaction between inputs exists in the process of synaptogenesis in the central nervous system (CNS).

The contralateral cerebral cortex is the predominant sprouting source following lesions of the ipsilateral cerebral cortex. It was found that newly formed projections from the contralateral SM are organized in the same manner as those in the normal ipsilateral SM–rubral projections. Three types of specificity have been investigated in this study, as diagramatically illustrated in Figure 3. Figure 3(a) shows topographical specificity as it is found in the normal ipsilateral cerebrorubral projections. RN neurons innervating the upper spinal segments (C-cells, see previous section), which are located in the dorsomedial portion of the nucleus, received EPSPs predominantly from the lateral part of the contralateral SM (forelimb region), whereas RN cells innervating the lower spinal segment (L-cells), which are located in the ventrolateral portion, received EPSPs predominantly from the medial area of the contralateral SM (hindlimb region). However, this topographical specificity is modifiable with additional lesions. In some kittens, the forelimb area of the contralateral SM was destroyed in addition to the ipsilateral cerebral ablation. In these kittens, the remaining hindlimb region of the contralateral SM projects not only onto L-cells but also onto C-cells, indicating expansion of the projective area. Organizational specificity with respect to excitatory versus inhibitory connections of the newly formed connections (Figure 3[b]) was found to be similar to that of the normal ipsilateral corticorubral projections. In the normal

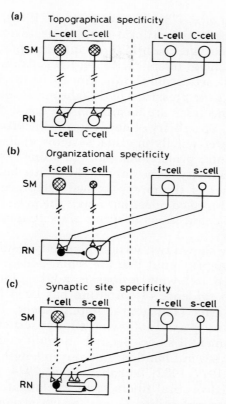

Figure 3. Specificity of connections in the newly formed cerebrorubral projections. (a) topographical specificity for somatotopy: (SM) sensory–motor cortex; (RN) red nucleus; (L-cell) cells innervating lumbosacral spinal cord; (C-cell) cells innervating cervicothoracic spinal cord. Dashed vertical lines, midlines; shaded cells, lesions. (b) organizational specificity with respect to excitatory versus inhibitory connections. (f-cell) fast-conducting pyramidal tract cell; (s-cell) slow-conducting pyramidal tract cell; Open circles, excitatory neurons; filled circles, inhibitory neurons. (c) same as (b) but for specificity of synaptic location on the somadendritic membrane of the RN cell.

cerebrorubral projections, fast-conducting pyramidal tract fibers connect to inhibitory interneurons in the RN region, whereas slow-conducting corticofugal fibers excite RN cells directly. The conduction velocity of fibers mediating the new corticorubral EPSPs in kittens with the ipsilateral cerebral lesions was in the range of 10 to 20 m/sec, which is in the range of slow-conducting pyramidal tract fibers or the normal excitatory corticorubral fibers. For several reasons (Tsukahara *et al.*, 1975a; Tsukahara *et al.*, 1983) it appears that, in the newly formed corticorubral projections, fast-conducting corticofugal fibers innervate the inhibitory interneurons, whereas slow-conducting corticofugal fibers excite the RN cells directly, as in the normal ipsilateral corticorubral projections. The specificity of synaptic location seems to be preserved in that the newly formed excitatory corticorubral connections are formed on the distal dendrites of RN cells (Figure 3[c]). Specificity of newly formed neuronal connections has been investigated chiefly in visual systems such as the retinotectal or retinocollicular projections. In these visual systems, however, topographical specificity is the only kind that has been investigated. In contrast, studies of the newly formed cerebrorubral map have clarified hitherto unasked questions about the preservation of specificity of neuronal connections in terms of excitatory and inhibitory connections.

Our results have shown two sorts of plasticity resulting from early damage to RN synaptic input that are remarkable increases beyond plasticity observed following lesions in adults (Tsukahara, 1981). First, whereas no evidence of sprouting has been found after SM lesions in adult cats (Tsukahara, unpublished), three sprouting sources have been observed following similar lesions performed at the early developmental stage. Second, in adult cats, corticorubral fibers sprout only several hundred microns in length after IP lesions (Murakami *et al.*, 1977, 1982; Tsukahara *et al.*, 1974, 1975a), whereas newly formed corticorubral fibers seem to elongate a considerable distance, up to several milimeters, after early damage of the ipsilateral cortex.

The degree and extent of formation of the contralateral corticorubral projection depends on the age of the animal at the time of the cerebral lesions. In order to evaluate the age dependency of sprouting of contralateral cerebrorubral fibers, recordings were made from kittens operated on at different times after birth. The degree of development of the contralateral cerebrorubral projections was estimated as a ratio of the number of RN cells in which EPSPs of the contralateral CP were detected to the number of sampled RN neurons in each chronic kittens with the ipsilateral cerebral lesions. The ratio of each chronic kitten was plotted against the time of the cerebral ablation, as is shown in Figure 4. It was found that the probability of appearance of detectable EPSPs of the contralateral CP is highest in kittens operated on at 17 days of age, after which it gradually decreases.

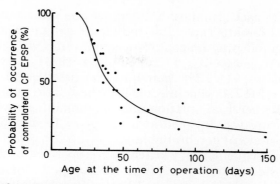

Figure 4. Age dependency of the appearance of contralateral CP EPSPs. Ordinate: ratio of the number of RN neurons in which EPSPs were recorded to the total number of sampled RN cells in each cat. Abscissa: age of cat at which the ipsilateral cerebral cortex was destroyed.

Effect of Ganglioside Application on Synaptic Plasticity

Gangliosides are characteristic acidic glycolipids in plasma membranes and are especially abundant in nerve cells of the brain. It has been suggested that they promote neurite growth in the CNS (Rapport & Gorio, 1981). We examined the effect of ganglioside application on sprouting and synaptogenesis of cerebrorubral fibers.

Bovine brain matter was homogenized in 10 volumes of cold acetone to remove neutral lipids and water, the homogenate was filtered by centrifugation, and the residue was dried at room temperature. The acetone-dried powder thus obtained was successively treated with 10 volumes each of chloroform–methanol mixtures in volume ratios of 1:1, 1:2, and 2:1 at room temperature. After adding 13 l of chloroform and 7.5 l of 0.74% KCl to the extraction solution, the lower phase was subjected to extraction with 7.5 l of a mixture of 0.5% KCl, methanol, and chloroform in a volume ratio of 49:48:1. The residue obtained by evaporation of the upper phase was dissolved in 500 ml of 0.5 N NaOH in methanol and incubated 20 minutes at 37°C, neutralized with 450 ml of 0.5 N acetic acid, and evaporated. The residue was dissolved in water, dialyzed against water, and lyophilized (crude gangliosides). The crude gangliosides were dissolved in a chloroform–methanol mixture in a 1:1 volume ratio and fractionated over a column of 100 g of DEAE–Sephadex A–25 (4 cm x

30 cm). After each ganglioside fractions was subjected to analytical thin-layer chromatography, the individual ganglioside was detected with resorcinol spray reagent. The gangliosides were determined to be 26.5% GM_1, 39% GD_{1a}, 17.3% GD_{1b}, 14.3% GT_{1b}, and 3.1% others (GQ_{1b}, proteins, etc.). The gangliosides (dissolved in 0.01 M phosphate buffer, pH 7.4) were injected into the gelatin sponge, which was inserted after cerebral ablation into the remaining cavity. The ganglioside mixture was injected at a dosage of 10 mg/day for 10 days after the ipsilateral cerebral ablation.

In this experiment, eight kittens were operated and treated with the ganglioside mixture from 79 to 135 days after birth. Two kittens were injected with the buffer for 10 days after the cerebral ablation as a control experiment. As shown in Figure 4, a larger proportion of the RN cells did not produce the EPSPs of the contralateral CP in the untreated kittens in which the ipsilateral cerebral cortices were chronically ablated at more than 2 months after birth. In contrast, the probability of appearance of the EPSPs of the contralateral CP was clearly higher, from 50–86%, in the ganglioside-treated kittens following cerebral ablation at 79 to 135 days of age (Figure 5, open squares). Intraventricular injection of the phosphate buffer alone seemed to produce no significant effect on sprouting of new contralateral cerebrorubral fibers (Figure 5, stars). Therefore, gang-

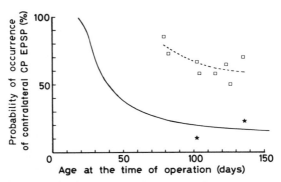

Figure 5. Effect of ganglioside administration on the appearance of new EPSPs induced by stimulation of the contralateral CP after destruction of the ipsilateral cerebral cortex. Ordinate: ratio of the number of RN neurons in which EPSPs were recorded to the total number of sampled RN cells in each cat. Abscissa: age of cat at which ipsilateral cerebral cortex was destroyed. Open squares, ganglioside-adminis-trated kittens after lesions of the ipsilateral cerebral cortex. Stars, phosphate-buffer-injected kittens following the cerebral destruction. Solid line represents the time course of the appearance of the newly appearing contralateral CP EPSPs in untreated cats with the ipsilateral cerebral ablation (see Figure 4).

lioside application appears to have a facilitatory effect on sprouting and formation of functional synapses in the kitten RN.

Oderfeld-Nowak and her colleagues have shown that chronic ganglioside administration facilitates the regrowth of new cholinergic nerve terminals in the rat hippocampus after restricted septal lesions (Oderfeld-Nowak, Wójcik, Ulas, & Potempska, 1981; Wójcik, Ulas, & Oderfeld-Nowak, 1982) by measuring the recovery of activity of cholinergic enzymes. Our findings on the effect of chronic ganglioside administration on growth and synaptogenesis of corticofugal fibers adds evidence on the facilitatory factor of synaptic plasticity in the CNS.

Nerve growth factor has been the only purified and well-characterized factor for survival, differentiation, and growth of neurons. Gangliosides are a family of glycolipids, and many species of ganglioside molecules have been detected (Rapport, 1981). Identification of the factor that is responsible for the facilitatory effects and investigation of the mechanisms for these effects in further detail is a likely subject for research.

Acknowledgments

The authors express their appreciation to Yoshitaka Nagai, Dep. of Biochemistry, Faculty of Medicine, University of Tokyo, Ken Ei Tan, Division of Biochemistry, Institute of Biological Sciences, Mitsui Pharmaceuticals, Inc. (MPI) and Akira Awaya, New Product Planning Department of MPI for their helpful discussions about ganglioside preparation and encouragement through this study.

References

Betz, W. J., Caldwell, J. H., & Ribchester, R. R. (1980). The effects of partial denervation at birth on the development of muscle fibers and motor units in rat lumbrical muscle. *The Journal of Physiology, 303*, 265–279.

Castro, A. (1978). Projections of superior cerebellar peduncle in rats and the development of new connections in response to neonatal hemicerebellectomy. *Journal of Comparative Neurology, 178*, 611–628.

Cotman, C. W., & Lynch, G. S. (1976). Reactive synaptogenesis in the adult nervous system; the effect of partial deafferentation on new synapse formation. In S. Barondes (Ed.), *Neuronal recognition* (pp. 69–108). New York: Plenum.

Fujito, Y., Tsukahara, N., Oda, Y., & Yoshida, M. (1982). Formation of functional synapses in the adult cat red nucleus from the cerebrum following cross-innervation of forelimb flexor and extensor nerves. II. Analysis of newly-appeared synaptic potentials. *Experimental Brain Research, 45*, 13–18.

Fujito, Y., Tsukahara, N., & Yoshida, M. (1980). Synaptic plasticity of the red nucleus in chronically hemicerebellectomized or hemispherectomized kittens. *Neuroscience Letters Supplement, 4*, S42.

Guillery, R. W. (1972). Experiments to determine whether retinogeniculate axons can form translaminar sprouts in the dorsal lateral geniculate nucleus of the cat. *Journal of Comparative Neurology, 146*, 407–420.

Hickey, T. L. (1975). Translaminar growth of axons in the kitten dorsal lateral geniculate nucleus following removal of one eye. *Journal of Comparative Neurology, 161*, 359–382.

Hicks, S. P., & D'Amato, C. J. (1970). Motor sensory and visual behavior after hemispherectomy in newborn and mature rats. *Experimental Neurology, 29*, 416–438.

Kawaguchi, S., Yamamoto, T., Samejima, A., Itoh, K., & Mizuno, N. (1979). Morphological evidence for axonal sprouting of cerebellothalamic neurons in kittens after neonatal hemicerebellectomy. *Experimental Brain Research, 35*, 511–518.

Leong, S. K. (1976). An experimental study of the corticofugal system following cerebral lesions in the albino rats. *Experimental Brian Research, 26*, 235–247.

Leong, S. K., & Lund, R. D. (1973). Anomalus bilateral corticofugal pathways in albino rats after neonatal lesions. *Brian Research, 62*, 218–221.

Lim, K. H., & Leong, S. K. (1975). Aberrant bilateral projections from the dentate and interposed nuclei in albino rats after neonatal lesions. *Brain Research, 96*, 306–309.

Lund, R. D. (1978). *Development and plasticity of the brain.* New York: Oxford University Press.

Lund, R. D., & Lund, J. S. (1971). Synaptic adjustment after deafferentation of the superior colliculus of the rat. *Science, 171*, 804–807.

Lund, R. D., & Lund, J. S. (1976). Plasticity in the developing visual system: The effects of retinal lesions made in young rats. *Journal of Comparative Neurology, 169*, 133–154.

More, R. Y., Björklund, A., & Stenevi, U. (1971). Plastic changes in the adrenergic innervation of the rat septal area in response to denervation. *Brain Research, 33*, 13–35.

Murakami, F., Katsumaru, H., Saito, K., & Tsukahara, N. (1982). A quantitative study of synaptic reorganization in red nucleus neurons after lesion of nucleus interpositus of the cat: an electron microscopic study involving intracellular injection of horseradish peroxidase. *Brain Research, 242*, 41–53.

Murakami, F., Tsukahara, N., & Fujito, Y. (1977). Analysis of unitary EPSPs mediated by the newly-formed corticorubral synapses after lesion of the nucleus interpositus of the cerebellum. *Experimental Brain Research, 30*, 233–243.

Nah, S. H., & Leong, S. K. (1976a). Bilateral corticofugal projection to the red nucleus after neonatal lesions in the albino rat. *Brain Research, 107*, 433–436.

Nah, S. H., & Leong, S. K. (1976b). An ultrastructural study of the anomalus corticorubral projection following neonatal lesions in the albino rat. *Brain Research, 111*, 162–166.

Oderfeld-Nowak, B., Wójcik, M., Ulas, J., & Potempska, A. (1981). Effects of chronic ganglioside treatment on recovery processes in hippocampus after brain lesions in rats. In M. M. Rapport and A. Gorio (Ed.), *Gangliosides in neurological and neuromuscular function, development, and repair* (pp. 197–209.) New York: Raven.

Raisman, G. (1969). Neuronal plasticity in the septal nuclei of the adult rat. *Brain Research*, *14*, 25–48.

Rapport, M. M. (1981). Introduction to the biochemistry of gangliosides. In M. M. Rapport & A. Gorio (Ed.), *Gangliosides in neurological and neuromuscular function, development, and repair* (pp. xv–xix). New York: Raven.

Rapport, M. M., & Gorio, A. (Ed.) (1981). *Gangliosides in neurological and neuromuscular function, development, and repair*. New York: Raven.

Steward, O., Cotman, C. W., & Lynch, G. S. (1973). Re-establishment of electrophysiologically functional entorhinal cortical inputs to the dentate gyrus deafferented by ipsilateral entorhinal lesions: Innervation by the contralateral entorhinal cortex. *Experimental Brain Research*, *18*, 396–414.

Tsukahara, N. (1981). Synaptic plasticity in the mammalian central nervous system. *Annual Review of Neuroscience*, *4*, 351–379.

Tsukahara, N. & Fujito, Y. (1976). Physiological evidence of formation of new synapses from cerebrum in the red nucleus neurons following cross-union of forelimb nerves. *Brain Research*, *106*, 184–188.

Tsukahara, N., & Fujito, Y. (1981). Neuronal plasticity in the newborn and adult feline red nucleus. In H. Flohr & W. Precht (Ed.), *Lesion-induced neuronal plasticity in sensorimotor systems* (pp. 64–74). Heidelberg: Springer-Verlag.

Tsukahara, N., Fujito, Y., Oda, Y., & Maeda, J. (1982). Formation of functional synapses in adult cat red nucleus from the cerebrum following cross-innervation of forelimb flexor and extensor nerves. I. Appearance of new synaptic potentials. *Experimental Brain Research*, *45*, 1–12.

Tsukahara, N., Fujito, Y., & Kubota, M. (1983). Specificity of the newly-formed corticorubral synapses in the kitten red nucleus. *Experimental Brain Research*, *51*, 45–56.

Tsukahara, N., Hultborn, H., & Murakami, F. (1974). Sprouting of corticorubral synapses in red nucleus neurons after destruction of the nucleus interpositus of the cerebellum. *Experientia Basel*, *30*, 57–58.

Tsukahara, N., Hultborn, H., Murakami, F., & Fujito, Y. (1975a). Electrophysiological study of formation of new synapses and collateral sprouting in red nucleus neurons after partial denervation. *Journal of Neurophysiology*, *38*, 1359–1372.

Tsukahara, N., & Kosaka, K. (1968). The mode of cerebral excitation of red nucleus neurons. *Experimental Brain Research*, *5*, 102–117.

Tsukahara, N., Murakami, F., & Hultborn, H. (1975b). Electrical constants of neurons of red nucleus. *Experimental Brain Research*, *23*, 49–64.

Willshaw, D. J. (1981). The establishment and the subsequent elimination of polyneuronal innervation of developing muscle: Theoretical considerations. *Proceedings of the Royal Society of London B*, *212*, 233–252.

Wójcik, M., Ulas, J., & Oderfeld-Nowak, B. (1982). The stimulating effect of ganglioside injections on the recovery of choline acetyltransferase and acetylcholinesterase activities in the hippocampus of the rat after septal lesions. *Neurosicence*, *7*, 495–499.

4

Multiple Effects of Lesions on Brain Structure in Young Rats

Mark R. Rosenzweig,
Edward L. Bennett, and Marie Alberti

Introduction

Experiments with mammalian subjects are providing illuminating indications of how the brain works and how it responds to injury. For example, after young rats sustain cortical lesions, their ability to learn and solve problems is diminished; but we have previously shown that living in an enriched laboratory environment reduces their functional impairment. This is true whether the lesions are inflicted neonatally (Will, Rosenzweig, & Bennett, 1976), after weaning (Will, Rosenzweig, Bennett, Hebert, & Morimoto, 1977), or postpubertally (Will & Rosenzweig, 1976; Rosenzweig, 1980). These experiments also revealed some unexpected effects of cortical lesions on brain structure and suggested additional questions that we have explored further. After briefly reviewing work that is reported elsewhere, we proceed to the newer studies.

Some Historical Background

Our research and that of several others in this volume can be seen in the double perspective of trying to understand regional functions of the brain and also trying to understand and aid rehabilitation after

49

brain lesions. A pioneer in both of these directions was the American psychologist Shepard Ivory Franz (1874–1933). He was the first to combine the techniques of making localized brain lesions with Thorndike's (1898) techniques for measuring animal learning (Franz, 1902). He hoped in this way to localize sites in the brain that were particularly responsible for learning and for memory. Karl S. Lashley became interested in this problem during postdoctoral research with Franz in 1917, and it became the theme of Lashley's life work.

At the time that Lashley worked with him, Franz was director of the Government Hospital for the Insane in Washington D.C. (now St. Elizabeth's hospital), and one of his major concerns was the rehabilitation of brain-injured patients, including veterans of the First World War. Franz attempted to persuade the federal government to launch a massive program of research and application in rehabilitation, and it was a major source of regret to him that he failed in this effort (Franz, 1932; Woodworth, 1934).

Neither Franz nor Lashley nor their students and successors were able to find particular parts of the mammalian brain that were responsible for learning or that stored memories. In part this failure has been attributed to the difficulty, if not impossibility, of determining whether impairments caused by lesions involve failures of learning and memory rather than deficits of perception or motivation (Isaacson, 1976). Others have concluded that the search was doomed to failure because learning and memory storage take place within the same neural circuits that mediate the responses being studied, so that it would not be possible to abolish learning and memory for a response without abolishing the response itself (e.g., Lynch, 1976). But even if one accepts these conclusions, it still remains true that the search for sites of learning and memory has led to many important discoveries about the functions of the brain. Consider, for example, only the work of some of Lashley's students, postdoctoral trainees, and collaborators: H. Klüver, C. Jacobson, D. O. Hebb, D. Krech, A. Riesen, and K. Pribram. But it may be that the many unsuccessful attempts to find brain sites of learning did not prove the impossibility of the quest. Research by Richard F. Thompson and his collaborators indicates that the hippocampus plays an important role in modulating learning and that deep cerebellar nuclei may be essential for learning of skeletal muscular responses (Clark, McCormick, Lavond, Baxter, & Thompson, 1982; Thompson, in press). A group in England has confirmed the evidence indicating an essential role for deep cerebellar nuclei in learning (Yeo, Hardiman, Glickstein, & Steele, 1982). So even though Lashley eventually became pessimistic about his long "search for the engram" (Lashley, 1950), others continue the quest enthusiastically.

Two studies of animal models of rehabilitation after brain injury had long intrigued us. One was an experiment of Schwartz (1964), who reported that of rats that had sustained cortical lesions neonatally, those assigned to complex laboratory living conditions performed better as adults on the Hebb–Williams maze than those kept under standard laboratory conditions. In fact, the brain-lesioned rats with enriched experience did better than intact animals from colony living conditions. This was of special interest to us because we had been finding since the late 1950s that enriched experience produces measurable changes in brain chemistry and brain anatomy (e.g., Bennett, Diamond, Krech, & Rosenzweig, 1964; Bennett & Rosenzweig, 1971; Globus, Rosenzweig, Bennett, & Diamond, 1973; Rosenzweig & Bennett, 1978; Rosenzweig, Krech, Bennett, & Diamond, 1962). Other workers have replicated some of these findings, have demonstrated effects of differential experience on other brain measures, and have employed such effects in other contexts (e.g., Cummins, Walsh, Budtz-Olsen, Konstantinas, & Horsfall, 1973; Ferchmin & Eterovic, 1980; Greenough, 1976; Mirmiran & Uylings, 1983; Pearlman, 1983; Szeligo & Leblond, 1977). Considering the report of Schwartz in conjunction with such results, it seemed worth testing whether these cerebral effects might provide a mechanism for the improved performance of brain-lesioned animals with enriched living conditions. The other intriguing study was that of Ward and Kennard (1942), who reported that low doses of stimulant drugs improved the rate and final level of recovery after lesions of the motor cortex in monkeys. We had found that stimulant drugs can enhance the cerebral effects of environmental enrichment (Bennett, Rosenzweig, & Wu, 1973; Rosenzweig & Bennett, 1972). Based on this and studies such as that of Ward and Kennard, we had suggested investigating the efficacy of combining an enriched environment and a stimulant drug to promote recovery of function (Bennett et al., 1973, p. 327). This was a line of investigation that we proposed when Bruno Will came to our laboratories in 1974 for a period of research, and it was not long before the research was producing results.

Our Earlier Work on This Problem

The first step was an attempt to replicate the single experiment of Schwartz (1964). For this experiment (Will et al., 1976), some neonatal rats were given lesions in the occipital cortex and others had only sham operations. At weaning, some of each group were placed in the enriched condition (EC). This was a large cage holding 10–12 rats of the same sex; the six or so stimulus objects were changed each day from a large pool of objects. Other rats were assigned to the impoverished condition (IC). This was a small cage holding a single animal; there was food and water ad libitum, but no stimulus objects. When rats were subsequently tested in the Hebb–Williams maze, we found that lesioned EC rats performed significantly better than lesioned IC rats. The lesioned EC rats performed about as well as intact IC rats. Examination of the brains of the subjects of this experiment revealed that neonatal lesions in the occipital cortex had caused significant decrease in growth of the cerebral hemispheres.

The experiment of Schwartz and our replication had shown that enriched experience improved performance after neonatal lesions, but could similar beneficial results of experience be found after lesions inflicted on older animals? To investigate this question, we performed similar experiments, but with cortical lesions inflicted on 30-day-old rats (Will et al., 1977) or on postpubertal rats (Will & Rosenzweig, 1976). We found significant beneficial effects of postoperative enriched experience on Hebb–Williams maze scores in these experiments, just as we had with the neonatally lesioned animals. Use of a stimulant drug did not increase the beneficial effect of enriched experience on recovery, at least under the conditions of our experiment (Will et al., 1977). The effects of enriched experience in counteracting the behavioral deficits caused by cortical lesions were obtained with rats of both sexes and of two strains, so considerable generality was shown for effects of postoperative experience on learning ability. Believing that similar effects might also be found in other species, including human, we called attention to our results at the 1978 Congress of the International Rehabilitation Medicine Association (Rosenzweig, 1980).

Examination of the brains of the experimental animals revealed some unexpected effects (Will et al., 1977). Whereas others had also found that localized cortical lesions in neonates restrict the subsequent growth of the entire cortical mantle (so that it is clearly smaller upon naked-eye inspection) (Isaacson, Nonneman, & Schmaltz, 1968; Nonneman, 1970), rodents given lesions after about 2 weeks of age did not appear to show such effects. We found, however, that a lesion in the occipital cortex of a postweaning rat leads to small but significant losses of weight in other cortical regions. Moreover, this reflects not just a diminution in size of cells but also an actual loss in cell number, as was demonstrated by a significant decrease in DNA (Will *et al.*, 1977). Since each cell is believed to possess a quantal amount of DNA, loss of DNA is a clear indication of loss of cells. Perhaps, then, the behavioral impairments caused by the lesion might be due not only to the direct loss of cells but also to the secondary loss of cells in other regions of the cortex. There was also an indication that the enriched environment might offer some protection against this remote (or distal) loss of cells, because such loss was somewhat smaller in EC than in IC rats, although this difference did not reach statistical significance.

The results of the experiments reported in our 1976–1977 studies suggested several questions about the cerebral effects of lesions that we tried to answer in subsequent research. The main questions were the following:

1. Since all the experiments had involved lesions in the occipital cortex, are the effects specific to this region or can lesions in other cortical regions also cause remote losses of cells and of tissue volume? If so, do the magnitudes of remote losses vary with the site at which the lesion is made? That is, are some regions more effective than others in provoking distal losses?

2. How do the magnitudes of remote losses vary among cortical regions? Are some regions more susceptible to such losses than others? Also, are such losses found as well in noncortical parts of the brain or only in the cerebral cortex?

3. How do the magnitudes of remote losses vary with the sizes of lesions inflicted? Is there a direct relation, or is it possible that lesions of quite different sizes provoke similar amounts of distal loss?

4. How do the magnitudes of remote losses vary with the time after the lesion is inflicted? Do they reach full size rather quickly or do they continue to develop over months?

5. Since enriched experience improves problem-solving behavior of rats with occipital cortex lesions, is it possible that it does so, in part at least, by inhibiting the remote loss of brain tissue?

Procedures

A brief description of the experimental procedures will help to understand the results. All animals in these experiments were males of the Berkeley S_1 strain, and the lesions were made at approximately 30 days of age.

In order to make cortical lesions of standard sizes and locations in laboratory rats, each animal was anesthetized, the skull was exposed, and a trephine was used to remove a disc of bone on each side of the brain. Trephines of larger or smaller diameters were used according to the size of lesion desired. Depending on the experiment, the skull was removed over either the anterior motor region, the dorsomedial somatosensory region, or the posterior occipital region of the cortex; Figure 1 shows the positions of these regions within which circular lesions were made. The exposed cortical tissue was removed by means of a fine suction tube with cortex being aspirated down to the underlying white matter. According to the experimental designs, some animals sustained relatively large lesions (approximately 65 mg of cortical tissue removed from the two bilateral sites combined), whereas others had smaller lesions (ranging down to approximately 20 mg removed). Control animals underwent a sham-lesion procedure in which the cortex was exposed but no tissue was removed.

After 5 to 7 days of recovery, the animals were placed in pre-assigned environmental conditions: EC, IC, or standard colony (SC). Some experiments included groups sacrificed approximately 36 and 94 days postlesion, and others included groups sacrificed approximately 36, 100, and 200 days postlesion.

At sacrifice, the brain was dissected into several standardized samples: the occipital, somatosensory, and motor regions of the dorsal

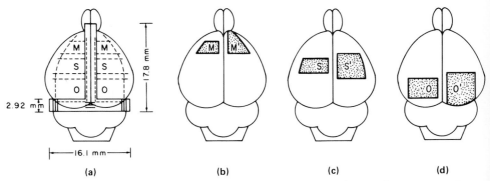

Figure 1. Dorsal views of the rat brain, showing regions dissected in our experiments. (a) brain with calibrated plastic T square used to delimit the following areas of cerebral cortex: anterior motor (M) area; dorsomedial somatosensory (S) area; and posterior occipital (O) area. (b–d) On the left hemisphere of each brain is indicated the standard area that we usually employed (M, S, O), and on the right hemisphere is indicated the modified enlarged region (M′, S′, O′) used for dissection of both lesioned and sham-lesioned brains when a particular area contained a cortical lesion.

cortex; the ventral cortex (in some cases this included the hippocampus and in other cases the hippocampus was dissected separately); the cerebellum and medulla taken together; and the remaining brain. The use of a calibrated plastic T square to delimit the dorsal cortical areas as well as other dissection procedures are described in detail in Bennett and Rosenzweig (1981). Distinct from the sections we normally took, we dissected an enlarged sample of whatever area the lesion was placed in, so that we could be certain that the lesion was contained within the sample dissected. Each tissue sample was weighed to the nearest 0.1 mg and then stored in a freezer at −15°C for subsequent chemical analysis. In some experiments, some or all of the samples were analyzed for RNA and DNA according to procedures developed in our laboratories (Morimoto, Ferchmin, & Bennett, 1974).

Results

The results of the further experiments largely confirmed the earlier ones, and they also furnished several surprises.

GENERALITY OF THE REMOTE-LOSS EFFECT

Lesions in the motor or somatosensory cortical areas were found to cause remote loss of tissue, so there is nothing unique about the occipital cortex in this respect. In fact, a lesion of given size produced greater loss in other regions of the cortex if it was situated in the motor or somatosensory cortex than if it was located in the occipital area; this can be seen in the data of Table 1. Since the total weight of the motor area, as defined for these experiments, was only about 55 mg, we wanted to restrict lesions there to about 20 mg in order to be certain not to go beyond the boundaries of this area; in fact, the motor area lesions averaged 17 mg. (The lesion size was determined by subtracting the weight of a lesioned area from that of the corresponding area in sham-lesioned controls at the time of sacrifice.) But motor cortex lesions of 17 mg made at 30 days of age resulted in a loss of weight of 11.4% of the rest of the cerebral cortex outside the boundaries of the motor area. In contrast, lesions that averaged 22 mg in the occipital cortex resulted in a loss of only 4.6% of the weight of all the cortex outside the occipital area. In fact, lesions averaging 66 mg

TABLE 1

Percentage of Change in Brain Weights at Approximately 100 Days Postlesion[a]

Site of lesion	Lesion size (mg)	n (pairs)	Total cortex − lesion area	Cerebellum + medulla	Remaining subcortex	Total brain − lesion area
Motor cortex	17	14	−11.4**	−3.2	−4.6	−6.9*
Somato-sensory cortex	19	12	−6.2*	−0.1	−3.5	−3.6
	54	9	−13.7**	−3.1	−6.3*	−8.2*
Occipital cortex	22	38	−4.6**	−1.2	−3.1**	−3.1**
	46	43	−8.9**	−1.1	−2.9	−4.7**
	65	58	−9.7**	−1.0	−2.7	−4.8**

[a]Based on final weights of brain areas of lesioned animals versus the baseline of sham-lesioned animals. Average weights of sham-lesioned animals were the following: Total cortex minus lesion area, depending on the site of the lesion, 600–650 mg. Cerebellum plus medulla, 440 mg. Remaining subcortex, 550 mg. Total brain minus lesion area, 1590–1640 mg.
*$p < .01$. **$p < .001$.

in the occipital cortex resulted in a loss of only 9.7% of all the cortex outside the occipital area, which is less than the 11.4% loss caused by the 17-mg motor cortex lesions.

BRAIN REGIONS DIFFER IN SUSCEPTIBILITY TO REMOTE LOSS

Regions of the brain differ considerably in their susceptibility to loss of tissue resulting from localized lesions inflicted in the cortex. The occipital region of the cortex is especially susceptible to such loss when a lesion is made in another area of the cortex. On the other hand, the somatosensory area seems to be relatively immune to remote loss. As can be seen in Table 2, a lesion in the motor area produced twice as large a percentage loss in the more distant occipital area as it did in the adjacent somatosensory area. In experiments on effects of differential environmental experience on changes in cortical tissue weight and neurochemistry, we have also found the occipital region to be especially sensitive and the somatosensory area relatively unaffected. Greenough, Volkmar, and Juraska (1973) also found the branching pattern of dendrites to be more sensitive to environmental influences in the occipital area than in other cortical

TABLE 2

Losses of Tissue Weight in the Occipital and Somatosensory Cortices
Approximately 100 Days after Lesions in Other Cortical Areas

| | | | Site of distal loss | | | |
| | | | Occipital | | Somatosensory | |
Site of lesion	Lesion size (mg)	n (pairs)	Sham weight (mg)	Loss (%)	Sham weight (mg)	Loss (%)
Motor cortex	17	14	68.6	10.9***	50.3	5.0
Somato-sensory cortex	19	12	86.7	9.1**	—	—
	54	9	85.8	21.7***	—	—
Occipital cortex	22	38	—	—	58.0	2.6*
	48	43	—	—	57.4	5.6***
	66	43	—	—	55.8	2.1

$*p < .05.$ $**p < .01.$ $***p < .001.$

regions. In the present experiments, the ventral cortex also showed distal loss, but when the hippocampus was assayed separately (as is seen in Tables 4 and 5), it showed no loss in either weight or DNA. We had previously found the hippocampus to be unresponsive on these measures to differential environmental experience.

Outside of the cerebral cortex, the remote losses are considerably smaller than those observed in the cortex; this can be seen in Table 1. Of the two samples into which the noncortical tissue was divided in these experiments, the cerebellum plus medulla showed remote tissue losses only about half as large as those in the remaining sub-cortex, and only some of the latter attained statistical significance. Thus different brain regions differ considerably in their suscep-tibilities to remote effects of lesions placed elsewhere in the brain.

REMOTE LOSS VARIES WITH EXTENT OF LESION,
AT LEAST EARLY IN THE POSTLESION PERIOD

In the occipital cortex we made lesions of three different sizes at 30 to 33 days of age, removing approximately 25, 45, or 65 mg of tissue from the two hemispheres combined. And in the somatosensory cortex we made lesions of two different sizes: approximately 20 or 55 mg. Results at approximately 90 days postlesion appear in Table 1. In both areas the smallest lesions resulted in only about half as much remote loss as did the next larger lesion when loss was measured in terms of weight of the total cortex minus the area in which the lesion was made. But in the occipital cortex, going from lesions of approximately 45 mg to lesions of approximately 65 mg did not lead to much further increase in remote loss of tissue weight, at least at 90 days postlesion. However, the relative magnitudes of remote losses resulting from lesions of different sizes was found to vary as a function of time after the lesion was made. Therefore, any attempt to compare extents of remote losses is inadequate and potentially misleading unless the time course is studied, so let us turn next to that question.

TIME COURSES OF REMOTE LOSSES

In some experiments involving lesions made in the occipital cortex at about 30 days of age, animals were sacrificed either approximately 36 or approximately 94 days postlesion. In some experiments with lesions made in the motor or somatosensory cortices at about 30 days of age, groups were sacrificed at approximately 36, 100, or 200 days postlesion.

Figure 2 shows distal losses in these experiments, measured in terms of loss of weight of the total cortex minus the region in which the lesion was made. Most of the curves continue to rise as a function of time; that is, the remote loss continued to increase for months after the lesion was inflicted. Morover, for both the occipital and the somatosensory cortices in which there were lesions of different sizes, the curves reporting the effects of the larger lesions rise more rapidly than the curves for the smaller lesions. In this regard, recall that in the preceding section we saw that at about 90 days postlesion, the remote losses caused by 45- or 65-mg lesions scarcely differed in magnitude. In Figure 2, however, we see that at about 30 days the remote effects of the 45-mg lesions were clearly smaller than those of the 65-mg lesions. In the case of the somatosensory cortex, the curve for the effects of the 20-mg lesions still appears to rise 200 days postlesion.

These curves suggest the possibility that a lesion in a given region of the cortex will cause a certain eventual amount of remote tissue

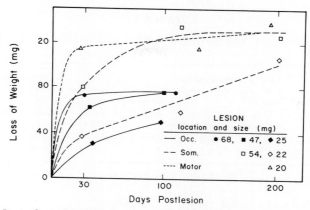

Figure 2. Loss of weight in the total brain outside of the region in which a lesion had been made. Bilateral lesions of various sizes were made in anterior or motor, dorsomedial or somatosensory (Som.), or posterior or occipital (Occ.) areas of the cerebral cortex. Groups of animals were sacrificed after various postlesion durations, approximately 30, 100, or 200 days. Each point is based on at least nine lesion versus control pairs of rats.

loss regardless of the extent of the tissue originally removed or damaged, but that the total loss develops more rapidly in the case of large lesions than in the case of small ones.

Figure 2 also shows, as we already saw in connection with Table 2, that lesions of the somatosensory and motor areas lead to much larger distal losses of tissue than do lesions of the occipital area.

In some experiments the remote loss was measured not only in terms of weight of tissue but also in terms of total DNA. These were some of the experiments in which relatively small (24 mg) and medium (47 mg) lesions were made in the occipital cortex; some of the animals were sacrificed at about 37 days postlesion, and others were sacrificed at about 96 days postlesion. DNA was assayed in two brain regions in these experiments: in all of the dorsal cortex outside the occipital region and in all of the ventral cortex including the hippocampus. The results presented in Table 3 show that at 37 days postlesion there were significant remote losses of DNA in animals that had sustained the larger lesions, but the remote losses in animals with small occipital lesions did not reach statistical significance. At 96 days postlesion, however, there were significant remote losses of DNA in animals with smaller occipital lesions as well as in those that had sustained the larger lesions. Just as we saw in the case of tissue weight, the remote loss of DNA also evolves more rapidly toward its

TABLE 3

Percentage of Change in Total DNA in Cerebral Cortical Areas
after Lesions in the Occipital Cortex[a]

		37 days postlesion				96 Days postlesion		
Lesion size (mg)	n (pairs)	Dorsal − occip.[b]	Ventral[c]	Total − occip.[d]	n (pairs)	Dorsal − occip.	Ventral	Total − occip.
24	36	−3.7*	−0.8	−2.5*	38	−7.4**	−1.6	−4.1*
47	34	−11.0**	−4.9*	−7.5**	36	−13.5**	−7.0**	−9.4**

[a]Based on brain area weights of brain-lesioned animals versus the baseline of sham-lesioned animals.
[b]All of the dorsal cortex outside the occipital region.
[c]The ventral cortex including the hippocampus.
[d]The sum of Dorsal − occip. and Ventral.
*$p < .01$. **$p < .001$.

final state in the case of a larger lesion than following a smaller lesion. It should also be noted that finding significant remote losses of DNA in these experiments confirms our initial report of this effect (Will *et al.*, 1977). Although transneural degeneration is well known to occur in certain neural tracts, we had not expected localized cortical lesions to lead to loss of cells distributed throughout the cerebral cortex.

DOES ENRICHED POSTLESION EXPERIENCE HELP TO PROTECT AGAINST DEVELOPMENT OF REMOTE LOSSES?

In our 1977 study, we had noted that losses of tissue weight and of DNA in the dorsal cortex were slightly larger in animals assigned postlesion to IC than in those assigned to EC. We therefore asked whether EC might help to protect against the development of remote losses of cerebral tissue. Further experiments were then undertaken to test this possibility. In these experiments, relatively large lesions were made in the occipital cortex and the animals were assigned to either IC or EC; half the subjects were sacrificed after 29 days in the different environments and half after 88 days. At sacrifice, the samples of brain tissue were weighed as usual, and some of the samples were later analyzed for DNA. The results for tissue weight are presented in Table 4, and those for DNA are given in Table 5. In each table, relative effects of lesions can be seen by comparing lesioned and sham-lesioned among both EC animals (EC–L vs. EC–S) and IC animals (IC–L vs. IC–S). To compare both EC–L and IC–L against the same baseline, we also show values for EC–L versus IC–S; the question of baseline is important to the comparison of effects. In the same tables, effects of differential environments can be seen both among lesioned rats (EC–L vs. IC–L) and sham-lesioned controls (EC–S vs. IC–S).

The relative magnitudes of remote lesion effects among rats placed in EC or IC depend on the baseline that is used for comparison. If the effects of brain lesions in rats placed in EC are measured against the

TABLE 4

Effects of Occipital Cortical Lesions and Postlesion Environments on Brain Weights

Brain region[a]	Weight of region in IC–S[b] (mg)	Lesion effects (% difference)			Environmental effects (% difference)	
		EC–L vs. EC–S	IC–L vs. IC–S	EC–L vs. IC–S	EC–L vs. IC–L	EC–S vs. IC–S
29 days EC or IC, 46-mg lesions, $n = 18$ per condition						
Somatosensory	55	−8.2***	−7.6**	−2.8	5.2*	5.8*
Ventral	146	−13.9***	−5.6	−4.3	1.4	11.1***
Hippocampus	97	3.1	0.9	4.5	3.5	1.3
Total cortex	546	−10.3***	−7.6***	−2.7	5.3**	8.5***
Total brain	1424	−5.2***	−3.1**	0.1	3.4**	5.7***
88 days EC or IC, 48-mg lesions, $n = 18$ per condition						
Somatosensory	57	−8.9***	−4.4*	−5.5**	−1.1	3.7
Ventral	164	−11.8***	−9.3**	−7.1**	2.4	5.3*
Hippocampus	106	0.3	−1.1	1.9	3.0	1.6
Total cortex	584	−9.4***	−9.6***	−5.0***	5.0***	4.9***
Total brain	1559	−4.4***	−5.7***	−2.3*	3.6***	2.2*

[a] Somatosensory cortex, ventral cortex excluding hippocampus, hippocampus, total cortex minus occipital area, total brain minus occipital area.

[b] (IC) impoverished environment; (EC) enriched environment; (L) lesioned animal; (S) sham-lesioned animal.

*$p < .05$. **$p < .01$. ***$p < .001$.

TABLE 5

Effects of Occipital Cortical Lesions and Postlesion Environments on Total DNA in Brain

Brain region[a]	IC–S[b] (μg)	Lesion effects (% difference)			Environmental effects (% difference)	
		EC–L vs. EC–S	IC–L vs. IC–S	EC–L vs. IC–S	EC–L vs. IC–L	EC–S vs. IC–S
29 days EC or IC, 46-mg lesions, $n = 18$ per condition						
Somatosensory	55	−5.0	−4.7	−4.6	0.0	0.5
Ventral	161	−16.4***	−1.7	−5.8	−4.1	12.6**
Hippocampus	97	6.9	−1.1	4.6	5.8	−2.1
Total cortex	551	−9.1***	−5.9**	−4.0*	2.1	5.6**
88 days EC or IC, 48-mg lesions, $n = 18$ per condition						
Somatosensory	57	−4.2	−1.5	−5.7*	−4.3	−1.5
Ventral	175	−11.8***	−8.6**	−8.6*	0.0	3.6
Hippocampus	100	0.4	−2.7	0.6	3.4	0.2
Total cortex	579	−8.9***	−9.8***	−7.0***	3.1	2.1

[a] Somatosensory cortex, ventral cortex excluding hippocampus, hippocampus, total cortex minus occipital area.

[b] (IC) impoverished environment; (EC) enriched environment; (L) lesioned animal; (S) sham-lesioned animal.

*$p < .05$. **$p < .01$. ***$p < .001$.

baseline of intact control rats in EC (EC–L vs. EC–S), then both losses in tissue weight (shown in Table 4) and losses in DNA (Table 5) are found to be somewhat larger than the comparable losses observed in the IC rats (IC–L vs. IC–S). For example, in the top entries in Table 4, for loss of weight of somatosensory cortex, the EC–L versus EC–S comparison shows a loss of 8.2% ($p < .001$), whereas IC–L versus IC–S shows a slightly smaller loss of 7.6% ($p < .01$). In the next set of values in Table IV, those for the ventral cortex, the comparable effects are more clearly different, −13.9% ($p < .001$) for EC–L versus EC–S and only −5.6% (not statistically significant) for IC–L versus IC–S. These results contradict the nonsignificant indication of the 1977 study that remote losses might be smaller among EC animals than among IC animals.

It could be argued, however, that the remote losses in both EC and IC animals should be measured against the same baseline. If we look then at the percentage effect for EC–L versus IC–S in the somatosensory cortex in Table 4, we find only a very small effect—2.8%—not statistically significant and clearly smaller than the IC–L versus IC–S loss. In 9 out of 10 cases in Table 4, the EC–L versus IC–S values are less negative than the corresponding IC–L versus IC–S values. Thus measuring the losses from the common baseline of the IC–S values suggests that enriched experience does inhibit the remote loss.

Which of the two apparently contradictory conclusions should be accepted—that enriched postlesion experience does or does not restrict distal loss of brain tissue? Actually, as we mentioned in describing the column headings in Table 4, there are two main kinds of effect in these tables: lesion effects and environmental effects. So if we try to use the same baseline (IC–S) to measure distal losses in both EC–L and IC–L animals, the EC–L versus IC–S results are actually a combination of positive environmental effects and negative lesion effects. Therefore the fact that EC–L versus IC–S differences are more positive than IC–L versus IC–S differences does not mean that enriched experience is limiting remote losses, but only that a different, environmental effect is being added algebraically to the lesion effect and is producing a smaller sum; the lesion effect is still present in full force.

This recalls a question that has previously been considered in regard to behavioral recovery after damage to the brain: Is there an interaction between lesion effects and environmental effects or are they simply additive? Our examination of our own research and that of others revealed some findings showing that complex experience may have even greater effect in brain-lesioned than in control animals, whereas other findings indicated comparable effects between lesioned and control animals (Will et al., 1977); none of the behavioral work indicated lesser effects of enriched experience in brain-lesioned than in normal animals. When we consider the environmental effects on brain weights in Table 4, however, we see that most of these effects are smaller in the lesioned rats (EC–L vs. IC–L) than in the sham-lesioned controls (EC–S vs. IC–S). If this lesser responsiveness to enriched experience among brain-lesioned animals is confirmed by further research, it could be considered a tertiary effect of localized brain lesions. That is, in addition to the primary or direct loss of the ablated tissue, there is also a progressive secondary or remote loss of brain tissue (as demonstrated earlier), and now we have indications that the lesioned brain may also show less structural benefit than the intact brain from experience in a relatively complex environment.

Discussion

The kinds of remote loss that we have shown here to follow localized damage to cortical tissue are not, of course, the only kinds to occur. For example, several investigators have shown that cutting a neural tract may cause sprouting of dendrites on intact portions of the neurons, which may lead to abnormal connections (e.g., Schneider, 1973). It has also been shown that cortical lesions interrupt intracortical noradrenergic fibers that course through the rat cortex from the frontal poles in a caudal direction (Morrison, Molliver, & Grzanna, 1979). Because of this direction, anterior lesions affect this system much more strongly than do posterior lesions of the cortex.

Like Franz and Lashley, although we do most of our investigations with laboratory rodents, we hope that some of our studies will suggest mechanisms that may also be found in other species, including humans, and we hope that some of our results will stimulate research that can be applied to alleviating human dysfunction. It is quite possible that some of the findings of this study apply to humans as well as to laboratory rats. In this regard, we note that Geschwind (1974, pp. 481–482) has cited clinical evidence suggesting that surgical removal of frontal cortical tissue in patients sets into motion a progressive and long-continued loss of cortical tissue in other regions of the brain, and that this damage can, in the course of time, become severe. This may reflect the remote loss of tissue that we can study directly in experiments like the present series. Thus the investigation in animal subjects of the reactions of the brain to localized damage may help us understand some complexities and limitations to rehabilitation in human patients, just as, on the other hand, the findings of the beneficial effects of postlesion enriched experience in animals have encouraged some studies of rehabilitation in people. Let us consider a few other aspects of both negative and positive processes that may occur during the postlesion period.

The fact that localized lesions cause remote cell loss is a further complication to the attempt to use the lesion method to map functions of the brain. If removing tissue from region A is found to affect function M, this may occur because the lesion in A led to loss of cells in region C, which is actually more closely related to function M. It would then be necessary to investigate the anatomical consequences in C (and perhaps elsewhere in the brain) of making a lesion in A. But this may represent more than a nuisance or barrier to mapping functions. If damage to cortical region A leads to a loss in C, then perhaps there are neural circuits involving *A* as well as *C* that play roles in function *M*.

The findings of this chapter have indicated that localized lesions in the brains of young rats initiate a progressive and long-continuing degeneration of neural tissue, and that a contrary building of neural tissue is produced in response to experience in a relatively complex environment. That these two processes are relatively independent is further indicated by their different time courses. We have indicated (Bennett, Rosenzweig, & Diamond, 1970) that cerebral differences between young animals assigned to EC or IC environments tend to reach their maximum after about 30 days and then to decline; the brain values of the EC animals tend to remain stable after about a month, whereas those of the IC animals gradually catch up. But the distal effects of brain lesions tend to increase over a few months, especially after smaller lesions, as we saw in Figure 2 and some of the other results presented earlier. The different time courses of the lesion effects and environmental effects can be seen by comparing the relative magnitudes in the upper and lower halves of Table 4. Many of the lesion effects are smaller in the upper half, which reports effects after 29 days, than in corresponding values in the lower half of Table IV, which gives results after 88 days; contrarily, the environmental effects tend to be larger in the upper half than in the corresponding lower half of the table.

These different time courses lead to a further phenomenon when EC–L is compared with IC–S and the environmental and lesion effects are pitted against each other. In the upper half of Table 4, the two effects are almost equal after 29 days of differential experience, so the difference values in the EC–L versus IC–S column tend to be small and none of them is significant. But in the lower half, after 88 days of differential experience in which the positive environmental (EC vs. IC) effects have declined and the negative lesion effects have grown, the EC–L versus IC–S differences are clearly negative, and each is statistically significant. Much the same picture is also seen in Table 5.

The fact that remote loss of cells is more rapid after larger lesions than after smaller ones may be one reason why single-stage lesions cause greater impairment than do multiple-stage lesions that add up to the same amount of direct damage. (For discussion of effects of single-stage versus multiple-stage lesions, see Finger, 1978.) That is, we suggest that the more abrupt secondary as well as primary losses may be harder to adjust to than the same total loss of tissue that occurs more gradually.

Functional recovery after localized cortical lesions is all the more remarkable when one realizes that it occurs despite the spreading and progressive loss of brain tissue that our studies have demonstrated. We have seen that enriched experience does not prevent this distal loss and that the lesioned brain may in fact be less responsive anatomically to enriched experience than is the intact brain. Nevertheless, experiments in our laboratories and elsewhere (e.g., Will & Eclancher, Chapter 18, this volume) have demonstrated that postlesion experience is effective in promoting rehabilitation. These positive findings concerning rehabilitation are both a source of hope and a challenge to discover their mechanisms.

FURTHER QUESTIONS

The findings presented in this chapter suggest many further questions for investigation. Here are a few:

1. What is the developmental course of the remote-lesion effects? We have found that even though localized cortical lesions inflicted in the first few postnatal days cause much more drastic distal effects than do lesions inflicted in 30-day-old rats, the latter effects are not negligible. Would the same be true of lesions inflicted in adults, or after a certain age are there no longer significant remote effects of localized cortical lesions?

2. We have investigated the distal effects using only the rather gross measures of tissue weight and DNA content. What effects will be found in terms of nerve cell anatomy and ultrastructure? What kinds of brain cell participate in the remote losses?

3. Can treatments be devised to minimize or even prevent distal losses following localized brain lesions? If this can be done, it might mitigate importantly the long-term functional effects caused by brain lesions.

Conclusions

A localized cortical lesion inflicted during the first week or two of life in a rat results in a severe restriction of growth of the cortical mantle that is observable upon naked-eye inspection of the adult brain. Although such gross effects are not caused by lesions inflicted later in life, a postweaning lesion confined to one area of the cortex causes measurable loss of weight and of DNA in other cortical regions; such losses reach the order of 10%. The remote loss of DNA indicates that cells not only lose volume but that many actually die as a result of distant lesions.

Three main regions of the dorsal cortex of the rat were investigated—anterior or motor, dorsomedial or somatosensory, and posterior or occipital—both as the site of lesions and as a region that might be affected by lesions inflicted elsewhere. Lesions in each region were found to cause loss of DNA and tissue weight in the other dorsal cortical regions and also in the ventral cortex; small losses were also found in noncortical regions of the brain. Lesions in the anterior and dorsomedial regions were more effective in producing loss elsewhere than were lesions in the posterior cortex. In susceptibility to losses as a result of lesions inflicted elsewhere, the occipital region was more sensitive than were the other cortical regions.

Larger lesions produced larger amounts of remote loss than did smaller lesions, at least during the month or more that followed production of the lesion. But as time elapsed, the remote losses continued to grow more markedly after small than after large lesions; that is, the effects of larger lesions appeared to reach asymptote more quickly. The results suggested that a lesion of a given region of the cortex causes a certain eventual amount of remote loss, almost regardless of the size of the lesion.

Postlesion experience in an enriched environment was not found to counter the development of remote loss of tissue weight or DNA. Enriched experience does lead to an increase in weight of cortical tissue among the lesioned rats, but this effect may be smaller than among intact controls. Thus the lesioned rats have been shown in these experiments to lose brain tissue in two and possibly three ways: through direct removal of tissue, through secondary or remote loss in regions outside the one in which the lesion was inflicted, and possibly through reduced responsiveness to experiential induction of growth of brain tissue. Thus, although we have found that enriched postlesion experience promotes performance after brain lesions, this beneficial effect cannot be attributed to a reduction in remote effects of the lesion.

These experiments have revealed further complications that beset attempts to use localized brain lesions to map the functions of brain regions. The present findings of secondary and tertiary effects of localized cortical lesions make all the more remarkable the facts that

functional recovery often occurs and that it can be promoted by
postlesion experience.

Acknowledgments

This research received support from Easter Seal Foundation Grant R7736, National
Institute of Mental Health Grant 1RO1 MH26704, and from the Office of Energy Research, Office of Health and Environmental Research, U.S. Department of Energy
under Contract no. DE-ACO3-76SF00098.

We wish to thank Kenneth Chin for aid in making the brain lesions and maintaining
the animals and Hiromi Morimoto for the analyses of nucleic acids.

Preliminary reports of some of the present experiments have been presented in
Rosenzweig, Bennett, Morimoto, and Hebert (1978) and in Rosenzweig (1983).

References

Bennett, E. L., Diamond, M. C., Krech, D., & Rosenzweig, M. R. (1964). Chemical and
    anatomical plasticity of brain. *Science, 146*, 610–619.
Bennett, E. L., & Rosenzweig, M. R. (1971). Chemical alterations produced in brain by
    environment and training. In A. Lajtha (Ed.), *Handbook of neurochemistry* (Vol. 6,
    pp. 173–201). New York: Plenum.
Bennett, E. L., & Rosenzweig, M. R. (1981). Behavioral and biochemical methods to
    study brain responses to environment and experience. In R. Lahue (Ed.), *Methods
    in neurobiology* (Vol. 2, pp. 101–141). New York: Plenum.
Bennett, E. L., Rosenzweig, M. R., & Diamond, M. C. (1970). Time courses of effects of
    differential experience on brain and behavior. In W. C. Byrne (Ed.), *Molecular
    approaches to learning and memory* (pp. 55–88). New York: Academic Press.
Bennett, E. L., Rosenzweig, M. R., & Wu, S. Y. C. (1973). Excitant and depressant drugs
    modulate effects of environment on brain weight and cholinesterase. *Psychophar-
    macologia, 33*, 309–328.
Clark, G. A., McCormick, D. A., Lavond, D. G., Baxter, K., & Thompson, R. F. (1982).
    Effects of electrolytic lesions of cerebellar nuclei on conditioned behavioral and
    hippocampal neuronal responses. *Society for Neuroscience Abstracts, 8*, 22.
Cummins, R. A., Walsh, R. N., Budtz-Olsen, O. E., Konstantinos, T., & Horsfall, C. R.
    (1973). Environmentally-induced changes in the brains of elderly rats. *Nature, 243*,
    516–518.
Ferchmin, P. A., & Eterovic, V. A. (1980). Fours hours of enriched experience are
    sufficient to increase cortical weight of rats. *Society for Neuroscience Abstracts, 6*,
    857.
Finger, S. (1978). Lesion momentum and behavior. In S. Finger (Ed.), *Recovery from
    brain damage: research and theory*. New York: Plenum Press.
Franz, S. I. (1902). On the functions of the cerebrum: The frontal lobes in relation to the
    production and retention of simple sensory-motor habits. *American Journal of
    Physiology, 8*, 1–22.

Franz, S. I. (1932). Autobiography. In C. Murchison (Ed.), *A history of psychology in autobiography* (Vol. 2, pp. 89–113). Worcester, MA: Clark University Press.

Geschwind, N. (1974). Late changes in the nervous system: An overview. In D. G. Stein, J. J. Rosen, & N. Butters (Eds.), *Plasticity and recovery of function in the central nervous system* (pp. 467–508). New York: Academic Press.

Globus, A., Rosenzweig, M. R., Bennett, E. L., & Diamond, M. C. (1973). Effects of differential experience on dendritic spine counts in rat cerebral cortex. *Journal of Comparative and Physiological Psychology, 82*, 175–181.

Greenough, W. T. (1976). Enduring brain effects of differential experience and training. In M. R. Rosenzweig & E. L. Bennett (Eds.), *Neural mechanisms of learning and memory* (pp. 255–278). Cambridge, MA: MIT Press.

Greenough, W. T., Volkmar, F. R., & Juraska, J. M. (1973). Effects of rearing complexity on dendritic branching in frontolateral and temporal cortex of the rat. *Experimental Neurology, 41*, 371–378.

Isaacson, R. L. (1976). Experimental brain lesions and memory. In M. R. Rosenzweig & E. L. Bennett (Eds.), *Neural mechanisms of learning and memory* (pp. 521–543). Cambridge, MA: MIT Press.

Isaacson, R. L., Nonneman, A. J., & Schmaltz, L. W. (1968). Behavioral and anatomical sequelae of damage to the infant limbic system. In R. L. Isaacson (Ed.), *The neuropsychology of development.* New York: Wiley.

Lashley, K. S. (1950). In search of the engram. *Symposia of the Society for Experimental Biology, 4*, 454–482.

Lynch, G. (1976). Some difficulties associated with the use of lesion techniques in the study of memory. In M. R. Rosenzweig & E. L. Bennett (Eds.), *Neural mechanisms of learning and memory* (pp. 544–546). Cambridge, MA: MIT Press.

Mirmiran, M., & Uylings, H. B. M. (1983). The environmental enrichment effect upon cortical growth is neutralized by concomitant pharmacological suppression of active sleep in female rats. *Brain Research, 261*, 331–334.

Morimoto, H., Ferchmin, P. A., & Bennett, E. L. (1974). Spectrophotometric analysis of RNA and DNA using cetyltrimethylammonium bromide. *Analytical Biochemistry, 62*, 436–448.

Morrison, J. H., Molliver, M. E., & Grzanna, R. (1979). Noradrenergic innervation of cerebral cortex: Widespread effects of local cortical lesions. *Science, 205*, 313–316.

Nonneman, A. J. (1970). *Anatomical and behavioral consequences of early brain damage in the rabbit.* Unpublished doctoral dissertation, University of Florida.

Pearlman, C. (1983). Impairment of environmental effects on brain weight by adrenergic drugs in rats. *Physiology & Behavior, 30*, 161–163.

Rosenzweig, M. R. (1980). Animal models for effects of brain lesions and for rehabilitation. In P. Bach-y-Rita (Ed.) *Recovery of function: Theoretical considerations for brain injury rehabilitation* (pp. 127–172). Bern, Switzerland: Hans Huber.

Rosenzweig, M. R. (1983). Learning and multimodal convergence. In E. Horn (Ed.), *Multimodal convergence in sensory systems. Fortschritte der Zoologie, Vol. 28.* (pp. 303–324). Stuttgart/New York: Gustav Fischer Verlag.

Rosenzweig, M. R., & Bennett, E. L. (1972). Cerebral changes in rats exposed individually to an enriched environment. *Journal of Comparative and Physiological Psychology, 80*, 304–313.

Rosenzweig, M. R., & Bennett, E. L. (1978). Experiential influences on brain anatomy and brain chemistry in rodents. In G. Gottlieb (Ed.), *Studies on the development of behavior and the nervous system* (Vol. 4, pp. 289–327). *Early influences.* New York: Academic Press.

Rosenzweig, M. R., Bennett, E. L., Morimoto, H., & Hebert, M. (1978). Lesions in occipital cortex of rat lead to secondary loss of cells in other cortical regions. *Society for Neuroscience Abstracts, 4,* 478.

Rosenzweig, M. R., Krech, D., Bennett, E. L., & Diamond, M. C. (1962). Effects of environmental complexity and training on brain chemistry and anatomy: A replication and extension. *Journal of Comparative and Physiological Psychology, 55,* 429–437.

Schneider, G. E. (1973). Early lesions of the superior colliculus: Factors affecting the formation of abnormal retinal connections. *Brain, Behavior and Evolution, 8,* 73–109.

Schwartz, S. (1964). Effect of neonatal cortical lesions and early environmental factors on adult rat behavior. *Journal of Comparative and Physiological Psychology, 57,* 72–77.

Szeligo, F., & LeBlond, C. P. (1977). Response of the three main types of glial cells of cortex and corpus callosum in rats handled during suckling or exposed to enriched, control and impoverished environments following weaning. *Journal of Comparative Neurology, 172,* 247–264.

Thompson, R. F. (in press). Neuronal substrates of learning and memory: A dual process theory. In G. S. Lynch, J. L. McGaugh, & N. Weinberger (Eds.), *Neurobiology of learning and memory.* New York: Guilford.

Thorndike, E. L. (1898). Animal intelligence: An experimental study of the associative processes in animals. *Psychological Monographs, 2*(8).

Ward, A. A., Jr., & Kennard, M. A. (1942). Effect of cholinergic drugs on recovery of function following lesions of the central nervous system in monkeys. *Yale Journal of Biology and Medicine, 15,* 189–228.

Will, B. E., & Rosenzweig, M. R. (1976). Effets de l'environment sur la récuperation fonctionelle après lésions cérébrales chez des rats adultes. *Biology of Behaviour, 1,* 5–16.

Will, B. E., Rosenzweig, M. R., & Bennett, E. L. (1976). Effects of differential environments on recovery from neonatal brain lesions, measured by problem-solving scores. *Physiology and Behavior, 16,* 603–611.

Will, B. E., Rosenzweig, M. R., Bennett, E. L., Hebert, M., & Morimoto, H. (1977). Relatively brief environmental enrichment aids recovery of learning capacity and alters brain measures after postweaning brain lesions in rats. *Journal of Comparative and Physiological Psychology, 91,* 33–50.

Woodworth, R. S. (1934). Shepard Ivory Franz. *American Journal of Psychology, 46,* 151–152.

Yeo, C. H., Hardiman, M. J., Glickstein, M., & Steele, I. R. (1982). Lesions of cerebellar nuclei abolish the classically conditioned nictitating membrane response. *Society for Neuroscience Abstracts, 8,* 22.

II

Behavioral Biology

5

A New Perspective for the Interpretation of Early Brain Damage

*Robert L. Isaacson
and Linda Patia Spear*

Introduction

A major premise of this chapter is that the behavioral and mental consequences of brain damage are related to alterations in the functioning of remaining brain systems. This type of interpretation is quite different from some traditional approaches wherein the effects of a brain lesion are viewed from the perspective of the functional significance of the absence of the damaged brain structure. We believe that the approach of examining the effects of brain damage within the context of altered functioning of residual brain areas (e.g., Isaacson, Hannigan, Springer, Ryan, & Poplawsky, 1983; Isaacson, 1984) is equally applicable to the study of individuals with brain insults sustained at any point in the life span. Although the behavioral and mental changes following brain damage may also be related to alterations in remaining brain systems, with early damage it is important to consider that the residual systems may be functionally quite different early in life than in adulthood. A similar interpretation can be made for lesions in elderly animals (e.g., Isaacson & Hannigan, 1983). In neither the young nor the old will the effects of the lesion-induced reactions on surviving brain systems necessarily be the same as in the adult, the usual animal subject.

It is clear that one of the dynamic factors that contributes to the effects of *any* central nervous system lesion is the age at which the damage occurs. Age, together with the environmental demands placed on the animal and its past history of dealing with such demands, determine how remaining neural systems will change as a consequence of damage (Isaacson, 1975; Johnson & Almli, 1978). The effects of brain damage depend on lesion-induced changes in the remaining neural systems available to the animal for organizing adaptive behavior. Normal age-related changes in these systems may occur during the entire life span and may be involved in mediating adaptively relevant behaviors appropriate to the needs of the individual at each age. Thus, when considering the effects of brain damage sustained in infancy, it is important to consider that the surviving brain systems affected by brain damage may have different functional, biochemical, and anatomical characters at different ages. Obviously, a variety of other factors may also contribute to the specific effects of infant brain damage. For example, disruption of neural tissue early in life may alter growth patterns, neurogenesis, terminal proliferation, cell–cell contacts, and so on, through morphogenetic, hormonal, and neurochemical disruption of the residual systems. Although the focus of this chapter is on insult-induced secondary reactions and their potential to disrupt age-specific behaviors critical for adaptability at each age, this is just one critical aspect to be addressed when comparing brain damage sustained in infancy with that occurring in adulthood.

Before considering just how this thesis may apply to the very young animal, we describe some work illustrating that the effects of brain damage may be related to alterations in remaining brain tissue in adult animals. Then we summarize some of the critical needs and strategies for meeting these needs that are used by developing rat pups as a background from which to address the interpretation of early brain damage.

Secondary Reactions after Brain Damage in Adult Animals

Because the hippocampus is connected with diverse cortical, basal gangliar, hypothalamic, and other brain areas, the number of locations where possible secondary neural changes occur is correspondingly large. A complete understanding of all these lesion-induced changes may be difficult, if not impossible. Yet we have identified some specific changes that appear to be related to behavioral alterations that occur following brain damage in adults.

At about 7 days after radical bilateral hippocampectomy in adult rats, there is an enchanced endogenous phosphorylation of specific membrane proteins in the caudate nucleus and nucleus accumbens suggestive of an altered synaptic efficacy in these areas (Bär, Gispen, & Isaacson, 1981). The dynamic, and perhaps transient, nature of these changes is reflected by different patterns of phosphorylation when measured 28 days after surgery.

These reactive neural changes in the basal ganglia, which may reflect modifications in the regulatory state of specific synapses, seem to be related to the behavioral effects of hippocampal destruction. When the lesion-induced decrease in the dopaminergic activity of nucleus accumbens was counteracted by local or systemic injections of a dopamine agonist, 3,4-dihydroxyphenylamino-2-imidazoline (DPI), some of the deficits in spontaneous open-field behavior were attenuated (Hannigan, Springer, & Isaacson, 1984; Reinstein, Hannigan, & Isaacson, 1982). The effectiveness of DPI varied with the postoperative recovery period, although it did not relate in any simple manner to the time course of measured levels of dopamine or its metabolites. Even though dopamine utilization appeared normal 4 weeks after surgery, hippocampally lesioned rats still exhibited altered behavioral characteristics such as hyperactivity and altered grooming, and DPI continued to effectively attenuate these deficits at the 4th postoperative week. These data suggest that the forebrain dopaminergic systems are still abnormal with respect to receptor sensitivity and associated regulatory systems and emphasize that the dynamic responses of deregulated neural systems are under the complex control of many factors, ones not restricted to forebrain dopaminergic systems.

There is a close association among normal hippocampal function, neuroendocrine systems, and behavior, and several reviews have examined these relationships in detail (Bohus, 1975; McEwen, Gerlach, & Micco, 1975; McGowan-Sass & Timiras, 1975; Van Hartesveldt, 1975). Disruptions of the hippocampal formation can alter these associations, as is indicated by changes in pituitary–adrenal cyclicity (Frischette, Komisaruk, Edinger, Feder, & Siegel, 1980) and response to stress (Johnson and Moberg, 1980; Lanier, Van Hartesveldt, Weis, & Isaacson, 1975). Hippocampal influences are not limited to corticosteroids but also affect diverse hormone systems including the gonadal steroids and responsiveness to centrally acting pituitary peptides such as corticotropin (ACTH). For example, the excessive grooming induced by intracerebroventricular injections of $ACTH_{1-24}$ is attenuated by hippocampal lesions (Elstein, Hannigan, & Isaacson, 1981; Gispen & Isaacson, 1981), perhaps via an interaction with nucleus accumbens dopamine systems (Hannigan, Balaz, Springer, Ryan, & Isaacson, 1982; Ryan and Isaacson, 1983a; Wiegant, Cools, & Gispen, 1977). It may be of interest that several types of hormones have direct regulatory influences on portions of the basal ganglia that have been shown to be affected by hippocampal damage. Interactions of this nature have been demonstrated for peptide hormones (Delanoy, Kramarcy, & Dunn, 1982; Gispen & de Wied, 1980) and gonadal steroids (Alderson & Baum, 1981; Cubells & Joseph, 1981).

Furthermore, some behavioral effects of hippocampal lesions in rats can be attenuated by manipulations of hormonal systems the activities of which may be modified by the lesion. This is especially obvious after manipulations of the pituitary adrenal axis. For example, Iuvone and Van Hartesveldt (1976) found that the hyperactivity induced by hippocampal lesions in rats was correlated with decreased plasma corticosterone levels measured after behavioral testing. Furthermore, the reduction of corticosterone pharmacologically by a synthesis inhibitor also reduces the hyperactivity found after hippocampal destruction (Ryan & Isaacson, 1983b). Lovely (1975) showed that both facilitated acquisition and delayed extinction of shuttle-box avoidance behavior in hippocampal-lesioned rats was reduced following hypophysectomy. This finding is especially interesting because hypophysectomy is known to reduce the development of dopamine-receptor supersensitivity (Hruska & Pitman, 1982), an effect that could be related to the sequence of dopaminergic changes found after hippocampal lesions.

Sources of Potential Age-Related Differences in Secondary Reactions after Brain Damage

The interactions just described between neurotransmitter and neurohormonal systems may provide the groundwork for understanding the different sorts of behavioral change found after brain damage in the young, changes that may not resemble those found in the young adult. For example, after damage to the hippocampus, the secondary reactions in dopaminergic systems of the very young animal could be unusual because the functional characteristics of these systems may differ from those of the adult. Supporting the idea that such differences exist, Gaddy, Britt, Neill, and Haigler (1979) found that kainic acid injected into the striatum of older rats (69–127 days) produced greater damage than when injected into those of rats at age 48–49 days, and Campochiaro and Coyle (1978) found that 7-day-old rats were less sensitive to kainic acid than were 21-day-old animals. These differences may be due to increased glutaminergic innervation of the striatum with aging or experience. The increasing ontogenetic influence of neurohormones and sexual hormones on neurotransmitter release from terminals could also be a factor in the greater sensitivity to kainic acid later in life.

In the early postnatal period, the dopaminergic systems of the basal forebrain are subject to different forms of regulation than are found in later life. Even though dopamine may be acting as a neurotransmitter as early as gestational Day 18 in the rat according to measures on the basis of Ca^{++}- and K^{+}-evoked dopamine-release capabilities in synaptosomal preparations (Nomura, Yotsumoto, & Segawa, 1981), depolarization produces relatively little dopamine release at this age. Furthermore, presynaptic cholinergic modulation of dopamine release is minimal or nonexistent in the 1st week after birth. Both muscarinic and nicotinic receptors play a role in dopamine modulation in the striatum. These receptors mature at different times. There is a rapid onset of muscarinic binding 7 days after birth (Coyle & Yamamura, 1976), whereas nicotinic binding peaks about 13 days following birth (Wade & Timiras, 1980). Therefore, any lesion that affects the dopaminergic modulation of basal activities, as thought to occur after hippocampal lesions, will be producing its effects on systems that are not subject to the usual, adult types of regulation. The systems are different from those of the prototypical adult.

Paralleling these neurobiological differences, behavioral responses related to food intake, elimination, arousal, and stress are also quite different at different ages, and are subject to different environmental influences. Even the simple act of moving an infant animal away from its mother or from its littermates can induce signs of profound stress. Stimuli of various sorts produce specialized reactions in young animals that are quite divergent from those of the adult. The stimuli mean different things to young animals in the sense that their brains and bodies are set to respond in different ways from those of the prototypical adult. The brain and body develop in synergistic fashion to provide the physiological functions and behaviors that are the hallmarks of particular ages. The behaviors of young animals are not aberrant from, nor are they poor-quality imitations of, the ideal adult response.

The brains of animals and people vary with genetic endowment, age, and experience. These three factors are inexorably intertwined and a complete unraveling of the contributions is probably impossible. However, the net effect of the interactions among these factors, under usual circumstances, is to produce a brain that is appropriate to the particular requirements of life at different ages. The young brain is suited to the needs of the young animal relative to the demands of the environment. Although this argument has elements of circularity, we believe that in evolution animals with brains inappropriate to their usual environmental and internal needs failed to thrive or to withstand selection pressures. Therefore, it would be a mistake to consider the infant brain as an immature adult brain with severe limitations on its functional capacities, one that exists only as a basis for the creation of the ideal adult brain, but rather as a functionally complete entity perfectly suited for the management of both internal and external demands. This approach is reminiscent of that of Adolph (1968) as revived by Oppenheim (1980).

In essence we support the view of Johnson and Almli (1978) that the understanding of the effects of brain damage depends on understanding the behavioral capacities at the time of the lesion. Beyond this, we believe that it is essential to understand the state of the brain's various systems and the nature of the changes occurring in these systems at the time of damage. When investigating brain damage sustained early in life, one needs to consider that the functional characteristics of the brain areas damaged, and the functional efficacy and modulatory influences of surviving brain systems, may be different early in life than they are in adulthood. Therefore, to understand the brain's activities at any age we must understand behavior and its relationship to satisfaction of the needs of the organism. Consequently, we next consider some behavioral abilities of young animals relative to the specific demands placed on them by their environment.

Needs and Behavioral Strategies
of Young Animals

THE NEONATAL PERIOD: THE FIRST POSTNATAL WEEK

The primary goals of the neonate are to survive and thrive. In so doing, the newborn rat pup exhibits an exquisite series of behavioral strategies that meet these fundamental requirements through the intake of nutrients, conservation of energy, and maintenance of an appropriate body temperature.

Suckling is the sole means by which the neonatal rat pup normally receives nutrients. The act of suckling requires a series of specialized behaviors: the pup searches the mother's ventral surface with wide, sweeping movements of the head to locate a nipple, probes with its snout to ease grasping of the teat, and treads and paddles with fore- and hindlimbs to align the body appropriately. Odor cues appear to be critical for locating and attaching to a nipple; for example, pups will not attach to a washed nipple (e.g., Teicher & Blass, 1976). Once attached to the nipple, other behaviors become necessary for the pup to extract milk efficiently during letdowns. When the pup senses that a milk letdown is imminent, it extends its body and increases negative pressure on the nipple. These responses facilitate the rapid influx of milk down the esophagus (e.g., Drewett, Statham, & Wakerley, 1974). The urge to suckle is very strong in these animals. Even in the absence of milk letdown, pups will continue to suckle for hours on the teats of an anesthetized dam. Indeed, termination of a suckling bout in pups of this age appears to be regulated by the mother, who terminates a suckling bout when her internal body temperature reaches a critical hyperthermic level (e.g., Woodside & Leon, 1980).

When the dam is absent, the pups' behavior in the nest seems to be directed largely toward conserving body temperature. When the mother leaves the nest, pups quickly form a huddle with siblings, a strategy that decreases both body heat loss and oxygen consumption in pups (Alberts, 1978). As the temperature of the environment changes, so do the movements of individual pups, thus changing the characteristics of the huddle, especially the surface-to-volume ratio (Alberts, 1978). The behaviors involved include forelimb treading and hindlimb paddling movements, as well as probing and rooting with the snout and head.

Neonatal rat pups are poikilothermic and, although this is seemingly due to the immaturity of regulatory processes, there may be some adaptive benefits of poikilothermia for the neonate as well. For example, poikilothermia may serve to prolong suckling-bout duration. The critical hyperthermic level at which the dam terminates suckling might be reached more rapidly if pups were homeothermic. The achievement of homeothermia would also require a substantial expenditure of energy for heat production.

Unnecessary energy expenditure is also reduced by the minimization of locomotor activity. The inheritance of locomotor activity is characterized by a pattern of nearly complete dominance for low activity in neonatal mice (Henderson, 1978). This suggests that low activity may be adaptive. Indeed, neonatal rats are largely inactive except for movements directed toward suckling and huddling. When exposed to a cooler environment (e.g., if inadvertently displaced outside of the nest or if the mother leaves the nest), the pup may be active for a short period of time as its body temperature drops rapidly, but it then becomes immobile (see Whishaw, Schallert, & Kolb, 1979). This activity may result in the formation of a huddle or a return to the nest site if the pup is not far from the nest, the homing response. Both of these responses appear to be directed more by temperature gradients than olfaction (e.g., Alberts, 1978; Johanson, 1978, 1979).

The sensitivity of the olfactory system in rat pups increases with age (Alberts & May, 1980) and, although olfaction seems critical for nipple attachment in the early postnatal period (e.g., Teicher & Blass, 1976), it is not used as a source of distal sensory information until later in ontogeny. This points to an important distinction between the maturation of a sensory system and the maturation of its functional uses. It appears that odors are used as signals for nipple attachment early in life, but only later as directional signals. It is likely, but not certain, that the differences in the uses of sensory information are dictated by changes in central neural mechanisms.

The brief burst of activity induced by separation from the nest is quickly followed by immobility. Even so, the behavior of the pup is not completely passive when it is isolated. Neonatal pups respond to isolation by emitting ultrasonic vocalizations. Thus, even the neonatal pup is able to detect that it is outside of the nest, a discrimination that is at least partially based on alterations in tactile and thermal cues (Oswalt & Meier, 1975). Pup-emitted ultrasounds elicit and direct pup retrieval on the part of the dam (Allin & Banks, 1971; Smotherman, Bell, Starzec, Elias, & Zachman, 1974). Pups also emit calls when subjected to rough handling and when being retrieved. The calls may serve to inhibit aggression on the part of the dam (Sales & Smith, 1978). Ultrasonic calling reaches its peak around the end of the 1st or the beginning of the 2nd postnatal week. It declines rapidly after the 2nd postnatal week and becomes virtually absent by weaning (Allin & Banks, 1971; Noirot, 1968; Okon, 1972). Neonates seem to rely on the mother for transportation, using ultrasounds to elicit and direct retrieval. This seems to have several benefits for the young. They expend little energy in locomotor movements that, because the pup is deaf, blind, and limited in its ability to use odors or follow thermal gradients except at very close ranges, would be as likely to move the pup away from the nest as toward it.

Despite the fact that neonatal rat pups normally expend little energy on body movements, they do have extensive motor capacities. Under certain conditions, rat pups can emit an impressive series of behavioral responses, indicating a high degree of motor maturity. For instance, milk cannulated into the mouth of deprived pups (e.g., Hall, 1979), novel odors (Gard, Hard, Larsson, & Petersson, 1967) shock (Collier & Bolles, 1980; Stehouwer, Haroutunian, & Campbell, 1980), and stroking with a paint brush (Pederson, Williams, & Blass, 1982) induce rolling, curling, paddling, pivoting, locomoting, and wall climbing in neonatal rat pups. Indeed, 3-day-old rat pups, when infused with milk intraorally, will walk and run with the torso held up off the floor (Caza & Spear, 1982), behaviors that are rarely reported in developmental surveys until a week or 10 days later in ontogeny. This pattern of generalized whole-body activation seen in response to sensory stimulation is similar to those induced in neonates by administration of monoamine agonists such as clonidine (Kellogg & Lundborg, 1972), L-dopa (Kellogg & Lundborg, 1972), amphetamine (Sobrian, Weltman, & Pappas, 1975), and quipazine (Spear & Ristine, 1981). Therefore, although neonates seldom move, this is not due to inadequacies of their motor mechanisms but rather to infrequent activation of existing motor systems.

The marked behavioral activation seen under these experimental conditions may be related to normal interactions in the nest. When the mother enters the nest, she stimulates the pups by vigorously licking, stepping on, and retrieving them (Hofer, 1975). This stimulation, through activating monoaminergic systems, may arouse the pups to a level that is necessary for the initiation of suckling. Pederson *et al.* (1982) argue that neonates must be stimulated in such a fashion to learn the variety of suckling-related cues (e.g., odors, tactile cues) associated with the dam's teats.

THE INFANT RAT PUP: POSTNATAL DAYS 8–14

The rat pup during the second postnatal week has some of the same needs, and strategies for meeting those needs, as the neonate. During this period, the sensory capacities and range of movements of the infant show further development.

Suckling remains the only natural means of nutrient intake for infant rats. Until the end of the second postnatal week, there are few internal controls that regulate the attachment and maintenance of suckling behavior. For instance, food deprivation only begins to have an influence on teat-attachment latency in 11- to 13-day-old animals (Hall, Cramer, & Blass, 1977).

Infant rat pups are still largely poikolothermic, with thermally neutral zones (ambient temperature inducing minimal oxygen consumption) nearly as high as those of the neonate (Thompson & Moore, 1968). Infant rats still spend a great deal of their time huddling (Alberts, 1978). However, by the middle of the 2nd postnatal week, rat pups are much more resistant to the effects of cold ambient temperatures, as measured in terms of drops in body temperature (Whishaw et al., 1979). Moreover, an ambient temperature of only 27–28°C elicits maximal oxygen consumption in neonates, whereas 12-day-old rat pups do not exhibit maximal oxygen consumption until ambient temperatures reach 15°C or cooler (Thompson & Moore, 1968). Around 10 days of age, shivering begins to be observed (Whishaw et al., 1979) and fur growth begins; both provide an increased resistance to cool temperatures.

At this time the rat pups' sensitivity to odors (Alberts and May, 1980) and social stimuli increases. For example, although alterations in thermal cues are most important for the induction of ultrasounds or huddling in neonatal rats, variations in social cues (olfactory and tactile) predominate in eliciting these behaviors during the second postnatal week (Alberts, 1978; Hofer & Shair, 1980). Also, it is during the second postnatal week that infant rats first begin to orient reliably toward odor cues from the home nest (Altman & Sudarshan, 1975; Gregory & Pfaff, 1971; Johanson, 1978).

During the 2nd postnatal week, the pup's repertoire of emitted behaviors increases substantially. They crawl, walk, groom, and begin to run, exhibiting moderate amounts of vigorous and effective locomotion (Altman & Sudarshan, 1975; Blank, Hard, & Larsson, 1967; Bolles & Woods, 1964). In the second half of this week, pups begin to explore areas of the cage other than the nest site (Bolles & Woods, 1964; Rosenblatt & Lehrman, 1963). These short excursions may be possible because, at this time, body temperature is less affected by the ambient temperature. As a consequence, the animals are able to sustain locomotor movements for an extended period of time (Whishaw et al., 1979). Their improved olfactory capabilities may help them to return to the nest with greater success, even though they still are frequently retrieved by the dam. Nursing outside of the nest also begins and becomes progressively more common near the end of the second and into the third postnatal week (Rosenblatt & Lehrman, 1963).

When confronted with potent sensory stimuli, neonates during the 1st week of life exhibit a generalized increase in a number of different behaviors. During the second postnatal week, these same stimuli induce more specific behaviors, one of the most prominent being wall climbing. Rat pups of this age (but not older) frequently wall climb in response to shock (e.g., Barrett, Caza, Spear, & Spear, 1982; Misanin, Haigh, Hinderliter, & Nagy, 1973; Stehouwer & Campbell, 1980), milk (referred to by Hall, 1979, as "aversive behavior"), and temperatures relatively high above nest temperature (Johanson & Hall, 1980). Age-specific wall climbing is also emitted in response to catecholaminergic agonists such as clonidine (Reinstein & Isaacson, 1977; Spear & Brick, 1979), apomorphine (Reinstein, McClearn, & Isaacson, 1978; Shalaby & Spear, 1980), and amphetamine (Barrett *et al.*, 1982). These drugs induce this behavior from approximately 7–14 days after birth, with little, if any, wall climbing being induced thereafter.

THE PREWEANLING RAT PUP: POSTNATAL DAYS 15–21

Although milk production of the dam reaches peak levels at 15 days postpartum, by 16 to 18 days postnatal this source of nutrients is insufficient to provide all of the caloric needs of the growing litter (Babicky, Parizek, Ostadobvar, & Kolar, 1973; Galef, 1981). Therefore, the pup must seek outside sources of nutrients. At this time, a variety of internal controls that serve to regulate suckling also emerge. For example, cholecystokinin (Blass, Beardsley, & Hall, 1979), glucose loading (Geiselman, Vanderweele, Dray, Ewing, & Cryder-Mooney, 1980), extracellular or intracellular dehydration (Bruno, Craigmyle, & Blass, 1982), and stomach loading (Hall & Rosenblatt, 1977) act to depress or terminate nipple attachment at about 15–20 days of age, but not earlier. Internal controls of food intake, which seem similar to those affecting adult food ingestion, become effective at the time when the pup begins to have a variety of sources of nutrients.

During the 3rd week of life, the preweanling rat pup must often go searching both for solid food and for the dam, who becomes less likely to initiate nursing bouts. Indeed, the dam even begins to evade nursing approaches made on the part of the pups (Rosenblatt & Lehrman, 1963). The transition to independent feeding may be accelerated by intolerance to lactose and subsequent learned aversions to milk (Galef, 1981). Progressive lactase deficiency in preweanling mammals may lead to lactose intolerance and gastrointestinal distress associated with milk ingestion (Lieberman & Lieberman, 1978). Although the dam initiates fewer suckling bouts, in the wild she meets the nutritive needs of her pups by providing food caches within the burrow. These food caches are essential for the pups because it is not until the periadolescent period that pups first leave the burrow (Galef, 1981).

At this time, the pups are quite active in exploring the home area. Although they, like adults, sleep and huddle a great deal, when awake they charge about the cage, exploring and playing (the amount of play, however, will increase until well after weaning). Their eyes and ears are now open, enriching their perception of the environment. Their thermoregulatory neutral zone is still higher than room temperature (Thompson & Moore, 1968), but they are able to withstand larger drops in ambient temperature without suffering a loss in body temperature than are younger animals.

The behavior of the preweanling rat pup is markedly influenced by the environment in ways that are not completely understood. When isolated for several hours or more in a novel environment, the activity of rat pups has been observed to show a rapid ontogenetic increase to a peak around 15 days of age and then to decline gradually until 30 days of age (Campbell & Mabry, 1972; Campbell, Lytle, & Fibiger, 1969). Rat pups tested in the nest or in a novel environment in the presence of an anesthetized adult or of home cage odors do not exhibit this marked ontogenetic peak in locomotor activity (Randall & Campbell, 1976; Campbell & Raskin, 1978). It has been suggested that this hyperactivity may be a result of novelty-induced fear or stress reaction (see Campbell & Raskin, 1978) or may be related to food deprivation (Moorcroft, 1981). In shorter-duration tests, home nest odors induce hyperactivity when isolated pups are tested in a relatively large arena (Barrett, Caza, Spear, & Spear, 1981; Buelke-Sam & Kimmel, 1980; Pappas, Vickers, Buxton, & Pusztay, 1982) but hypoactivity when they are tested in a small apparatus (Barrett et al., 1982; Sosis & Spear, in preparation). Thus, locomotor activity omitted by preweanling rat pups seems to be influenced by a variety of factors, including presence or absence of familiar cues, deprivational state, and size of the apparatus.

There is no doubt that preweanling rat pups are influenced by odors and other cues associated with the home nest. Beginning at 14 days postpartum and continuing until 27 days postnatally, lactating rats have been reported to secrete a pheromone in the feces that is highly attractive to preweanling and weanling rat pups (Leon &

Moltz, 1972). This pheromone may induce the approach and consumption of maternal feces that contains other substances that aid in the survival of the young (Moltz & Lee, 1981). Release of pheromones at the nest site that are attractive to the pups could function to insure that the young stay near the nest even though their locomotor capacities permit them to wander far afield.

The preweanling seems to be at an age of transition in which it gradually evolves behavioral strategies that can be used in a later, more independent status. At this time, the pup may be extremely sensitive to cues that may serve to maintain its association with the dam in the face of emerging motor and sensory capabilities.

THE WEANLING RAT PUP: POSTNATAL DAYS 21–30

Much less is known of the natural behavior of the weanling rat than that of younger rat pups. Many developmental surveys test animals only up to the conventional age of artificial weaning, 21 days postnatally. One of the difficulties in assessing the "natural" behavior of weanling animals in the laboratory is that many laboratories wean litters by removing them from the dam at 21 days of age, well in advance of the date that the pups would be naturally weaned (see Galef, 1981; Ostadolova, Ribr, Babicky, Parizek, & Kohar, 1971).

It appears that the behavior of the weanling rat resembles that of the adult. Like adults, they no longer show the intense hyperactivity when isolated in a novel situation that was characteristic of the preweanling (Campbell & Mabry, 1972; Campbell et al., 1969). Their behavioral repertoire and sensory capabilities appear to be similar to the adult. Yet, they play more than adults. Play will continue to increase until the periadolescent period. The thermoregulatory neutral ambient temperature of 30-day-old animals (28 °C) approaches that of adults (Thompson & Moore, 1968). Weanlings continue to be especially sensitive to home nest odors and will continue to be responsive through 27 days of age (Leon & Moltz, 1972). This may serve to keep them near the nest.

THE PERIADOLESCENT PERIOD: POSTNATAL DAYS 30–42

During the periadolescent period (about Day 34 postpartum), rats in seminatural test conditions leave the burrow and begin to explore distant areas (see Galef, 1981). They begin to seek out food and to interact with conspecifics other than their own dams and littermates.

In novel testing situations, periadolescents are often reported to be hyperactive and to "hole poke" more than either younger or older animals (e.g., Lanier & Isaacson, 1977; Spear, Shalaby, & Brick, 1980). It is during the periadolescent period that the greatest amounts of conspecific social play behavior is exhibited (e.g., Baenninger, 1967; Meaney & Stewart, 1981; Panksepp, 1981). In laboratory learning tasks, periadolescents often have difficulty learning, or at least performing, complex tasks, perhaps because they are unable to focus attention on salient cues or contingencies. At the same time, they have little difficulty learning or performing the kind of goal-oriented tasks that require little more than a simple active response (see Spear & Brake, 1983, for further discussion and references). Spear and Brake (1983) have hypothesized that these transient behavioral alterations may be a function of a temporary decrease in the efficacy of mesolimbic dopamine projections occurring during the periadolescent period.

Galef (1981) has speculated about the possible adaptive value of the age-specific, species-typical behaviors of periadolescents. For example, the strong social tendencies of the periadolescent coupled with high levels of locomotor activity and exploration may be useful in searching for food. Play behavior may serve to inhibit aggressive behavior on the part of older novel conspecifics. Play behavior during periadolescence may also be necessary for the development of later social, sexual, or aggressive behavior. The rather poor performance of animals of this age in complex learning tasks used in laboratories may be merely a manifestation of age-specific response patterns that have overall adaptive significance.

It is at the end of the periadolescent period (approximately postnatal Day 40) that rats become sexually mature as defined by vaginal opening in females and presence of sperm in the seminiferous tubules in males (e.g., Clermont & Perry, 1957; Döhler & Wuttke, 1975). At this time the sexual hormones begin to become abundant and exert profound influences on both brain and behavior. They have both direct effects on certain brain regions and indirect effects, as when they modulate neurotransmission. Correlated with the development of these systems is the gradual transformation of periadolescent behaviors into those typical of the young adult.

Assessing the Effects of Early Brain Damage

The preceding survey of some of the behavioral milestones found early in the life of the rat reveals that there are important differences in how young animals fulfill needs that are critical for their survival and further development. The neonate is not a behaviorally impoverished organism with the capability of responding to but few stimuli. Rather, the neonate is a behaviorally competent individual with different ways of coping with its own particular environmental requirements and internal states. The importance of bodily temperature early after birth and the ultrasound vocalizations that the pups produce in response to temperature reductions are instances of these special characteristics of the very young animal. The same sort of special circumstances can be found throughout development and aging. We interpret this to mean that the structure, function, and behavioral contributions of the various brain systems are organized quite differently at different ages. The brains of young animals are not simply immature; rather, they are prepared to function appropriately for the situations they confront. It is within this framework that both the immediate and long-term consequences of early brain damage must be considered.

Within this context, it should be clear that the effects of lesions at one stage of life may be quite different from those at another. As an immediate effect, brain damage could disrupt the expression of the age- and species-specific behavior patterns. The effects of early brain damage must be considered within the context of the possible disruption of behaviors appropriate for that age. For instance, it would be expected that some forms of early brain damage might disrupt suckling behavior, a critical behavior of the neonate. If suckling is disturbed, nutritional input will be affected and overall development may be affected. Therefore, in this case the effects of an early insult to the brain when measured in adulthood may be related both to the effects of the lesion itself and to the effects of the insult on nutrient intake and subsequent brain growth.

Suckling is a useful model to illustrate the possible involvement of various brain systems in mediating age-specific behaviors. Although the precise brain systems involved in suckling are not established, the brain mechanisms subserving suckling behavior in infants do not appear analogous to those controlling adult feeding. For example, ventromedial hypothalamic lesions increase food intake in animals lesioned in adulthood (e.g., Anand & Brobeck, 1951) but do not induce hyperphagia in rats lesioned in the neonatal period until the animals reach 50–70 days of age (Hill, Almli, & Williams, 1978). Also, whereas lateral hypothalamic lesions induce aphagia in rats lesioned in adulthood, extensive lesions of this area in neonatal rat pups have little influence on food intake at any subsequent age, although such lesions produce transient growth retardation and an increase in nipple-attachment latency in suckling-latency tests. If the lesions are made 7 days after birth or later, however, these same lesions produce an immediate cessation of suckling (Almli, 1978). Beyond these lesion effects, internal stimuli that influence ingestion in adults (e.g., glucose or stomach loading or dehydration) have little impact on suckling behavior during the first 2 weeks of postnatal life.

Although lesions and manipulations of internal stimuli that influence ingestion in adults are generally ineffective in altering suckling behavior of neonates, the strong suckling propensity of neonates can be reduced by other types of manipulations. Electrolytic lesions of the anterior raphe nuclei (containing serotonergic nuclei that project primarily rostrally) have been reported to disrupt suckling in neonatal rat pups (Adrien, 1978). Similarly, we observed that intracisternal administration of the serotonergic neurotoxin 5,6-dihydroxytryptamine on postnatal Day 5 disrupted suckling behavior of rat pups to the extent that it was often necessary to hand-feed the pups for several days to maintain their viability (Isaacson, Fish, Lanier, & Dunn, 1977). Intact serotonergic systems seem critical for the maintenance of suckling in neonates.

Psychopharmacological work supports this suggestion. The serotonergic antagonists metergoline, methiothepin, and methysergide all block suckling behavior of rat pups 3–4 days after birth (Spear & Ristine, 1982). This effect seems to be centrally mediated, because intracisternal administration of small doses of these compounds block suckling of the neonates. The reduction in suckling induced by these antagonists does not appear to be a result of a debilitating effect of the drugs or to an alteration in body temperature. These effects appear to be at least somewhat specific to the serotonergic system, because opiate, dopaminergic, α-adrenergic, and β-adrenergic antagonists do not consistently produce any alteration in suckling behavior. However, the cholinergic antagonist scopolamine does reduce suckling behavior of neonates after peripheral or central administration (Spear & Ristine, 1982).

These effects of serotonergic antagonists on suckling behavior in neonates are different and in some ways opposite those reported later in ontogeny. For instance, Ristine and Spear (1981, 1982) observed that metergoline blocked suckling in rat pups 7–8 days of age or younger but *increased* suckling significantly in pups 23–24 days of age. This supports a prior report that serotonergic antagonists induce suckling in weanlings (Williams, Rosenblatt, & Hall, 1979). An intriguing possibility exists that an early maturing serotonergic system may stimulate suckling behavior in the neonate, whereas one or more other serotonergic systems maturing later in life may inhibit suck-ling. These other serotonergic systems may become functionally important when the animals begin to incorporate solid food.

This example indicates that the brain systems mediating infant behaviors may be different from those mediating adult-typical be-havior patterns, even when the ultimate goal of the behaviors is sim-ilar: food incorporation. This is another reason why it is difficult to predict the effects of early brain damage even when the behavioral effects of a certain type of lesion are considered in light of moti-vational effects rather than specific behaviors.

What kinds of behavioral or physiological effects can be expected after brain damage early in life? The answer is complicated and in some ways paradoxical. On one hand, we anticipate that critical age- and species-typical behaviors such as those described earlier would be neurologically protected and therefore relatively resistant to damage. On the other hand, we would also expect that if the damage is sufficient to produce noticeable symptoms early in life, it would have to be reflected by changes in these behaviors.

Although researchers rarely assess the effects of early brain damage on age-specific behaviors, from those examples that are available it appears that age-specific behaviors may be protected from insults to the forebrain. For example, Nonneman (1970) was unable to find any immediate effects of early neocortical or hippo-campal damage in rabbits as measured by suckling, homing, or other spontaneously occurring age- and species-typical behaviors. A sim-ilar result has been found in the hamster, in which extensive damage to the neocortex seems not to affect the unfolding of age- and species-typical behaviors[1] (Murphy, MacLean, & Hamilton, 1981). The mech-anisms responsible for the resistance of age-dependent behaviors to forebrain damage remain to be established, but it is likely that these behaviors are embedded in the brainstem and probably mediated by redundant neural networks. The protection of such basic behaviors is of adaptive significance because it fosters survival and procreation even after brain damage.

Later appearing age- and species-typical behaviors also may be resistant to disruption, although perhaps less so than the earliest appearing age-specific behaviors. The mechanisms responsible for

---

[1] In this study, additional midline cortical damage produced a disturbance of con-specific play. However, this effect could have been a consequence of the greater overall damage suffered by the animals and not of damage of the presumably limbic cortex of the midline.

this resistance may resemble the resistance of sexual behaviors of adult rats to the elimination of usual sensory input due to forebrain damage (Beach, 1967).

Brain lesions that fail to affect age- and species-typical behaviors cannot be assumed to be without effect. This only indicates that the damage is of insufficient amount or in the wrong location to overcome the built-in protection of such systems. According to our views, the nervous systems of animals at every age are suited to the reactions to specific stimuli and the execution of behaviors appropriate for them to meet the demands of the environment. Furthermore, part of the adaptive program is the protection of the critically important functions at each developmental period.

If the early brain damage is extensive enough to produce immediate behavioral symptoms, we would predict that these symptoms would be evident in a disruption of age-specific behaviors. Observable symptoms after such extensive damage in the first postnatal week might involve disruptions in behavioral thermoregulation and suckling. Brain damage occurring at later times may produce more numerous and specific symptoms including disturbances in ultrasound production, thermal responsivity, huddling, and—later in life—play, food search, and homing. With this behavioral differentiation, greater localization of lesion effects on specific behaviors might be found.

Because alterations in early age-specific behaviors induced by brain damage would alter the prospectus for future development, the symptoms of the damage evident at maturity would be difficult to predict on the basis of data obtained from animals lesioned in adulthood. Mental and behavioral development subsequent to brain damage will also vary from that found in the intact animal because of secondary changes produced in remaining systems. Even when brain damage occurs that is below some threshold for influencing age-specific behaviors, it still induces secondary reactions. As indicated, these will not be equivalent at different ages, and thus the evaluation of these consequences is difficult. Consequently, the constellations of behavioral and anatomical aberrations as they are elaborated over subsequent days, months, and years following early brain damage are likely, at all times of assessment, to vary considerably from the usual effects of damage later in life (for examples of such differences, see Goldman & Galkin, 1978, and Nonneman & Corwin, 1981). Comparability in the long-term effects of early and late brain damage will occur only when the final constellations of secondary alterations in structure and function are similar. The earlier the lesion, the less likely this will be.

In most cases in which sparing of function after early brain damage has been reported, the behaviors assessed to examine recovery are those behaviors that are altered after presumably comparable brain damage in adulthood. Yet the aberrations observed after infant brain damage are likely to be different from the consequences of brain damage sustained in adulthood. It is difficult to know what to look for in behavior and, at this point in our understanding of the impact of early brain damage on subsequent brain development and behavior, it may be premature to limit assessment to only a small number of measures. We anticipate that a thorough examination of behavioral and cognitive abilities after early brain damage would demonstrate aberrations, many subtle and perhaps unexpected.

Summary and Conclusions

At each developmental period the brain and its component systems are prepared to respond to certain internal and external stimuli and to execute those responses that are adaptive for immediate survival and future growth. It is not a matter of an immature, inadequate brain struggling to cope with environmental demands, but rather a well-organized brain competent to deal with the particular demands of the time.

A significant part of the behavioral consequences of brain damage at all ages is due to secondary reactions in remaining systems, but it must be recognized that the normal functional activities of all systems may vary with age. Early brain lesions may not produce immediate, or even long-term, effects that resemble those seen after comparable lesions in adulthood. Rather, insults early in life, if sufficiently devastating, have the potential to disrupt age- and species-specific behaviors of relevance to the animal at that point in its life span. Early in life these behaviors may be rather resistant to disruption after neural insults, due in part to redundant representations in the brain. Lesions that do disrupt these age-specific behavior patterns may produce long-term alterations in neural functioning in numerous brain regions. In order to assess the effects of early brain damage adequately, the development of age-specific behaviors must be carefully assessed.

The long-term effects of early brain damage will be particularly hard to assess because the mental and behavioral changes may not bear resemblance to the effects of comparable lesions later in life. It is not sufficient to use tests designed for the evaluation of comparable damage in young adults. The consequences of early damage can be manifested in ways that are quite unanticipated. This is due to the imposition of lesion-induced neural changes on remaining systems that are different from those of the adult and which, because of the early insult, will never resemble those of the intact adult.

The assumption that a significant part of the behavioral consequences of brain damage at all ages is due to secondary reactions in remaining systems, however, offers the hope that some intervention procedure, whether pharmacological, hormonal, or experiential, can ameliorate the behavioral handicaps produced by the damage. This exciting possibility has been examined in the case of adult animals with hippocampal damage and needs to be extended to animals receiving damage early in life. We expect the animals with damage inflicted at an early age to require different types of treatments, but there is the hope that successful intervention approaches can ultimately be found for many of the common types of early brain damage.

Acknowledgments

This work was supported in part by Grant 1R01MH35761 from the National Institute of Mental Health and a BRSG Grant S07RR07149-10 awarded by the Biomedical Research Support Grant Program Division of Research Resources, National Institutes of Health.

References

Adolph, E. F. (1968). *Origins of physiological regulations.* New York: Academic Press.

Adrien, J. (1978). Ontogenesis of some sleep regulations: Early postnatal impairment of the monoaminergic systems. *Progress in Brain Research, 48,* 393–403.

Alberts, J. R. (1978). Huddling by rat pups: Group behavioral mechanisms of temperature regulation and energy conservation. *Journal of Comparative Physiological Psychology, 92,* 231–245.

Alberts, J. R., & May, B. (1980). Development of nasal respiration and sniffing in the rat. *Physiology and Behavior, 24,* 957–963.

Alderson, L. M., & Baum, M. J. (1981). Differential effects of gonadal steroids on dopamine metabolism in mesolimbic and nigrostriatal pathways of male rat brain. *Brain Research, 218,* 189–206.

Allin, J. T., & Banks, E. M. (1971). Effects of temperature on ultrasound production by infant albino rats. *Developmental Psychobiology, 4,* 149–156.

Almli, C. R. (1978). The ontogeny of feeding and drinking: Effects of early brain damage. *Neuroscience and Biobehavioral Reviews, 2,* 281–300.

Altman, J., & Sudarshan, K. (1975). Postnatal development of locomotion in the laboratory rat. *Animal Behaviour, 23,* 896–920.

Anand, B. K., & Brobeck, J. R. (1951). Hypothalamic control of food intake in rats and cats. *Yale Journal of Biology and Medicine, 24,* 123–140.

Babicky, A., Parizek, J., Ostadolova, I., & Kolar, J. (1973). Initial solid food intake and growth of young rats in nests of different sizes. *Physiologica Bohemoslovia, 22,* 557–566.

Baenninger, L. P. (1967). Comparison of behavioral development in socially isolated and grouped rats. *Animal Behaviour, 15,* 312–323.

Bär, B. R., Gispen, W. H., & Isaacson, R. L. (1981). Behavioral and regional neurochemical sequelae of hippocampal destruction in the rat. *Pharmacology Biochemistry and Behavior, 14,* 305–312.

Barrett, B. A., Caza, P., Spear, L. P., & Spear, N. E. (1981, April). *Psychopharmacological effects of dl-amphetamine in the presence of odors from the home nest.* Paper presented at Eastern Psychological Association meetings, New York.

Barrett, B. A., Caza, P., Spear, N. E., & Spear, L. P. (1982). Wall climbing, odors from the home nest, and catecholaminergic activity in rat pups. *Physiology and Behavior, 29,* 501–507.

Beach, F. A. (1967). Cerebral and hormonal control of reflexive mechanisms involved in copulatory behaviour. *Physiological Reviews, 47,* 289–316.

Blank, A., Hard, E., & Larsson, K. (1967). Ontogenetic development of orienting behavior in the rat. *Journal of Comparative and Physiological Psychology, 63,* 327–328.

Blass, E. M., Beardsley, W., & Hall, W. G. (1979). Age-dependent inhibition of suckling by cholecystokinin. *American Journal of Physiology, 236,* E567–E570.

Bohus, B. (1975). The hippocampus and the pituitary–adrenal system. In R. L. Isaacson & K. H. Pribram (Eds.), *The hippocampus* (Vol. I, (pp. 323–354). New York: Plenum.

Bolles, R. C., & Woods, P. J. (1964). The ontogeny of behavior in the albino rat. *Animal Behaviour, 12,* 427–441.

Bruno, J. P., Craigmyle, L. S., & Blass, E. M. (1982). Dehydration inhibits suckling behavior in weanling rats. *Journal of Comparative Physiological Psychology, 96,* 405–415.

Buelke-Sam, J., & Kimmel, C. A. (1980). *Developmental locomotor activity in rats tested over clean vs. home cage bedding.* Paper presented at Society for Neuroscience meeting, Cincinnati.

Campbell, B. A., Lytle, L. D., & Fibiger, H. C. (1969). Ontogeny of adrenergic arousal and cholinergic inhibitory mechanisms in the rat. *Science, 166,* 637–638.

Campbell, B. A., & Mabry, P. D. (1972). Ontogeny of behavioral arousal: A comparative study. *Journal of Comparative Physiological Psychology, 81,* 371–379.

Campbell, B. A., & Raskin, L. A. (1978). Ontogeny of behavioral arousal: The role of environmental stimuli. *Journal of Comparative and Physiological Psychology, 92,* 176–184.

Campochiaro, P., & Coyle, J. T. (1978). Ontogenetic development of kainic acid neurotoxicity: Correlates with glutaminergic innervation. *Proceedings of the National Academy of Science, 75,* 2025–2029.

Caza, P., & Spear, L. P. (1982). Pharmacological manipulation of milk-induced behaviors in 3-day-old rat pups. *Pharmacology Biochemistry and Behavior, 16,* 481–486.

Clermont, Y., & Perry, B. (1957). Quantitative study of the cell population of the seminiferous tubules in immature rats. *American Journal of Anatomy, 100,* 241–260.

Collier, A. C., & Bolles, R. C. (1980). The ontogenesis of defense reactions to shock in preweanling rats. *Developmental Psychobiology, 13,* 141–150.

Coyle, J. T., & Yamamura, H. I. (1976). Neurochemical aspects of the ontogenesis of cholinergic neurons in the rat brain. *Brain Research, 118,* 429–440.

Cubells, J. F., & Joseph, J. A. (1981). Neostriatal dopamine receptor loss and behavioral deficits in the senescent rat. *Life Sciences, 28,* 1215–1218.

Delanoy, R. L., Kramarcy, N. R., & Dunn, A. J. (1982). $ACTH_{1-24}$ and lysine vasopressin selectively activates dopamine synthesis in frontal cortex. *Brain Research, 231,* 117–129.

Dühler, K. D., & Wuttke, W. (1975). Changes with age in levels of serum gonadotrophins, prolactin, and gonadal steroids in prepubertal male and female rats. *Endocrinology, 97,* 898–907.

Drewett, R. F., Statham, C., & Wakerley, J. B. (1974). A quantitative analysis of the feeding behavior of suckling rats. *Animal Behaviour, 22,* 907–913.

Elstein, K., Hannigan, J. H., Jr., & Isaacson, R. L. (1981). Behavioral effects of repeated intracerebroventricular injection of ACTH in hippocampally lesioned rats. *Behavioral and Neural Biology, 32,* 248–254.

Frischette, C. T., Komisaruk, B. R., Edinger, H. M., Feder, H. H., & Siegel, A. (1980). Differential fornix ablations and the circadian rhythmicity of adrenal corticoid secretion. *Brain Research, 195,* 373–387.

Gaddy, J. R., Britt, M. D., Neill, D. B., & Haigler, H. J. (1979). Susceptibility of rat neostriatum to damage by kainic acid: Age dependence. *Brain Research, 176,* 192–196.

Galef, B. G., Jr. (1981). The ecology of weaning: Parasitism and the achievement of independence by altricial mammals. In D. J. Guberick & P. H. Klopfer (Eds.), *Parental care in mammals* (pp. 211–241). New York: Plenum.

Gard, C., Hard, E., Larsson, K., & Petersson, V.-A. (1967). The relationship between sensory stimulation and gross motor behavior during the postnatal development in the rat. *Animal Behaviour, 15,* 563–567.

Geiselman, P. J., Vanderweele, D. A., Dray, S. M., Ewing, A. T., & Cryder-Mooney, E. (1980). Ontogeny of chemospecific control of ingestive behavior in the rat. *Brain Research Bulletin, 5*(Suppl. 4), 37–42.

Gispen, W. H., & de Wied, D. (1980). ACTH as neuromodulator: Behavioral and neurochemical aspects. In L. Battistin, G. Hashim, & A. Lajtha (Eds.) *Neurochemistry and clinical neurology,* New York: Alan R. Liss, Inc., 251–263.

Gispen, W. H., & Isaacson, R. L. (1981). ACTH-induced grooming in the rat. *Pharmacology and Therapeutics, 12,* 209–246.

Goldman, P. S., & Galkin, T. W. (1978). Prenatal removal of frontal association cortex in the fetal rhesus monkey: Anatomical and functional consequences in postnatal life. *Brain Research, 152,* 451–485.

Gregory, E. H. & Pfaff, D. W. (1971). Development of olfactory-guided behavior in infant rats. *Physiology and Behavior, 6,* 573–576.

Hall, W. G. (1979). The ontogeny of feeding in rats: I. Ingestive and behavioral responses to oral infusions. *Journal of Comparative and Physiological Psychology, 93,* 977–1000.

Hall, W. G., Cramer, C. P., & Blass, E. M. (1977). Ontogeny of suckling in rats: Transitions toward adult ingestion. *Journal of Comparative and Physiological Psychology, 91,* 1141–1155.

Hall, W. G., & Rosenblatt, J. S. (1977). Suckling behavior and intake control in the developing rat pup. *Journal of Comparative and Physiological Psychology, 91,* 1232–1247.

Hannigan, J. H., Jr., Balaz, M. A., Springer, J. E., Ryan, J. P., & Isaacson, R. L. (1982). Hippocampal lesions: Are the secondary dopaminergic changes following the lesion responsible for the decrease in ACTH-induced excessive grooming? *Neuroscience Abstracts, 8,* 371.

Hannigan, J. H., Jr., Springer, J. E., & Isaacson, R. L. (1984). Differentiation of basal ganglia dopaminergic involvement in behavior after hippocampectomy. *Brain Research, 291,* 83–91.

Henderson, N. D. (1978). Genetic dominance for low activity in infant mice. *Journal of Comparative and Physiological Psychology, 92,* 118–125.

Hill, D. L., Almli, C. R., & Williams, D. M. (1978). Ventromedial hypothalamic destruction in neonatal rats: Effects upon growth and consummatory behaviors. *Neuroscience Abstracts, 4,* 175.

Hofer, M. A. (1975). Studies on how early maternal separation produces behavioral change in young rats. *Psychosomatic Medicine, 37,* 245–264.

Hofer, M. A., & Shair, H. (1980). Sensory processes in the control of isolation-induced ultrasonic vocalization by 2-week-old rats. *Journal of Comparative and Physiological Psychology, 94,* 271–279.

Hruska, R. E., & Pitman, K. T. (1982). Hypophysectomy reduces the haloperidol induced changes in dopamine receptor density. *European Journal of Pharmacology, 85,* 201–205.

Isaacson, R. L. (1975). The myth of recovery from early brain damage. In N. R. Ellis (Ed.) *Aberrant development in infancy* (pp. 1–26). Hillsdale, NJ: Erlbaum.

Isaacson, R. L. (1984). Hippocampal damage: Effects on dopaminergic systems of the basal ganglia. In R. J. Bradley & J. R. Smythies (Eds.), *International review of neurobiology* (Vol. 25). New York: Academic Press.

Isaacson, R. L., Fish, B. S., Lanier, L. P., & Dunn, A. J. (1977). Serotonin reduction early in life and its effects on behavior. *Life Sciences, 21,* 213–222.

Isaacson, R. L., & Hannigan, J. H., Jr. (1983). The hippocampus and age-related disorders. In W. H. Gispen & J. Traber (Eds.), *Aging of the brain,* pp. 139–148. Amsterdam: Elsevier.

Isaacson, R. L., Hannigan, J. H., Jr., Springer, J. E., Ryan, J., & Poplawsky, A. (1983). Limbic and neurohormonal influences modulate the basal ganglia and behavior. In E. Endröczi, D. de Wied, L. Angelucci, & U. Scapagnini (Eds.), *Integrative neurohumoral mechanisms* (pp. 23–34). Amsterdam: Elsevier.

Iuvone, P. M., & Van Hartesveldt, C. (1976). Locomotor activity and plasma corticosterone in rats with hippocampal lesions. *Behavioral Biology, 16,* 515–520.

Johanson, I. B. (1978). Development of olfactory and thermal responsiveness in hypothyroid and hyperthyroid rat pups. *Developmental Psychobiology, 13,* 343–351.

Johanson, I. B. (1979). Thermotaxis in neonatal rat pups. *Physiology and Behavior, 23,* 871–874.

Johanson, I. B., & Hall, W. G. (1980). The ontogeny of feeding in rats: III. Thermal determinants of early ingestive responding. *Journal of Comparative and Physiological Psychology, 94,* 977–992.

Johnson, D., & Almli, C. R. (1978). Age, brain damage, and performance. In S. Finger (Ed.), *Recovery from brain damage* (pp. 115–134.) New York: Plenum.

Johnson, L. L., & Moberg, G. P. (1980). Adrenocortical responses to novelty stress in rats with dentate gyrus lesions. *Neuroendocrinology, 30,* 187–192.

Kellogg, C., & Lundborg, P. (1972). Ontogenetic variations in responses to L-DOPA and monoamine receptor-stimulating agents. *Psychopharmacologia, 23,* 187–200.

Lanier, L. P., & Isaacson, R. L. (1977). Early developmental changes in the locomotor response to amphetamine and their relation to hippocampal function. *Brain Research, 126,* 567–575.

Lanier, L. P., Van Hartesveldt, C., Weis, B. J., & Isaacson, R. L. (1975). Effects of differential hippocampal damage upon rhythmic and stress-induced corticosterone secretion in the rat. *Neuroendocrinology, 18,* 154–160.

Leon, M., & Moltz, H. (1972). The development of the pheromonal bond in the albino rat. *Physiology and Behavior, 8,* 683–686.

Lieberman, M., & Lieberman, D. (1978). Lactose deficiency: A genetic mechanism which regulates the time of weaning. *American Naturalist, 112,* 625–627.

Lovely, R. H. (1975). Hormonal dissociation of limbic lesion effects on shuttle box avoidance in rats. *Journal of comparative and physiological Psychology, 89,* 224–230.

McEwen, B. S., Gerlach, J. L., & Micco, D. J. (1975). Putative glucortocoid receptors in hippocampus and other regions of rat brain. In R. L. Isaacson & K. H. Pribram (Eds.), *The hippocampus* (Vol. I, pp. 285–322). New York: Plenum.

McGowan-Sass, B. K., & Timiras, P. S. (1975). The hippocampus and hormonal cyclicity. In R. L. Isaacson & K. H. Pribram (Eds.), *The hippocampus* (Vol. I, pp. 355–374). New York: Plenum.

Meaney, M. H., & Stewart, J. (1981). A descriptive study of social development in rat (*Rattus norvegicus*). *Animal Behaviour, 29,* 34–45.

Misanin, J. R., Haigh, J., Hinderliter, C. F., & Nagy, Z. M. (1973). Analysis of response competition in discriminated and nondiscriminated escape training of neonatal rats. *Journal of comparative and physiological psychology, 85,* 570–580.

Moltz, H., & Lee, T. M. (1981). The maternal pheromone of the rat: Identity and functional significance. *Physiology and Behavior, 26,* 301–306.

Moorcroft, W. H. (1981). Heightened arousal in the 2-week-old rat: The importance of starvation. *Developmental Psychobiology, 14,* 187–199.

Murphy, M. R., MacLean, P. D., & Hamilton, S. C. (1981). Species-typical behavior of hamsters deprived from birth of the neocortex. *Science, 213,* 459–461.

Noirot, E. (1968). Ultrasounds in young rodents. II. Changes with age in albino rats. *Animal Behavior, 16,* 129–134.

Nomura, Y., Yotsumoto, I., & Segawa, T. (1981). Ontogenetic development of high potassium- and acetylcholine-induced release of dopamine from striatal slices of the rat. *Developmental Brain Research, 1,* 171–177.

Nonneman, A. J. (1970). *Anatomical and behavioral consequences of early brain damage in the rabbit.* Unpublished Ph.D. dissertation, University of Florida.

Nonneman, A. J., & Corwin, J. V. (1981). Differential effects of prefrontal cortex ablation in neonatal, juvenile, and young adult rats. *Journal of comparative and physiological Psychology, 95,* 588–602.

Okon, E. E. (1972). Factors affecting ultrasound production in infant rodents. *Journal of Zoology London, 168*, 139–148.

Oppenheim, R. W. (1980). Metamorphosis and adaptation in the behavior of developing organisms. *Developmental Psychobiology, 13*, 353–356.

Ostadolava, I., Ribr, B., Babicky, A., Parizek, J., & Kohar, J. (1971). Transfer of [85]Sr from lactating rats to sucklings as affected by the size of the litter. *Physiologica Bohemoslovia, 20*, 397.

Oswalt, G. L., & Meier, G. W. (1975). Olfactory, thermal, and tactual influences on infantile ultrasonic vocalization in rats. *Developmental Psychobiology, 8*, 129–135.

Panksepp, J. (1981). The ontogeny of play in rats. *Developmental Psychobiology, 14*, 327–332.

Pappas, B. A., Vickers, G., Buxton, M., & Pusztay, W. (1982). Infant rat hyperactivity elicited by home cage bedding is unaffected by neonatal telencephalic dopamine or norepinephrine depletion. *Pharmacology Biochemistry and Behavior, 16*, 151–154.

Pederson, P. E., Williams, C. L., & Blass, E. M. (1982). Activation and odor conditioning of suckling behavior in 3-day-old albino rats. *Journal of Experimental Psychology (Animal Behavior Processes), 8*, 329–341.

Randall, P. K., & Campbell, B. A. (1976). Ontogeny of behavioral arousal: Effect of maternal and sibling presence. *Journal of comparative and physiological Psychology, 90*, 453–459.

Reinstein, D. K., Hannigan, J. H., Jr., & Isaacson, R. L. (1982). Time course of certain behavioral changes after hippocampal damage and their alteration by dopaminergic intervention into nucleus accumbens. *Pharmacology Biochemistry and Behavior, 17*, 193–202.

Reinstein, D. K., & Isaacson, R. L. (1977). Clonidine sensitivity in the developing rat. *Brain Research, 135*, 378–382.

Reinstein, D. K., McClearn, D., & Isaacson, R. L. (1978). The development of responsiveness to dopaminergic agonists. *Brain Research, 150*, 216–223.

Ristine, L. A., & Spear, L. P., (1981, November). *Effects of serotonergic and cholinergic antagonists on suckling behavior of neonatal, infant, and weanling rat pups.* International Society for Developmental Psychobiology, New Orleans.

Ristine, L. A., & Spear, L. P. (1982, October). *Parity of the maternal female influences suckling of weanling age offspring.* International Society for Developmental Psychobiology, Minneapolis.

Rosenblatt, J. S., & Lehrman, D. S. (1963). Maternal behavior of the laboratory rat. In H. L. Rheingold (Ed.), *Maternal behavior in mammals* (pp. 8–57). Wiley: New York.

Ryan, J. P., & Isaacson, R. L. (1983a). Intra-accumbens injections of ACTH induce excessive grooming in rats. *Physiological Psychology, 11*, 54–58.

Ryan, J. P. & Isaacson, R. L. (1983b) Suppression of corticosterone synthesis alters the locomotor behavior of hippocampally lesioned rats. *Society for Neuroscience abstracts, 9*, 1980.

Sales, G. D., & Smith, J. C. (1978). Comparative studies of the ultrasonic calls of infant murid rodents. *Developmental Psychobiology, 11*, 595–619.

Shalaby, I. A., & Spear, L. P. (1980). Psychopharmacological effects of low and high doses of apomorphine during ontogeny. *European Journal of Pharmacology, 76*, 451–459.

Smotherman, W. P., Bell, R. W., Starzec, J., Elias, J. W., & Zachman, T. A. (1974).

Maternal responses to infant vocalizations and olfactory cues in rats and mice. *Behavioral Biology, 12,* 55–66.

Sobrian, S. K., Weltman, M., & Pappas, B. A. (1975). Neonatal locomotor and long-term behavioral effects of *d*-amphetamine in the rat. *Developmental Psychobiology, 8,* 241–250.

Sosis, B. S. & Spear, L. P. The effects of the home environment and shock on catecholamine levels in the young rat. In preparation.

Spear, L. P., & Brake, S. C. (1983). Periadolescence: Age-dependent behavior and psychopharmacological responsivity in rats. *Developmental Psychobiology, 16,* 83–109.

Spear, L. P., & Brick, J. (1979). Cocaine-induced behavior in the developing rat. *Behavioral and Neural Biology, 26,* 401–415.

Spear, L. P., & Ristine, L. A. (1981). Quipazine-induced behavior in neonatal rat pups. *Pharmacology Biochemistry and Behavior, 14,* 831–834.

Spear, L. P., & Ristine, L. A. (1982). Suckling behavior in neonatal rats: Psychopharmacological investigations. *Journal of comparative and physiological Psychology, 96,* 244–255.

Spear, L. P., Shalaby, I. A., & Brick, J. (1980). Chronic administration of haloperidol during development: Behavioral and psychopharmacological effects. *Psychopharmacology, 70,* 47–58.

Stehouwer, D. J., & Campbell, B. A. (1980). Ontogeny of passive avoidance: Role of task demands and development of species-typical behaviors. *Developmental Psychobiology, 13,* 385–398.

Stehouwer, D. J., Haroutunian, V., & Campbell, B. A. (1980). Generalization of habituation to electrical stimulation of the forelimb in neonatal and preweanling rats. *Behavioral and Neural Biology, 29,* 203–215.

Teicher, M. H., & Blass, E. M. (1976). Suckling in newborn rats: Eliminated by nipple lavage, reinstated by pup saliva. *Science, 193,* 422–425.

Thompson, G. E., & Moore, R. E. (1968). A study of newborn rats exposed to the cold. *Canadian Journal of Physiology and Pharmacology, 46,* 865–871.

Van Hartesveldt, C. (1975). The hippocampus and regulation of the hypothalamic–hypophyseal–adrenal cortical axis. In R. L. Isaacson & K. H. Pribram (Eds.), *The hippocampus* (Vol. I, pp. 375–392). New York: Plenum.

Wade, P. D., & Timiras, P. S. (1980). Whole brain and regional [^{125}I]-alpha-bungarotoxin binding in developing rat. *Brain Research, 181,* 381–389.

Whishaw, I. Q., Schallert, T., & Kolb, B. (1979). The thermal control of immobility in developing infant rats: Is the neocortex involved? *Physiology and Behavior, 23,* 757–762.

Wiegant, V. M., Cools, A. R., & Gispen, W. H. (1977). ACTH-induced excessive grooming involves brain dopamine. *European Journal of Pharmacology, 41,* 343–345.

Williams, C. L., Rosenblatt, J. S., & Hall, W. G. (1979). Inhibition of suckling in weanling-age rats: A possible serotonergic mechanism. *Journal of Comparative and Physiological Psychology, 93,* 414–429.

Woodside, B., & Leon, M. (1980). Thermoendocrine influences on maternal nesting behavior in rats. *Journal of Comparative and Physiological Psychology, 94,* 41–60.

6

Early Brain Damage and Time Course of Behavioral Dysfunction: Parallels with Neural Maturation

C. Robert Almli

Introduction

One of the more intriguing and perplexing issues in the brain damage literature (animal experimental and human clinical) is the relationship between the organism's developmental status at the time brain damage is sustained and the resultant behavioral and physiological abnormality: the relationship between age at the time of brain damage and age-differential in sparing or recovery of function following neural insult.

Many laboratory and clinical studies yield results that suggest that brain damage sustained early in life is associated with greater sparing or recovery of function than is comparable brain damage sustained at maturity (e.g., Almli, 1978; Johnson & Almli, 1978; see other chapters, these volumes). In spite of the fact that there often is some degree of recovery following brain damage sustained at any age, the infant advantage for sparing and recovery of function has been stressed (the so-called Kennard principle). In fact, some researchers (e.g., Hans-Lucas Teuber, see Schneider, 1979) have suggested that it may be better to have brain damage early in life than later.

Does all of the research literature attest to the infant advantage with respect to recovery from brain damage? The answer, of course, is no (see other chapters, these volumes). There are many examples of damage to cortical, subcortical, and cerebellar regions in which infants (animals and human) appear to be as severely affected as adults (see Almli, 1978; Finger & Stein, 1982; Johnson & Almli, 1978). In addition, diffuse neural damage or dysfunction, such as that associated with early exposure to malnutrition or toxic agents, appears to more severely affect the infant brain than the adult brain (e.g., Renis & Goldman, 1980).

Thus the inconsistent state of the research literature on the age–brain damage relationship is readily apparent, and the critical variables that may underlie age differences in sparing or recovery of function following neural insult have not been determined. Some variables that have received consideration in this regard are cortical versus subcortical distinctions, differential timing of functional neural commitment, differential diaschisis (Von Monokow), and species differences (e.g., Almli, 1978; Finger & Stein, 1982; Johnson & Almli, 1978). These factors, although interesting, may share a common fundamental element, that is, the developmental growth status of the neural system at the time of neural insult (e.g., Almli, 1978; Goldman, 1974; Johnson & Almli, 1978).

Much of the research on the age–brain damage relationship has been limited to comparing the behavioral outcome of neural damage sustained by an infant group versus an adult group; that is, an infant brain is an infant brain (see Johnson & Almli, 1978). This research orientation ignores the fact that infancy is not a homogeneous or static state with regard to neural growth and organization; the developmental growth status of the neural system under study has only received limited research attention (e.g., Goldman, 1974; Johnson & Almli, 1978).

The lack of serious consideration of the growth issue in age–brain damage research is probably related, at least in part, to our lack of knowledge of neural growth and organization of mammals during postnatal ontogeny. In spite of years of research, our knowledge of postnatal brain growth is quite elementary and is often limited to brain-weight increase, neuropil expansion in selected regions, regional myelination, or regional neurochemistry (e.g., Jacobson, 1978). Furthermore, much of our more "detailed" knowledge of "normal" neural growth phenomena has actually been derived from denervation (neural damage) studies (e.g, Cotman & Lynch, 1976; Jacobson, 1978; Lund, 1978) for which a parallel process with normal development has been assumed or implied.

In spite of our limited knowledge of brain development, it is clear that there are tremendous age differences in the rate and extent of neural growth and organization during the early life of mammals (e.g., Almli, 1978; Jacobson, 1978). Thus, the factors that promote and support normal growth and organization of the developing nervous system, whatever they may be, may continue to be relatively more active following neural damage sustained during early life. In support of this notion, research indicates that the developing brain retains much of its enhanced growth capacity, in comparison to the adult, after neural damage. For example, it has been shown that denervation in some brain regions during early development is associated with greater axonal sprouting and synaptogenesis than is found for denervation later in life (e.g., Cotman & Lynch, 1976; Tsukahara, 1981).

Thus, if damage to a neural system is sustained preceding an important developmental period of neural growth and organization (e.g., dendritic, axonal, synaptic), then the enhanced growth capacity of the remaining neural tissue of that region may manifest itself in (1) the establishment of some approximation of the normal neural circuitry of the region and (2) the establishment of new neural circuitry not seen in intact animals (i.e., ectopic or abnormal). In the former case, the closer the approximation of the neural circuitry to normal, the greater the degree of functional preservation or return. In the latter case, the new neural circuitry could yield some degree of unique—for example, abnormal—behavioral function. Because both forms of neural circuitry would become established to varying degrees following brain damage sustained prior to critical growth phases, early brain damage would be simultaneously associated with alterations in behavioral performance reflecting instances of recovery of function, lack of recovery of function, and unique (or abnormal) forms of behavioral function. Systematic and in-depth behavioral testing would be required to uncover these brain damage outcomes, as was shown by Almli (1978), Goldman (1974), Milner (1974), and Schneider and Jhaveri (1974).

Within this context, we have been using the following as a working hypothesis: Age differences in the effects of brain damage are related to the growth status of the neural system under study and the amount of the neural system actually destroyed. This working hypothesis does not assume that all growth subsequent to brain damage is good growth, that is, growth leading to neural reorganization that essentially duplicates the normal developmental pattern of organization. Rather, growth subsequent to brain damage may result in only some degree of approximation of normal organization, as well as in the establishment of new or abnormal circuits (anomalous growth), as was demonstrated by Schneider and Jhaveri (1974) for superior colliculus–perception relationships in the hamster. In this sense, an infant growth advantage subsequent to early brain damage would be expected to yield complex effects upon behavior such as a trade-off of a lack of function for an abnormal function (e.g., Schneider & Jhaveri, 1974) or, as in the case of early language-cortex damage, a relative sparing or recovery of linguistic function with a concomitant attenuation of other cognitive processing (e.g., Milner, 1974). Thus, although early brain damage may be associated with enhanced sparing or recovery of function on some tasks, the infant advantage may not generalize to other behavioral tasks. In this sense, early brain damage may very well preclude normal development and, thus, normal behavioral function.

Much of the age–brain damage research can be interpreted as being consistent with this working hypothesis (e.g., Almli, 1978; Finger, 1978; Finger & Stein, 1982). In addition, this hypothesis could at least partially account for differences in recovery of function following brain damage between neural systems that differ in the timing of their developmental growth phases (e.g., cerebellum versus brainstem), and that differ in their lifelong capacity for growth (e.g., pyramidal versus aminergic tracts). The entire brain and its subsystems do not grow in a homogeneous fashion (e.g., Jacobson, 1978), and it seems reasonable to expect differential effects of brain damage between different neural systems and between different age groups. In addition, the difference between infants and adults for the debilitating effects of diffuse neural insult, such as that resulting from early malnutrition, would be expected to occur because of the overall reduction in the capacity for neural growth as a direct consequence of malnutrition, thereby resulting in a decreased capacity for establishment of appropriate types and numbers of neural circuits.

Age–Brain-Damage Relationship: The Lateral Hypothalamus

Our early research on the age–brain damage relationship (e.g., Almli, 1978) has yielded results that indicate that (1) there are age differences for the behavioral effects of damage to a variety of neural regions, (2) developmental neural growth and organizational processes may underlie the differential effects of brain damage sustained at different ages, and (3) although early brain damage may be associated with sparing or recovery of function on some behavioral measures, it may also be associated with abnormality on other behavioral measures. Our research has concentrated on the lateral hypothalamic area; thus, research on this neural area is emphasized in the present chapter.

EFFECTS OF DAMAGE TO THE LATERAL HYPOTHALAMUS

The lateral hypothalamic–medial forebrain bundle area (LHA–MFB) was chosen for in-depth study because of the vast quantity of brain-damage research conducted with this neural area in adult mammals. In adult mammals (the majority of studies using rats), bilateral destruction of the LHA–MFB results in immediate effects on a wide range of behaviors—including ingestive, sensory, and motor behaviors. Furthermore, these brain-damage effects have been replicated on a variety of species in numerous laboratories around the world, thereby attesting to the consistency of outcome of LHA–MFB destruction. In fact, LHA–MFB damage with adult rats is often used as an exercise in student laboratory courses and laboratory manuals. Thus the LHA–MFB area may represent an ideal neural system in which to study the age–brain damage relationship: (1) The behavioral effects of damage are immediate and can be studied continuously and longitudinally, (2) the effects of damage are consistent and replicable, (3) damage to this area produces multifaceted behavioral dysfunction in ingestive, sensory, and motor behavior, and (4) in adults, eventual "recovery" from damage to this area unfolds in a relatively stereotyped fashion.

In the following sections of this chapter, the effects of LHA–MFB lesions (electrolytic) sustained by rats at different ages throughout development are documented and compared. Then the time course for age differences in the effects of damage to this region are compared with morphological, biochemical, and electrophysiological indices of the developmental status of the LHA–MFB at the age that damage was sustained.

DESTRUCTION OF THE LHA–MFB IN ADULT RATS

A summary of the behavioral effects of LHA–MFB destruction in rats of different ages is presented in Table 1. Immediately following bilateral destruction of the LHA–MFB, adult rats become adipsic (do

TABLE 1

Effects of LHA–MFB Damage as a Function of Age[a]

Abnormality/deficit	Age at brain damage (days)			
	Adult	14–25	6–10	1–5
No suckling from dam	—	Yes	Yes	**Subtle**[b]
Ingestive deficits				
Aphagia	Yes[Rc]	Yes[R]	Yes[R]	**No**
Adipsia	Yes[R]	Yes[R]	Yes[R]	**No**
Residual Ingestive	Yes	Yes	Yes	**No**
Body-weight reduction				
Males	Yes	Yes	Yes	Yes
Females	Yes[R]	Yes[R]	Yes[R]	**Yes**
Motor abnormality				
Posture	Yes[R]	Yes[R]	**Subtle**	**No**
Gait	Yes[R]	Yes[R]	**Subtle**	**No**
Sensory neglect				
Visual	Yes[R]	Yes[R]	**No**[1d]	**No**
Auditory	Yes[R]	Yes[R]	**No**[1]	**No**
Olfactory	Yes[R]	Yes[R]	**No**[1]	**No**
Tactile	Yes[R]	Yes[R]	**No**[1]	**No**
Open-field activity				
Hypoactivity	Yes	Yes	**No**[2e]	**No**[2]

[a]The results in this table are summarized from Almli, 1978; Almli, Fisher, and Hill, 1979, Almli and Golden, 1974, 1976a, 1976b; Almli, Henault, Velozo, McGinley, and Truitt, 1981; Almli and Hill, 1984; Almli, Hill, McMullen, and Fisher, 1979; Almli and Weiss, 1974; Cox and Kakolewski, 1970; Lytle and Campbell, 1975; McMullen and Almli, 1980; Marshall and Teitelbaum, 1974; Oltmans and Harvey, 1976; Teitelbaum and Epstein, 1962; and Velozo and Almli, 1979.

[b]**Boldface** indicates effects of brain damage different from adult.

[c]R = recovery of function with time.

[d]1 = hyperreactive to sensory stimulation.

[e]2 = hyperactive in open field.

not drink water) and aphagic (do not eat food), and they will die without some form of nutritional maintenance by the experimenter, for example, gavage or special diets (Almli & Weiss, 1974; Teitelbaum & Epstein, 1962). With experimenter maintenance, most of the brain-damaged rats will eventually recover voluntary feeding and drinking behaviors after a period of weeks or months.

In spite of the fact that most animals recover voluntary ingestive behaviors following LHA–MFB damage, they continue to display relatively permanent (residual) deficits in responding to a wide variety of specific feeding and drinking tests (e.g., Almli & Weiss, 1974;

Teitelbaum & Epstein, 1962). In addition, males, but not females, display permanent body-weight reduction of 20 to 25% below control values (e.g., Cox & Kakolewski, 1970).

Damage to the LHA–MFB in adult rats also results in an immediate and persistent effect on sensory and motor behaviors. These brain-damaged rats fail to respond to multimodal sensory stimulation (e.g., tactile, olfactory), and this transient period of sensory neglect appears to be most severe during the period of adipsia and aphagia (McMullen & Almli, 1980; Marshall & Teitelbaum, 1974). Furthermore, LHA–MFB-damaged adult rats display reduced locomotor activity in the open field (hypoactivity) as well as abnormality of posture and gait (e.g., McMullen & Almli, 1980). The animals that show recovery of ingestive behaviors also show recovery from sensory and motor dysfunction following LHA–MFB destruction.

Thus, adult rats sustaining bilateral destruction of the LHA–MFB display severe and persistent dysfunction for ingestive behaviors, sensory responsivity, posture and gait, and locomotor activity. Although these animals may eventually show some degree of recovery of function on most measures, they are by no means normal: they continue to display residual deficits in ingestive behaviors, attenuated responsivity to the environment, and relatively low locomotor activity levels.

DESTRUCTION OF THE LHA–MFB IN 14- TO 25-DAY-OLD RATS

Bilateral destruction of the LHA–MFB of rats at 14 to 25 days of age results in ingestive, sensory, and motor behavioral deficits that are nearly identical in topography, severity, and persistence to the behavioral deficits produced with LHA–MFB destruction in adults (Almli, 1978; Almli & Golden, 1974; Lytle & Campbell, 1975). As presented in Table 1, comparisons of the effects of LHA–MFB damage between adults and rats at 14 to 25 days of age reveal no indication of an advantage for the younger juvenile or infant rats.

DESTRUCTION OF THE LHA–MFB IN 6- TO 10-DAY-OLD RATS

As occurs with older animals, LHA–MFB damage sustained by preweaning rats at 6 to 10 days of age results in cessation of suckling from the dam (requiring experimenter maintenance to sustain life) and in adipsia and aphagia once these rats are beyond the age of normal weaning (21 days). The adipsia and aphagia of these rats may persist for many months, although most rats eventually recover voluntary feeding and drinking behaviors. However, rats of the 6- to 10-day group display permanent residual feeding and drinking deficits in response to specific ingestive tests, and body-weight deficits of 20 to 25% are permanent for males, whereas females again recover to control body-weight levels. (Almli, 1978; Almli, Fisher, & Hill, 1979; Almli & Golden, 1974, 1976a; Lytle & Campbell, 1975; Velozo & Almli, 1979).

With regard to ingestive behaviors, LHA–MFB destruction at 6 to 10 days of age results in ingestive dysfunction nearly identical to that found with older animals (14 days and older). In spite of the fact that these preweaning pups use a different ingestive mode (suckling) at the time of brain damage, sucking from the dam and independent feeding and drinking behaviors are abolished for a period of months following brain damage. There are no indications of an advantage of sparing or recovery of function for ingestive behaviors even when LHA–MFB damage is sustained as early as the end of the 1st week of life.

In contrast to the effects on ingestive behaviors, LHA–MFB damage in 6- to 10-day-old rats results in obvious age-differential effects for sensory and motor behaviors. Rats sustaining LHA–MFB damage at 10 days of age display subtle posture and gait abnormalities, and these mild abnormalities are less persistent than those found in older animals (14 days and over) sustaining brain damage. Furthermore, when LHA–MFB damage is sustained by progressively younger rats, from 10 days of age down to 6 days of age, postural and gait abnormalities are not detectable. Thus the age of 6 to 10 days appears to be a transition period for the production of posture and gait abnormality following LHA–MFB damage. This is the first incidence of the infant rat showing an advantage following LHA–MFB damage.

An even more striking age difference is found for sensory orientation and locomotor activity measures following LHA–MFB damage at 6 to 10 days of age. Rats sustaining damage at this age do not display sensory neglect in response to multimodal sensory stimulation; in fact, just the opposite is the case. Rats sustaining LHA–MFB damage at 6 to 10 days of age are hyperresponsive to stimulation, especially tactile stimulation, for which they display an exaggerated, "startle" type of reaction. Furthermore, these rats do not display low locomotor activity levels in the open field; rather, they display elevated locomotor activity (hyperactivity relative to age-matched controls) that persists through at least 35 days of age.

When LHA–MFB damage is sustained by rats at 6 to 10 days of age, the first indication of an age difference for the effects of brain damage is found. In spite of the fact that the ingestive behavior deficits (short-term and long-term) are nearly identical to those of older rats sustaining LHA–MFB damage, the 6- to 10-day-old group display only subtle postural and gait dysfunction, and they do not display the typical sensory neglect or low locomotor activity levels found for rats sustaining brain damage at 14 days of age and older. However, only for the posture and gait measures is there a clear indication of enhanced sparing or recovery of function for the 6- to 10-day-old group. The sensory orientation and locomotor activity measures, although showing a rather dramatic age at brain damage difference, actually reveal a trade-off of one abnormal behavior pattern for another: hyperresponsivity to sensory stimulation in lieu of sensory neglect, and hyperactivity in lieu of hypoactivity. Thus, for this age group there is evidence for enhanced sparing or recovery of function (i.e., postural and gait measures) and also clear evidence that one type of abnormal behavior pattern is replaced by another (i.e., sensory orientation and locomotor activity measures).

DESTRUCTION OF THE LHA–MFB
IN 1- TO 5-DAY-OLD RATS

When LHA–MFB damage is sustained by rats at 1 to 5 days of age, additional age differences are found (Almli, 1978; Almli, Henault, Velozo, McGinley, & Truitt, 1981; Almli, Hill, McMullen, & Fisher, 1979; Velozo & Almli, 1979). Damage to the LHA–MFB in these neonates does not result in a complete cessation of suckling from the dam, nor does it ever result in adipsia or aphagia later in life. The brain-damaged rats do not require any form of experimenter maintenance to maintain survival or growth. However, these rats display attenuated (but not eliminated) suckling from the dam for a few days postlesion, and they show attenuated body-weight gains for the first 5–10 days following brain damage. Thereafter, the brain-damaged rats' growth rates approximate control levels. However, both male and female rats fail to regain their initial body-weight losses and they display permanent body-weight reduction of 20 to 25%. When tested for specific feeding and drinking behaviors as adults, these brain-damaged rats are in the low-normal range for a majority of the nine ingestive tests.

In response to sensory and motor testing, rats sustaining LHA–MFB damage at 1 to 5 days of age are hyperactive in the open field (like 6- to 10-day-old rats); however, they do not display any detectable dysfunction for posture, gait, or sensory orientation. The subtle posture and gait abnormalities of the 6- to 10-day group are not discernible in the 1- to 5-day group, and the hyperresponsivity to sensory stimulation of the later lesioned group is not displayed by the early lesioned group.

Thus, rats sustaining LHA–MFB damage at 1 to 5 days of age show evidence of an enhanced sparing or recovery of function for ingestive, sensory, postural, and gait measures when compared to older animals sustaining similar damage. The major behavioral abnormality of these neonatal brain-damaged rats is the elevated level of locomotor activity, which is similar to the 6- to 10-day-old group but very different from the hypoactivity of the 14-day-old and older groups. Finally, as it does in the older age groups, LHA–MFB damage results in reduced body weights for males. However, the body weights of females are also reduced, and this result is not found for any of the older age groups sustaining LHA–MFB damage.

SUMMARY OF EFFECTS OF LHA–MFB DAMAGE BY TIME OF LESION

Research on the effects of LHA–MFB damage as a function of the age at which damage is sustained reveals an interesting developmental time course for the effects of brain damage that could only be determined from systematic and longitudinal analysis. In the adult, LHA–MFB damage results in severe and persistent adipsia, aphagia, body-weight reduction (males), residual feeding and drinking deficits, multimodal sensory neglect, abnormality of posture and gait, as well as reduced levels of locomotor activity in the open field.

As presented in Table 1, there are obvious differences in the behavioral effects of LHA–MFB damage when such damage is sustained by rats at different ages from birth through adulthood. It is apparent from the results reported here that there is also no simple relationship between age at brain damage and the resultant behavioral abnormality. Although there are representative examples of an infant advantage for sparing of function (e.g., posture and gait) and perhaps recovery of function (e.g., ingestive behaviors in which brain-damaged rats younger than 5 days of age do not require experimenter maintenance for survival), there are also measures for which infants and adults are equally affected (male's body-weight reduction), or for which neonates are more affected than adults (female's body-weight reduction only for neonatal damage).

The results for other measures do not fit neatly into these categories. For example, on the sensory orientation measure, rats older than 14 days of age at the time of damage display sensory neglect, rats at 6 to 10 days of age at the time of damage show hyperresponsivity to sensory stimulation, and rats sustaining damage at 1 to 5 days of age display essentially normal sensory orientation. In the case of a neonate (1–5 days of age) versus adult comparison, or a neonate versus older infant comparison, the neonate shows an advantage for sparing of function on the sensory orientation measure. However, a comparison of older infant (6–10 days of age) versus adult represents a comparison of sensory hyperreactivity to sensory neglect, respectively, two qualitatively distinct abnormalities with no obvious infant advantage.

Also a complex issue is the relationship between age at brain damage and locomotor activity levels. In rats older than 14 days of age, LHA–MFB damage results in reduced locomotor activity levels, whereas damage sustained at younger ages (10 days of age or earlier) results in hyperactivity. Thus, all age groups are abnormal on the locomotor activity measure following LHA–MFB damage, but there is a qualitative difference between the 1–10-day-old groups (hyperactivity) and the 14-day-old and older groups (hypoactivity).

Relationship between Development of the Lateral Hypothalamus, Brain Damage, and Behavioral Dysfunction

The LHA–MFB in adult animals is a complex neuropil consisting of neurons whose soma reside within the area, as well as numerous ascending and descending axonal projection systems (Millhouse, 1969). We have undertaken the study of the developmental growth of this region using anatomical (Golgi), electrophysiological, and neurochemical techniques. Both the anatomical and electrophysiological results reveal that 6 days of age and 14–25 days of age are important ages for changes in growth and organization of the LHA–MFB. As our studies show, the same two age periods appear to be critical ages for the production of ingestive and sensory behavioral abnormality (i.e., 6 days of age and older) and the full-blown behavioral symptomatology (i.e., 14 days of age through adulthood) following LHA–MFB damage.

The Golgi research (e.g., McMullen & Almli, 1979, 1981) has revealed that path neurons intrinsic to the LHA–MFB display little somatic or dendritic growth between the ages of birth and 5 days of age. From 5 and 6 days of age through approximately 14 to 21 days, both somatic and dendritic growth are rapid and extensive. At the end of this growth spurt, the LHA–MFB path neurons have essentially achieved their mature somatic volume and dendritic expansion. These morphological growth-rate changes are paralleled by changes in neuronal organizational processes as revealed by electrophysiological analysis.

Recordings from single neurons of the LHA–MFB made during ontogeny have revealed developmental changes in LHA–MFB neuronal responses (organization) to various forms of sensory stimulation. In the adult, individual neurons of the LHA–MFB respond to external sensory stimulation (e.g., olfactory, gustatory, tactile), internal sensory stimulation (e.g., changes in body fluid electrolyte or glucose concentration), or multimodal sensory stimulation, that is, both internal and external modes of sensory stimulation (e.g., Almli, McMullen, & Golden, 1976; Fisher & Almli, 1984). In contrast, LHA–MFB neuronal activity recorded in rats from birth through 5 days of age showed that almost all neurons respond to all forms of sensory stimulation (e.g., olfactory, gustatory, tactile, osmotic, glucose) applied to the animal; that is, the vast majority of neurons respond to multimodal sensory stimulation (external and internal). From 6 days of age through 14 to 25 days of age, there is a progressive decrease in the proportion of neurons responding to multimodal stimulation, with a simultaneous increase in the proportions of neurons responding only to external (e.g., olfactory sensitive) or only to internal (e.g., glucose sensitive) stimulation. Thus, by 14 to 25 days of age, LHA–MFB neurons have essentially matured with respect to their organizational responses to various forms of sensory stimulation.

These electrophysiological results indicate a developmental fine-tuning process of neural organization whereby the majority of the neonate's LHA–MFB neurons are modulated by multiple forms of sensory stimulation. As the animal ages, the neurons fine-tune in that they become selectively sensitive to a more unitary form of sensory stimulation. This developmental fine-tuning could be accomplished, for example, by the development of inhibitory inputs or synaptic elimination (e.g., Purves & Lichtman, 1980).

The time course for developmental changes in sensory-evoked potentials of LHA–MFB neurons precisely parallels the developmental morphological changes. The age period of attenuated neuronal growth is paralleled by the period of multimodal sensory responsivity of the neurons, and the age period of rapid growth of neurons is paralleled by rapid changes in the neuron's response mode (fine-tuning). The neurons are essentially mature by approximately 14 days of age, based on both the morphological and the electrophysiological growth criteria. Thus, important age periods determined for changes in neural growth and organization tend to precisely correspond to important age periods revealed for the differential effects of LHA–MFB damage (see Table 1).

Our preliminary neurochemical work has been concerned with the amine system (dopamine, norepinephrine, and serotonin) and alteration of regional brain amine levels in response to LHA–MFB damage sustained by rats at early ages. In adult rats, LHA–MFB damage results in depletion of telencephalic and striatal dopamine (~60–80%), norepinephrine (~30–50%), and serotonin (~30–40%) (e.g., Heller & Moore, 1965; Oltmans & Harvey, 1976). These amine depletions are associated with the severe and persistent behavioral deficits presented earlier (see "Adult," Table 1). Because of the very different behavioral effects of LHA–MFB damage seen in rats at 1 to 5 days of age, we thought it possible that LHA–MFB damage in neonatal rats might be associated with attenuated amine depletion levels.

The results of this study were clear. Damage to the LHA–MFB in neonatal rats was associated with amine depletions that were equivalent to those produced by LHA–MFB damage in adults, and the amine depletions appeared permanent (unchanged through 150 days of age). For 4-day-old rats sustaining LHA–MFB destruction, telencephalic and striatal dopamine was depleted by 60–83%, norepinephrine was depleted by 50%, and serotonin was depleted by 86% (Almli et al., 1981). In spite of the fact of equivalent amine depletion between brain-damaged neonates and adults, the neonates displayed no adipsia or aphagia, postural or gait abnormalities, or sensory neglect. However, the neonates did display reduced body weights and elevated locomotor activity levels. Thus the dopamine, norepinephrine, and serotonin depletion between neonates and adults was equivalent, but the postlesion behaviors were not. These results may indicate that preservation of some behavioral functions of neonates following LHA–MFB damage-induced amine depletion may be related to another developmental growth phenomenon: elaboration of postsynaptic receptors, often referred to as *denervation supersen-sitivity* in the adult-brain-damage literature (e.g., Ungerstedt, Ljungberg, Hoffer, & Siggins, 1975).

Conclusions

Research on the effects of LHA–MFB damage sustained by rats at different ages throughout development has revealed that there is no simple relationship between age at brain damage and behavioral outcome. This research has shown that early LHA–MFB damage may be associated with a relative infant advantage for sparing or recovery of function on some measures (e.g., posture and gait), whereas other measures may reveal no recovery of function, but rather a trade-off of one type of abnormality for another (e.g., locomotor activity). Fur-thermore, other measures (e.g., female's body weight) are more se-verely affected by neonatal damage than by adult damage. Finally, still other measures such as sensory orientation are differentially affected, depending on the age of the infant at the time of neural insult.

These varied results indicate that early brain damage may be asso-ciated with enhanced recovery of function on some measures, where-as other measures may reveal persistent abnormalities. Also, the finding that brain damage sustained at different infant ages may produce different behavioral outcomes (e.g., sensory orientation) sug-gests caution in treating the brain throughout infancy as a homoge-neous substrate. Thus, it appears that early brain damage may have a multidimensional effect upon the animal, and the resultant behav-ioral repertoire of the animal may be related to the patterns of neural circuits preserved and established subsequent to neural insult. The capacity to establish neural circuitry may very well be related to the growth status of the neural system at the time brain damage is sustained.

Although any relationship between neural growth capacity and the outcome of early brain damage is likely to be complicated, the pre-sent anatomical and electrophysiological measures show develop-ment timecourse changes in LHA–MFB neuronal characteristics that coincide with critical age-related differences in the effects of LHA–MFB destruction (see Table 1). From 1 to 5 days of age, LHA–MFB neurons display little if any somatic or dendritic growth, and the responsivity of these neurons is immature in that activity can be modulated by multiple forms of sensory stimulation. LHA–MFB damage sustained at such early ages is the least disruptive to the animal, compared with any other age group, at least with respect to survival without experimenter maintenance.

The earliest age at which LHA–MFB damage results in complete cessation of ingestive behavior and sensory abnormality (6 days of age) is the same age at which accelerated neuronal growth begins and the neuron's responsivity to sensory stimulation begins to organize by fine-tuning. Rapid neuronal growth and neuronal fine-tuning occur through the age of 14 days, at which time the neurons become basically mature. At this same age, the behavioral effects of LHA–MFB damage are now equivalent to those resulting from damage sustained by adults.

Although the relationship between development of LHA–MFB neuronal characteristics and age differences for the effects LHA–MFB damage presented here is admittedly simple, the results may suggest an important connection between the growth and organizational status of neurons associated with the damaged system and the behavioral outcome of brain damage. For LHA–MFB damage in the youngest age group (neonates), it is possible that the immature (small and multimodal) neurons bordering the damaged tissue may have continued their growth with subsequent establishment of some degree of approximation of normal neural circuitry and organization. This growth and organization would contribute to preservation of some degree of function following damage to the neural region. The animal's behaviors would hardly be normal, but an approximation of function would be preserved. This might explain why neonatal rats sustaining LHA–MFB damage are functional but not normal.

In an attempt to determine if the perilesion tissue is involved in the organization of function of neonatal rats sustaining LHA–MFB damage, we conducted the following study (Almli & Hill, 1984). At 1 day of age, rats sustained bilateral LHA–MFB damage, and then at 10 or 25 days of age they were subjected to a second operation during which the perilesion tissue of the first operation was destroyed. The results showed that damage of the perilesion tissue (but not other areas) at 10 or 25 days of age resulted in behavioral symptomatology equivalent to that which would have been seen had these rats undergone their initial bilateral LHA–MFB damage at 10 or 25 days of age (see Table 1). These results suggest that the perilesion tissue (local neurons and projection fibers) of the first operation (1 day of age) was involved in the organization (or reorganization) of function observed in neonatal rats following LHA–MFB damage. These results also sug-

114

gest that the neonate's capacity for neuronal growth and organization may be the basis of the postlesion approximation of function. Similar studies conducted with older rats yield results that indicate that the capacity for reorganization within the perilesion tissue is severely attenuated by the 10th day of life in rats (Almli & Golden, 1976b; Almli & Hill, 1984; McMullen & Almli, 1980). As shown earlier, the morphological and electrophysiological characteristics of LHA–MFB neurons are approaching mature levels by 10 days of age.

Thus the developmental growth and organizational status of the neural region under study may be of critical importance for age differences in response to brain damage, as well as for the differential degree of sparing or recovery of function seen following damage to different neural regions. Although much brain-damage research is targeted toward mechanisms such as axonal sprouting and denervation supersensitivity, it hardly seems likely that such mechanisms evolved to repair brain damage. These mechanisms are normal developmental growth processes, and the capacity for establishment of neural circuits following brain damage may very well be related to the developmental status of the neural system at the time brain damage is sustained. The generality of this notion will be determined by future research. However, it seems clear that if we are to gain a firm understanding of the relationship between age at brain damage and functional organization, it is important that we understand normal neural growth and organizational processes throughout development.

References

Almli, C. R. (1978). The ontogeny of feeding and drinking behaviors: Effects of early brain damage. *Neuroscience Biobehavioral Reviews, 2,* 281–300.

Almli, C. R., Fisher, R. S., & Hill, D. L. (1979). LHA destruction in infant rats produces consummatory deficits without sensory neglect or attenuated arousal. *Experimental Neurology, 66,* 146–157.

Almli, C. R., & Golden, G. T. (1974). Infant rats: Effects of lateral hypothalamic destruction. *Physiology and Behavior, 13,* 81–90.

Almli, C. R., & Golden, G. T. (1976a). Preweanling rats: Recovery from lateral hypothalamic damage. *Journal of Comparative and Physiological Psychology, 90,* 1063–1974.

Almli, C. R., & Golden, G. T. (1976b). Serial lateral hypothalamic destruction: Infancy and adulthood. *Experimental Neurology, 53,* 646–662.

Almli, C. R., Henault, M. A., Velozo, C. A., McGinley, P. A., & Truitt, E. B. (1981). Brain-damaged neonatal rats: Relationship between dopamine, norepinephrine, and serotonin and the development of open-field locomotor activity. *Neuroscience Abstracts, 7,* 891.

Almli, C. R., Hill, D. L., McMullen, N. T., & Fisher, R. S. (1979). Newborn rats: Lateral hypothalamic damage and consummatory-sensorimotor ontogeny. *Physiology and Behavior, 22,* 767–773.

Almli, C. R., & Hill, D. L. (1984). Unpublished manuscript.

Almli, C. R., McMullen, N. T., & Golden, G. T. (1976). Infant rats: Hypothalamic unit activity. *Brain Research Bulletin, 1,* 543–552.

Almli, C. R., & Weiss, C. S. (1974). Drinking behaviors: Effects of lateral preoptic and lateral hypothalamic destruction. *Physiology and Behavior, 13,* 527–538.

Cotman, C. W., & Lynch, G. S. (1976). Reactive synaptogenesis in the adult nervous system; the effect of partial deafferentation on new synapse formation. In S. Barondes (Ed.), *Neuronal recognition* (pp. 69–108). New York: Plenum.

Cox, V. C., & Kakolewski, J. W. (1970). Sex differences in body weight regulation in rats following lateral hypothalamic lesions. *Communications in Behavioral Biology, 5,* 195–197.

Finger, S. (Ed.) (1978). *Recovery from brain damage.* New York: Plenum.

Finger, S., & Stein, D. G. (1982). *Brain damage and recovery: Research and clinical perspectives.* New York: Academic Press.

Fisher, R. S., & Almli, C. R. (1984). Postnatal development of sensory influences on lateral hypothalamic neurons in the rat. *Developmental Brain Research, 12,* 55–75.

Goldman, P. S. (1974). An alternative to developmental plasticity: Heterology of CNS structures in infants and adults. In D. G. Stein, J. J. Rosen, & N. Butters (Eds.), *Plasticity and recovery of function in the central nervous system* (pp. 149–194). New York: Academic Press.

Heller, A., & Moore, R. Y. (1965). Effect of central nervous system lesions on brain monoamines in the rat. *Journal of Pharmacology and Experimental Therapeutics, 150,* 1–9.

Jacobson, M. (1978). *Developmental neurobiology.* New York: Plenum.

Johnson, D., & Almli, C. R. (1978). Age, brain damage, and performance. In S. Finger (Ed.), *Recovery from brain damage* (pp. 115–134). New York: Plenum.

Lund, R. D. (1978). *Development and plasticity of the brain.* New York: Oxford University Press.

Lytle, L. D., & Campbell, B. A. (1975). Effects of lateral hypothalamic lesions on consummatory behavior in developing rats. *Physiology and Behavior, 15,* 323–331.

McMullen, N. T., & Almli, C. R. (1979). Neuronal development in the medial forebrain bundle: A Golgi study of preoptic and hypothalamic neurons in the rat. *Federation Proceedings, 38,* 1397.

McMullen, N. T., & Almli, C. R. (1980). Serial lateral hypothalamic destruction with various interlesion intervals. *Experimental Neurology, 67,* 459–471.

McMullen, N. T., & Almli, C. R. (1981). Cell types within the medial forebrain bundle: A Golgi study of preoptic and hypothalamic neurons in the rat. *American Journal of Anatomy, 161,* 323–340.

Marshall, J. F., & Teitelbaum, P. (1974). Further analysis of sensory inattention following lateral hypothalamic damage in rats. *Journal of Comparative and Physiological Psychology, 86,* 375–395.

Millhouse, O. E. (1969). A Golgi study of the descending medial forebrain bundle. *Brain Research, 15,* 341–363.

Milner, B. (1974). Sparing of language functions after early unilateral brain damage. In E. Eidelberg & D. G. Stein (Eds.), Functional recovery after lesions of the nervous system. *Neuroscience Research Program Bulletin, 12,* 213–216.

Oltmans, G. A., & Harvey, J. A. (1976). Lateral hypothalamic syndrome in rats: A comparison of the behavioral and neurochemical effects of lesions placed in the lateral hypothalamus and nigrostriatal bundle. *Journal of Comparative and Physiological Psychology, 90,* 1051–1063.

Purves, D., & Lichtman, J. W. (1980). Elimination of synapsis in the developing nervous system. *Science, 210,* 153–157.

Renis, S., & Goldman, J. M. (1980). *The development of the brain.* Springfield, IL: Thomas.

Schneider, G. E. (1979). Is it really better to have your brain lesion early? A revision of the "Kennard principle." *Neuropsychologia, 17,* 557–583.

Schneider, G. E., & Jhaveri, J. R. (1974). Neuroanatomical correlates of spared or altered function after brain lesions in the newborn hamster. In D. G. Stein, J. J. Rosen, & N. Butters (Eds.), *Plasticity and recovery of function in the central nervous system* (pp. 65–109). New York: Academic Press.

Teitelbaum, P., & Epstein, A. N. (1962). The lateral hypothalamic syndrome: Recovery of feeding and drinking after lateral hypothalamic lesions. *Psychological Review, 69,* 74–90.

Tsukahara, N. (1981). Synaptic plasticity in the mammalian central nervous system. *Annual Review of Neuroscience, 4,* 351–379.

Ungerstedt, U., Ljungberg, T., Hoffer, B., & Siggins, G. (1975). Dopaminergic supersensitivity in the striatum. In D. B. Calne, T. N. Chase, & A. Barbeau (Eds.), *Advances in neurology* (Vol. 9, pp. 57–65). New York: Raven.

Velozo, C. A., & Almli, C. R. (1979). *Ontogenetic time-course of LH damage and consummatory-suckling deficits.* Paper presented at Eastern Psychological Association, Philadelphia.

7

Behavioral and Anatomical Studies of Rats with Complete or Partial Decortication in Infancy*

*Ian Q. Whishaw
and Bryan Kolb*

Introduction

Influenced by Kennard's (1936, 1938, 1940) studies, today's zeitgeist in neuropsychology is that early neocortical damage permits substantial sparing of function. Yet an examination of some research with both animal (Lawrence & Hopkins, 1976; Schneider, 1979) and human (Milner, 1975; Woods & Teuber, 1973) subjects suggests that early injury results in more severe effects than would be expected were this proposition absolute. We have been examining the behavior of rats subjected to early neocortical damage and have found some counterintuitive and paradoxical relationships between behavioral and anatomical changes that further limit the generality of the Kennard principle.

Our behavioral method involves giving every animal a comprehensive physical and behavioral examination, followed by various detailed tests. It derives from work with humans in which a test battery that assesses the function of specific regions of the cortex is given to

*This research was supported by grants from the Natural Sciences and Engineering Research Council of Canada. The authors thank Richard Dyck for assistance with the figures and Adria Allen for typing the manuscript.

117

each patient (Kolb & Whishaw, 1980) after a standard neurological examination has been administered (Denny-Brown, Dawson, & Tyler, 1982). Elsewhere we have justified (Kolb & Whishaw, 1983a) and described (Whishaw, Kolb, & Sutherland, 1983) the procedure for the rat. The approach is also based on the idea that the appropriate behaviors for study are those the rat displays spontaneously in its home environment or in simple models of that environment. Our experimental technique also involves the use of an ablation technique with damage inflicted on cortical sites similar to those indicated in Figure 1.

Sparing of Learned but Not Species-Typical Behavior

There can be little doubt that sparing of function follows partial decortication (e.g. Basser, 1962; Benjamin & Thompson, 1959; Goldman & Galkin, 1978; Kolb & Nonneman, 1978). In our studies of rats with neonatal frontal cortex ablations we were struck by their nearly normal performance on learning tasks (Kolb & Nonneman, 1976, 1978). For example, adult medial frontal-ablated rats were unable to wait more than 1 sec in a delayed-response task, but rats with often larger, neonatal excisions were as good as normal animals, delaying as long as 10 sec. Sparing was also related to age of surgery: 1–5-day ablations allowed complete sparing, 10–25-day ablations allowed less sparing, 25- and 60-day ablations allowed sparing on only some tasks, and later ablations allowed no sparing. Finally, there seemed to be an anatomical basis for sparing; degeneration in the dorsomedial nucleus of the thalamus was extensive in the adult- but not the infant-ablated animals (Kolb & Nonneman, 1978). But sparing was not uniform across all behaviors. When rats with identical infant ablations were given the entire behavioral test battery, many behaviors including maternal behavior, next building, swimming, food hoarding, and nail cutting were not spared at all (Kolb & Holmes, 1983; Kolb & Whishaw, 1981b, 1983a; Whishaw & Kolb, 1983a, 1983b; Whishaw, Kolb, Sutherland, & Becker, 1983). The most obvious difference between the behaviors that were spared and those that were not is that the former primarily involve learning, whereas the latter are innate and are largely species specific. Thus, as a work-

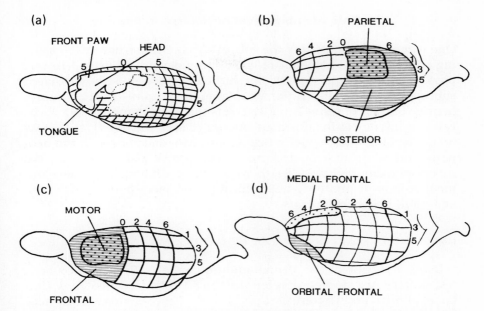

Figure 1. Representations of the brain areas damaged by different cortical ablations. (a) reconstruction of the motor (solid lines) and sensory (dotted lines) cortical areas in the rats. (b) extent of small (parietal) and large (posterior) ablations behind the bregmoidal landmark (0 point). (c) extent of motor-cortex and complete frontal ablations anterior to the bregmoidal landmark. (d) extent of medial and orbital frontal ablations in the prefrontal cortex.

ing hypothesis we have suggested that cognitive behaviors are different and more resilient to the effects of early brain injury than species-specific behaviors. The cognitive behaviors may have been spared either because they are subsumed by subcortical structures or because they are subsumed by residual neocortex. We felt that the first possibility required careful investigation, first because decorticated rats were reported to be as good as normal rats on many cognitive tasks (Oakley, 1979), and second because, counterintuitively, sparing in the infant-ablated rats occurred despite a 16% reduction in the expected size of the remaining neocortex. The second possibility also required investigation because forebrain neonatal noradrenaline depletion (see Kasamatsu, Pettigrew, & Ary, 1979; 1981; Walsh, 1981) blocked the sparing of function produced by neonatal ablations (Sutherland, Kolb, Whishaw, & Becker, 1982).

The Role of Subcortical Structures in Sparing

One way in which to study the role of subcortical structures in sparing is to study the behavior of rats totally devoid of cortex.[1] In this
preparation, any sparing that might be observed must be mediated
subcortically. With this rationale in mind we administered a comprehensive battery of tests (Table 1) to rats that were completely decorticated in infancy or in adulthood. As can be seen in Table 1, there was
no convincing evidence of a behavioral difference between the neo-
nate- and adult-decorticated groups (Kolb & Whishaw, 1981a). We
therefore examined whether there might be differences in development or in more qualitative aspects of performance between neonate-
and adult-decorticated rats.

EMERGING DEFICITS IN COMPLEX BEHAVIORS

Using a version of the Altman and Sudarshan (1975) development
test battery, we studied development in 13 rats decorticated within
hours of birth and 10 control rats (Table 2). There were no differences
for age of ear and eye opening or for the start of vibrissae movements
(about 14–15 days of age). The rate of development of postural support, locomotion, and dynamic postural adjustments were indistinguishable. The decorticated rats, however, were severely impaired
in placing reactions and in performances of complex locomotor behaviors. They showed no visual or tactile placing reactions, and when
suspended by the tail, they clasped their limbs together or clasped
their body, rather than extending their limbs to contact distant stimuli. The actual clasping of limbs did not begin until about Day 16,
and from then until about Day 30 it was common in decorticated and
normal rats. After Day 30 only decorticated rats showed this behavior. There was, however, evidence that limb posture was abnormal as
early as Day 1. When suspended by the tail, the decorticated rats held
their limbs about 1 cm closer together than did the control rats, and
this distance decreased until clasping began. The development of
complex locomotor behavior in our control rats was identical to that

[1]People seem to believe that the brainstem can assume functions of the forebrain. In a
widely publicized editorial, Lewin (1980, p. 1232) phrased the question, presumably
tongue in cheek, by asking, "Is your brain really necessary?" His question was formed
after a neurologist observed that some people with hydrocephalus accompanied by an
extremely thin neocortex suffered no obvious psychological or intellectual impairments. An explanation was that because the condition originated early, subcortical
structures had saved functions normally controlled by the neocortex.

TABLE 1

Chronic Behaviors of Neonatal and Adult Decorticates[a]

Behavior	Neonate decorticate	Adult decorticate
Feeding		
Aphagia	ok	ok[b]
Paw and digit use	X	X
Tongue use	X	X
Chronic body weight	X	X
General activity		
Running wheel	X	X
24-hour video recording	ok	ok
Light/dark tilt box	ok	ok
Grooming		
Sequence	X	X
Distribution on body	X	X
Posture	X	X
Toenail cutting[c]	X	X
Swimming	X	X
Hoarding	X	X
Male sexual behavior	X	X
Learning		
Shock avoidance (passive)	ok	ok
Shock-prod burying	X	X
Spatial reversal	X	X
Morris water task	X	X

[a]Kolb and Whishaw, 1981a.
[b]An "X" denotes behavior significatly different from controls. An "ok" indicates behavior not significantly different from controls.
[c]Whishaw, Kolb, Sutherland, and Becker, 1983.

described by Altman and Sudarshan (1975), but development was so poor in decorticated rats that it could be considered absent. The behaviors we found to be impaired in developing decorticated rats are also impaired in rats ablated in adulthood (Hicks & D'Amato, 1975; Kolb & Whishaw, 1981a, 1983a; Vanderwolf, Kolb, & Cooley, 1978; Whishaw, Schallert, & Kolb, 1981).

ENVIRONMENTAL CONSTRAINTS ON MOTOR
ABNORMALITIES

Although in these studies decorticated rats showed characteristic abnormalities, occasionally their behavior was surprisingly normal. This suggested that factors other than just the lesions (e.g., the condi-

TABLE 2

Performance of Developing Neonate-Decorticated Rats[a]

Behavior	Neonatal performance[b]	Adult performance
Sensory		
Ears open	ok	ok
Eyes open	ok	ok
Vibrissae move	ok	ok
Support		
Elevation of head	ok	ok
Elevation of forelimbs	ok	ok
Elevation of hindlimbs	ok	ok
Locomotion		
Pivoting	ok	ok
Crawling	ok	ok
Walking	ok	ok
Postural adjustment		
Righting on a surface	ok	ok
Righting in midair	ok	ok
Geotatic reactions	ok	ok
Cliff avoidance	ok	ok
Placing reactions		
Forelimb placing	X	X
Forelimb clasping when suspended	X	X
Hindlimb clasping when suspended	X	X
Complex locomotion		
Beam walking	X	X
Ascending a wire mesh	X	X
Descending a wire mesh	X	X
Ascending a rope	X	X
Descending a rope	X	X

[a]Locomotor test battery from Altman and Sudarshan, 1975.
[b]An "X" denotes an impairment of a behavior that develops normally in controls. An "ok" indicates normal development.

tions in which the observations were made) were important for understanding their dysfunctions and hence other aspects of the cortex's contribution to the control of movement. In further studies in adult-decorticated rats, we found normal-length grooming sequences during spontaneous home-cage grooming, but when grooming was elicited by wetting the fur, grooming sequence length was abbreviated. In cold (18 °C) water, the rats swam well and with exaggerated vigor and frequently inhibited forelimb movements in the normal way, but in warm (37 °C) water, they swam poorly and paddled with all four limbs. To eat small pieces of food, they sat up and used their forepaws as do normal rats, but they frequently dropped the food. They did not use their forepaws to eat large pieces of food. Thus, it seemed that in a narrow range of stimulus conditions, decorticated rats could make movements resembling those of normal rats. We have argued, therefore, that to describe their deficit it is necessary to construct a behavioral profile of their abilities by using many different stimulus conditions (Whishaw, Nonneman, & Kolb, 1981).

If neonatal decortication does not permit sparing, it still might extend the range of stimulus conditions in which more normal-like behavior appears. To investigate this, we constructed behavioral profiles of eating and swimming in 6 rats decorticated on the day of birth, 6 littermate control rats, and 6 rats decorticated at 60 days of age. When adult, the rats were deprived of food for 24 hours and tested in their home cage. In one test they were given two 4–5-g Purina chow pellets, and in the second they were given 20 Purina pellet fragments weighing a mean of 0.3 g each. The impairments of the infant- and adult-decorticated rats were indistinguishable. Typically the control rats sat on their haunches and held the food in their forepaws. Usually they ate an entire pellet at a sitting, frequently manipulating it with their paws and biting pieces from it. Decorticated rats ate the large food pellets in a different way. They pushed the food with their mouth, held it down with one paw, or pushed it under their body. Rats in neither group held the pellet with both paws for more than about 10% of the feeding time. When given small food pellets, rats in both groups picked up the food with their forepaws for more than 90% of the feeding time. Nevertheless, whenever they attempted to manipulate the food, it fell from their paws. We repeated these experiments with food pellets of a number of different sizes, but always to the same effect. Thus, in this test the range of stimulus conditions in which more normal-like behavior appeared was not different for the two groups.

A study of swimming led to the same conclusion. Rats swim with a characteristic motor pattern: Their back is nearly horizontal in the water, their forepaws are tucked up beneath the chin, and they propel themselves with vigorous thrusts of the back limbs. During ontogeny, swimming is well developed by 10 days of age, but forepaw immobility develops gradually up to 25 days of age (Schapiro, Salas, & Vukovich, 1970). Motor cortex ablation or decortication spares swimming but abolishes forepaw inhibition (Vanderwolf et al., 1978). Thus, it was our expectation that forelimb inhibition might fail to develop in the decorticated rats. This was the case when the rats were tested in a narrow alley. When they were tested in a large circular pool (145-cm diameter), immobility began to develop at about 12 days of age and was almost perfect by 25 days (Figure 2). In this situation, it was also perfect in adult-decorticated rats. The only deficit we were able to detect occurred when the animals turned; they paddled with the forepaw contralateral to the direction of the turn (Figure 2). Normal rats made small rotary or skulling movements of the paws to aid their turns. Changing water temperature did not change performance in the two groups of decorticated rats. In fact, animals in both groups swam well provided that they were not near the edge. This experiment showed that the swimming deficit of decorticated rats was not as simple as was originally thought. Deficits only appeared in situations in which the rats were insufficiently motivated to swim (warm water), were distracted from directed swimming by proximal walls (straight alley), or were performing more complex navigational maneuvers (turning). Together these different manipulations showed that the recalcitrant deficit of neonatal- and adult-decorticated rats was the loss of inhibition in one limb when turning, which was perhaps due to the loss of the ability to make small rotary movements of the distal portions of the limbs. Thus the

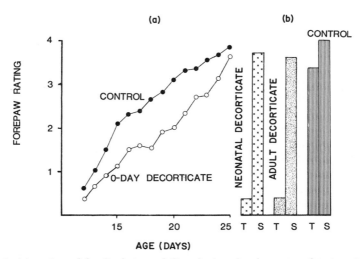

Figure 2. (a) rating of forelimb immobility during development of swimming in control and decorticated rats. (b) rating of forelimb immobility in the limb contralateral to a turn (T) and in the same limb when swimming in a straight line (S). Rating: 1 = one limb immobile for one stroke cycle; 2 = both limbs immobile for one stroke cycle; 3 = both limbs usually immobile; 4 = both limbs always immobile.

profile analysis permitted an accurate description of the deficit embedded in the complex behaviors (eating, swimming) that we examined, and it also pointed to the fact that the most persistent deficits
were in the use of the paws and limbs, a finding that is consistent
with other research (Lawrence & Hopkins, 1976; Lawrence & Kuypers, 1968a, 1968b).

CUE SPECIFICATION CAN DISTINGUISH CORTICAL FROM SUBCORTICAL LEARNING

   Complex tasks provide many cues, and hence the opportunity for
many strategies for their solution. Not to fall into what Goltz (1892,
pp. 603–604) described as the trap of the serial ablation technique of
finding "centers fleeing before the cutting knife with astounding
speed and crowding together in the remaining tissue as uncomfort-
ably as fish in a pond that is drying out," it is necessary to specify the
cues used by an animal to solve a problem. Cue specification has been
importantly involved in distinguishing cortical from subcortical visual functions (Bauer & Cooper, 1967; Goodale, 1983) and can contribute to the understanding of the functions of different neuroaxis
levels (Satinoff, 1978). Cue specification can also be used to see
whether neonatal decortication permits an animal to use cues that an
adult-decorticated rat cannot use. We studied cue use in learning
tasks, since decorticated rats are relatively proficient at learning
(Oakley, 1979). Performance of neonatal and adult decorticates was
compared in two spatial tasks: spatial reversals in the Grice box (see
Kolb & Whishaw, 1981a, 1981b; Kolb, Sutherland & Whishaw,
1983c), and the Morris water task (Morris, 1981).
   In the Grice box, the animals were required to run correctly for 10
consecutive trials to one side of the box, and then to make a number
of reversals. Both groups of decorticated rats were impaired but able
to acquire the initial response and make reversals (Figure 3[b]). In
the Morris water task, the animals were required to find a platform
hidden just beneath the surface in a large pool of water made opaque
with powdered milk. Because the platform could not be seen, there
were no local cues, and because the animals' starting position was
varied from trial to trial, they were unable to use positional cues.
Neither the infant, nor adult-decorticated rats showed any ability to
learn to find the platform (Figure 3[a]). We believe that in the Grice
box the decorticated rats use olfactory or body-position cues to solve

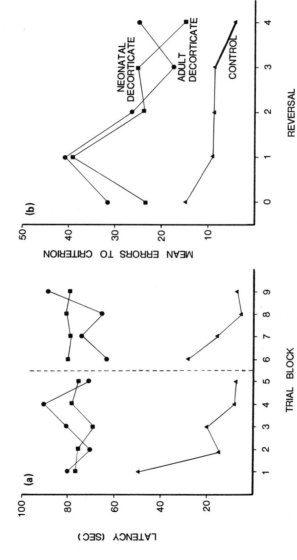

Figure 3. Performance of neonate- (■) and adult- (●) decorticated and control (▼) rats in two learning tasks. (a) Decorticated rats are unable to learn the water task, which requires that they use distal cues. (b) They are able to learn reversals in the Grice box, which allows the task to be solved using proximal cues. Dotted line in (a) is point at which target was moved. Trial block = four trials. Reversal criteria = 9/10 correct in a daily session.

the task; nevertheless, the early lesion does not seem to confer an advantage. In the Morris task, the animals must use distal visual cues and some type of cognitive mapping strategy; nevertheless, the early lesion does not save the ability to use such cues. We conclude that neonatal decortication does not enhance learning ability on tasks that provide cues that a decorticated animal can use, nor does it save the ability to use cues that are characteristically used by the neocortex.

SUBCORTICAL SPARING

To this point our studies have demonstrated that subcortical structures do not save functions of the neocortex. But we must still ask whether decorticated rats are better at things that they can do if decortication takes place in infancy. In some tasks they seem better, even though their deficits are similar qualitatively. For example, the lordosis posture is exaggerated and prolonged in adult-decorticated female rats, but not in neonate-decorticated female rats (Carter, Witt, Kolb, & Whishaw, 1982). This normalcy may be due to more efficient subcortical functioning, a phenomenon we call subcortical sparing. Subcortical sparing is striking in two other behaviors: tongue protrusion and sensory–motor orienting. Adult-decorticated rats show impaired tongue protrusion and dexterity (Castro, 1972, 1975; Kolb & Whishaw, 1983b; Whishaw & Kolb, 1983a). However, we have found that, as adults, rats decorticated within hours of birth show enhanced tongue protrusion but not enhanced accuracy or manipulation, when compared to adult-decorticated rats (Whishaw & Kolb, Figure 4). Similarly, in a test of sensory-motor behavior that requires that they remove small pieces of adhesive paper placed on the radial (inward and relatively hairless) aspect of the forelimb (Schaller, Upchurch, Lobaugh, Farrar, Spirduso, Gilliam, Vaughn, & Wilcox, 1982), the neonate-decorticated rats were impaired with respect to control rats but performed significantly better than adult-decorticated rats (Figure 5). In fact, in the tests of threshold, the neonate-decorticated rats removed stimulus objects of all sizes, whereas the adult-decorticated rats failed to remove the three smallest stimuli altogether.

A final consideration, with respect to the possibilities of subcortical sparing, is that of anatomical change. If subcortical structures can save the functions of an ablated neocortex, it might be expected that

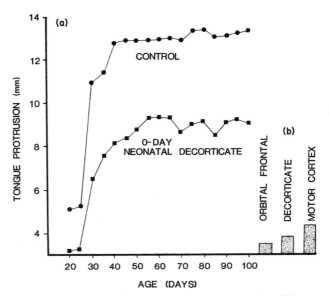

Figure 4. (a) tongue protrusion distance in maturing control and decorticated rats. (b) protrusion in adult-ablated rats. The test required the rat to protrude its tongue through the cage mesh to lick mash from a ruler.

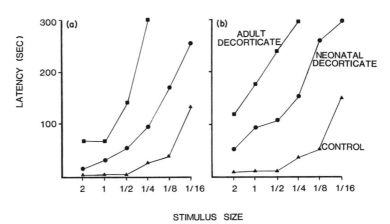

Figure 5. Mean latency of contol and decorticated rats to contact (a) and remove (b) different size stimuli from the radial portion of the forelimb. 1 = 1.3-cm diameter circular piece of adhesive tape.

the brainstem would show some increase in size. Such change can be detected by measurement of gross dimensions (Diamond, Kretch, & Rosenzweig, 1964) and weighing. We compared the brains of infant- and adult-decorticated rats and found that neonatal decortications actually produce smaller and lighter brains (Figure 6). Microscopic examination did show changes in the topography of subcortical nuclei, so that many areas were difficult to identify, but there was no clearly visible enhancement of growth, and in fact subcortical nuclei frequently appeared to be shrunken (Kolb, Sutherland, & Whishaw, 1983a).

We derive several conclusions from this series of studies.

1. Rats are able to develop into adulthood without a neocortex, and when adult, they survive in the simple environment of the animal colony.
2. Behavioral impairments observed during development of neonate-decorticated rats are also observed following adult decortication.
3. Subcortical structures do not save functions of the neocortex,

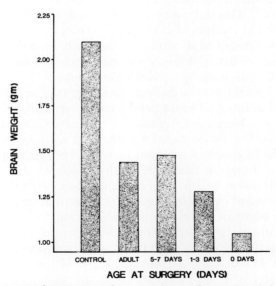

Figure 6. Brain weights in control rats and rats that received decortications at different ages. All measures were taken at least 1 year postsurgery.

    even if decortication is performed as early as a few hours after birth.

4. Sparing of function following subtotal decortication must require neocortical circuitry, either alone or in combination with subcortical structures.

5. There is a harmony between the behavioral and anatomical results: Subcortical structures do not save functions of the neocortex and there is no neurogenesis to provide the cells to support new responsibilities.

6. The absence of compensation after neocortex loss, even in infancy, implies that the neocortex has unique functions.

The Role of Cortical Structures in Sparing

The studies of completely decorticated rats demonstrate that sparing following subtotal neocortical ablations must be mediated by residual neocortex. But it has also become clear that sparing is not inevitable, and that costs may accompany benefits. Obviously, if residual neocortex is assuming new functions, it must combine them with the functions it normally controls or else give up some control of those functions. The only way to determine whether the neocortex gives up efficient control of certain behaviors in order to accommodate other behaviors is to study the animals on a large number of tests on which relative efficiency of performance can be compared. Using exactly this paradigm, Kolb and Holmes (1983) studied rats that received motor cortex damage in adulthood or at 4 days of age. The neonatal ablations in fact produced abnormalities not seen after adult ablations. Because the residual neocortex was comparatively reduced in size by the neonatal ablations, it seemed possible to conclude that the function of residual neocortex was disrupted. Perhaps the sparing of function that follows the neonatal ablations resulted from reorganization within the remaining neocortex that in turn displaced or crowded out behavioral functions that are ordinarily undisturbed by equivalent ablations in adulthood. In humans, the functions of an intact hemisphere have been found to be crowded by invading functions from a neonatally damaged hemisphere (Dennis & Whitaker, 1976; Kohn & Dennis, 1974; Milner, 1974; Woods & Teuber, 1973).

CORTICAL CROWDING

Perhaps one of the most curious phenomena encountered in the human neuropsychological literature is the disability in learning displayed by many schoolage children. If the hypothesis that they suffer from some type of early brain damage is admitted (see Kolb & Whishaw, 1980), the enduring impairments they display in acquiring such skills as reading are difficult to understand in the context of sparing. The fact that they display many other abnormalities, including short-term memory deficits, impaired coding, and increased incidence of lef-handedness (Whishaw & Kolb, 1984), is also difficult to understand. Why is it that they do not display sparing of function? Why is it that they display so many different kinds of impairment? An explanation that has been suggested in the literature a number of times is that they have undergone early brain injury that has resulted in crowding of other functions (Hebb, 1942; Rudel & Teuber, 1971; Schneider, 1979).

It is generally accepted that if sparing is to occur, it will be greater with early ablations. The possibility that crowding occurs must, however, lead to a reconsideration of this proposition: Earlier may in fact be worse. Experimental support for this conclusion comes from the work of Schneider (1970), who reported deleterious effects of aberrant connections in hamsters receiving neonatal superior colliculus ablations. The effect also has generality beyond the superior colliculus of the hamster (Schneider & Jhaveri, 1974). Gramsbergen (1982) has found greater impairments in cerebellar hemispherectomized rats that received surgery at 5 and 10 days of age than in rats that received surgery at 30 days of age. We have found greater impairments with infant posterior cortex damage than occurs with adult damage (Kolb & Holmes, 1983; Kolb, Whishaw, & Holmes, 1983). Furthermore, the principle that earlier is worse seems to apply to humans. Woods (1980) reports that children with lateralized lesions show greater impairments on the Wechsler intelligence scale if their damage occurs before, as compared with after, the 1st year of life.

In other experiments we have attempted to develop an animal model of early infant damage that might be useful in studying and understanding the phenomena that appear to occur after early brain damage in humans. These experiments have been undertaken with animals that received posterior cortex damage. The studies suggest

that posterior cortex damage has far-reaching consequences for behavior that are not seen to such a degree after prefrontal cortex ablations. First, there appear to be certain ages at which damage to the
posterior cortex results in a series of changes that are so severe that
the animals do not survive. Figure 7 shows the probability of surviving decortication performed at different ages (Kolb & Whishaw,
1981a). Survival in the first 4 days of life was a virtual certainty,
whereas survival from 8 days through the juvenile period was unlikely. The young rats recovered from hypothermic anesthesia quickly and within 24 hours, milk was visible in their stomach, indicating
successful reattachment to the nipple. Older rats began to recover
from anesthesia, but then respiration progressively slowed and they
died within hours of surgery. The finding was counterintuitive because the principle of developmental encephalization (Teitelbaum,
1971) suggests that adult ablations should be the most debilitating.

The cause of this infant death was not anesthesia, because many
anesthetic combinations produced the same effect (Kolb & Whishaw,
1981a). It was also not surgery per se, because frontal lesions can be
made at any age with impunity. Death seems to be produced by
posterior decortication, because we have found that even very small
posterior ablations produce death at these ages in as many as 50% of
the animals. We think that the cause of death is diaschisis; that is,
shock to distant neural elements resulting from removal of their innervation. Perhaps this age is critical for the formation of connec-

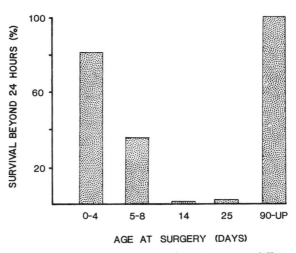

Figure 7. Percentage of animals surviving decortication at different ages.

tions made by the posterior neocortex with many other areas of the brain, so that denervation at just this time produces widespread neural shock and subsequent death. Certainly there is supporting evidence that this is a critical period in development. First, many new behaviors undergo rapid maturation at this time (Altman & Sudarshan, 1975). Second, ablations before about 4 days of age produce little subcortical gliosis and degeneration by comparison with ablations made after 4 days of age (Kolb & Nonneman, 1978; Kolb, Sutherland, & Whishaw, 1983b). The latter point is important, for it strongly suggests that it is the loss of these connections that provides the anatomical basis for the occurrence of shock.

Two other lines of evidence also suggest that the posterior cortex, particularly the posterior parietal cortex, is an area that produces profound abnormalities when damaged at any early age. The first evidence is behavioral. Using a methodology similar to that used for frontal-ablated rats, we examined rats with small posterior parietal cortex ablations on a broad battery of tests, including some that animals with equivalent adulthood ablations performed normally. The results were surprising: The rats were impaired at tests of both cognitive and species-typical behavior that animals with equivalent removals in adulthood performed normally. For example, rats with adult ablations are impaired at limb placement over difficult terrain, and at acquisition of spatial reversals. They are not impaired at performance of the radial arm maze, opening of latch puzzles, grooming, manipulation of the forepaws, tongue extension, or food hoarding (Kolb & Whishaw, 1983b). The rats with parietal excisions in infancy were not impaired at the acquisition of spatial reversals, but they were impaired at the acquisition of the radial arm maze and food hoarding, and they showed deficits similar to those observed in adults in limb placement on a narrow beam (Kolb, Whishaw & Holmes, 1983). In short, rats with parietal lesions in infancy showed sparing on some tasks that are normally found to be impaired following adult lesions, but they were impaired at tasks that are not normally disrupted by equivalent adult lesions. The second source of evidence is anatomical. The adult brain weight of rats that received parietal ablations on the 1st day of age was profoundly reduced compared with animals that received comparable ablations at 7 days of age or in adulthood (Figure 8). In fact, the brain weight of this group was comparable with that of rats that received entire neocortex removal at 5 days of age. The reduction in brain weight was attributable to shrinkage in both the remaining neocortex and the brainstem. The change was also greater than that observed after frontal ablations at the same age (Kolb & Whishaw, 1981b).

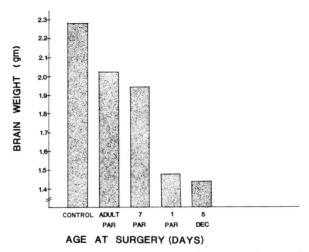

Figure 8. Brain weights in control rats and rats that received cortical ablations at different ages. All measures were taken at least 1 year postsurgery. (PAR) parietal; (DEC) decorticated.

Conclusions

The rat has not been thought of as an ideal species for the study of the effects of early brain injury in humans. This may be because it has been assumed that there is little in common between the recovery of function expected of the rat and the often persistent disabilities characteristic of humans who have suffered early brain injury. Our investigations suggest that there is room for generalization. First recovery from neocortical damage is dependent on the remaining neocortex. Second, recovery seems better in some, but not other, classes of behavior. Third, recovery can be partly dissociated from anatomical changes. Fourth, early brain damage may result in neocortical shrinkage and widely generalized behavioral impairments, both uncharacteristic of similar adult brain damage. If the mechanisms underlying these phenomena can be understood in the rat, they may reveal some important insights into the effects of early brain injury in humans.

References

Altman, J., & Sudarshan, K. (1975). Postnatal development of locomotion in the laboratory rat. *Animal Behavior, 23,* 896–920.

Basser, L. (1962). Hemiplegia of early onset and the faculty of speech with special reference to the effects of hemispherectomy. *Brain, 85,* 427–460.

Bauer, J. H., & Cooper, R. M. (1967). Effects of posterior cortical lesions on a brightness discrimination task. *Journal of Comparative and Physiological Psychology, 58,* 84–92.

Benjamin, R. M., & Thompson, R. F. (1959). Differential effects of cortical lesions in infant and adult cats on roughness discrimination. *Experimental Neurology, 1,* 305–321.

Carter, C. S., Witt, D. M., Kolb, B., & Whishaw, I. Q. (1982). Neonatal decortication and adult female sexual behavior. *Physiology & Behavior, 29,* 763–766.

Castro, A. J. (1972). The effects of cortical ablations on tongue usage in the rat. *Brain Research, 45,* 251–253.

Castro, A. J. (1975). Tongue usage as a measure of cerebral cortical localization in the rat. *Experimental Neurology, 44,* 343–352.

Dennis, M., & Whitaker, H. A. (1976). Language acquisition following hemidecortication: Linguistic superiority of the left over the right hemisphere. *Brain and Language, 3,* 404–433.

Denny-Brown, D., Dawson, D. M., & Tyler, H. R. (1982). *Handbook of neurological examination and case recording.* Cambridge: Harvard University Press.

Diamond, M. C., Kretch, D., & Rosenzweig, M. S. (1964). The effects of an enriched environment on the histology of the rat cerebral cortex. *Journal of Comparative Neurology, 123,* 111–119.

Goldman, P. S., & Galkin, T. W. (1978). Prenatal removal of frontal association cortex in the fetal rhesus monkey: Anatomical and functional consequences in postnatal life. *Brain Research, 152,* 451–485.

Goltz, G. M. (1892). Der Hund ohne Gosshern. *Pfügers Archiv fur die Gesamte Physiologie, 51,* 570–614.

Goodale, M. A. (1983). Vision as a sensorimotor system. In T. E. Robinson (Ed.), *Behavioral contributions to brain research.* London: Oxford University Press.

Gramsbergen, A. (1982). The effects of cerebellar hemispherectomy in the young rat. I. Behavioral sequelae. *Behavioral Brain Research, 6,* 85–92.

Hebb, D. O. (1942). The effect of early and late brain injury upon test scores, and the nature of normal adult intelligence. *Proceedings of the American Philosophical Society, 85,* 265–292.

Hicks, S. P., & D'Amato, C. J. (1975). Motor–sensory cortex–corticospinal system and developing locomotion and placing in rats. *American Journal of Anatomy, 143,* 1–42.

Kasamatsu, T., Pettigrew, J. D., & Ary, M. (1979). Restoration of visual cortical plasticity by local microperfusion of norepinephrine. *Journal of Comparative Neurology, 185,* 163–182.

Kasamatsu, T., Pettigrew, J. D., & Ary, M. (1981). Cortical recovery from effects of monocular deprivation: Acceleration with norepinephrine and suppression with 6-hydroxydopamine. *Journal of Neurophysiology, 45,* 254–266.

Kennard, M. A. (1936). Age and other factors in motor recovery from percentral lesions in monkeys. *American Journal of Physiology, 115,* 138–146.

Kennard, M. A. (1938). Reorganization of motor function in the cerebral cortex of monkeys deprived of motor and premotor areas in infancy. *Journal of Neurophysiology, 1,* 477–496.

Kennard, M. A. (1940). Relation of age to motor impairment in man and in subhuman primates. *Archives of Neurology & Psychiatry, 44,* 377–397.

Kohn, B., & Dennis, M. (1974). Selective impairments of visuo–spatial abilities in infantile hemiplegics after right hemidecortication. *Neuropsychologia, 12,* 505–512.

Kolb, B., & Holmes, C. (1983). Neonatal motor cortex lesions in the rat: Absence of sparing of motor behaviors and impaired spatial learning concurrent with abnormal cerebral morphogenesis. *Behavioral Neuroscience, 97,* 697–709.

Kolb, B., & Nonneman, A. J. (1976). Functional development of the prefrontal cortex in rats continues in adolescence. *Science, 193,* 335–336.

Kolb, B., & Nonneman, A. J. (1978). Sparing of function in rats with early prefrontal cortex lesions. *Brain Research, 151,* 135–148.

Kolb, B., Sutherland, R. J., & Whishaw, I. Q. (1983a). Abnormalities in cortical and subcortical morphology after neonatal neocortical lesions in rats. *Experimental Neurology, 79,* 223–244.

Kolb, B., Sutherland, R. J., & Whishaw, I. Q. (1983b). Neonatal hemidecortication or frontal cortex ablation produces similar behavioral sparing but opposite effects on morphogenesis of remaining cortex. *Behavioral Neuroscience, 97,* 154–158.

Kolb, B., Sutherland, R. J., & Whishaw, I. Q. (1983c). A comparison of the contributions of the frontal and parietal association cortex to spatial localization in rats. *Behavioral Neuroscience, 97,* 13–27.

Kolb, B., & Whishaw, I. Q. (1980). *Fundamentals of human neuropsychology.* San Francisco: Freeman.

Kolb, B., & Whishaw, I. Q. (1981a). Decortication in rats in infancy or adulthood produced comparable functional losses on learned and species-typical behaviors. *Journal of Comparative and Physiological Psychology, 95,* 468–483.

Kolb, B., & Whishaw, I. Q. (1981b). Neonatal frontal lesions in the rat: Sparing of learned but not species-typical behavior in the presence of reduced brain weight and cortical thickness. *Journal of Comparative and Physiological Psychology, 95,* 863–879.

Kolb, B., & Whishaw, I. Q. (1983a). Problems and principles in cross-species generalizations. In T. E. Robinson (Ed.), *Behavioral contributions to brain research.* London: Oxford University Press.

Kolb, B., & Whishaw, I. Q. (1983b). Dissociation of the contributions of the prefrontal, motor and parietal cortex to the control of movement in the rat. *Canadian Journal of Psychology. 37,* 211–232.

Kolb, B., Whishaw, I. Q., & Holmes, C. (1983, June). *Neonatal ablation of the posterior parietal cortex of rats is more debilitating than similar injury in adulthood.* Paper presented at the Canadian Psychological Association, Winnipeg.

Lawrence, D. G., & Hopkins, D. A. (1976). The development of motor control in the rhesus monkey: Evidence concerning the role of corticomotoneuronal connections. *Brain, 99,* 235–254.

Lawrence, D. G., & Kuypers, H. G. J. M. (1968a). The functional organization of the motor system in the monkey: I. The effects of bilateral pyramidal lesions. *Brain, 91,* 1–14.

Lawrence, D. G., & Kuypers, H. G. J. M. (1968b). The functional organization of the motor system in the monkey: II. The effects of lesions of the descending brain-stem pathways. *Brain, 91,* 15–36.

Lewin, R. (1980). Is your brain really necessary? *Science, 210,* 1232–1234.

Milner, B. (1974). Sparing of language function after early unilateral brain damage. *Neurosciences Research Progress Bulletin, 12,* 213–217.

Milner, B. (1975). Psychological aspects of focal epilepsy and its neurosurgical management. *Advances in Neurology, 8,* 299–321.

Morris, R. G. M. (1980). Spatial localization does not require the presence of local cues. *Learning and Motivation, 12*, 239–260.

Oakley, D. A. (1979). Cerebral cortex and adaptive behavior. In D. A. Oakley & H. C. Plotkin (Eds.), *Brain, behavior and evolution.* London: Methuen.

Rudel, R. G., & Teuber, H.-L. (1971). Spatial orientation in normal children and in children with early brain injury. *Neuropsychologia, 9*, 401–407.

Satinoff, E. (1978). Neural organization and evolution of thermal regulation in mammals. *Science, 201*, 16–22.

Schallert, T., Upchurch, M., Lobaugh, N., Farrar, S. B., Spirduso, W. W., Gilliam, P., Vaughn, D., & Wilcox, R. E. (1982). Tactile Extinction: Distinguishing between sensorimotor and motor asymmetries in rats with unilateral nigrostriatal damage. *Pharmacology Biochemistry and Behavior, 16*, 455–462.

Schapiro, S., Salas, M., & Vukovich, K. (1970). Hormonal effects on ontogeny of swimming ability in the rat. Assessment of central nervous system development. *Science, 168*, 147–150.

Schneider, G. E. (1970). Mechanisms of functional recovery following lesions of visual cortex or superior colliculus in neonate and adult hamsters. *Brain Behavior and Evolution, 3*, 295–323.

Schneider, G. E. (1979). Is it really better to have your brain lesion early? Revision of the Kennard principle. *Neuropsychologia, 17*, 557–584.

Schneider, G. E., & Jhaveri, S. R. (1974). Neuroanatomical correlates of spared or altered function after brain lesions in the newborn hamster. In D. G. Stein, J. J. Rosen, & N. Butters (Eds.), *Plasticity and recovery of function in the central nervous system.* London: Academic Press.

Sutherland, R. J., Kolb, B., Whishaw, I. Q., & Becker, J. B. (1982). Cortical noradrenaline depletion eliminates sparing of spatial learning after neonatal frontal cortex damage in the rat. *Neuroscience Letters, 32*, 125–130.

Teitelbaum, P. (1971). The encephalization of hunger. In E. Stellar & J. M. Sprague (Eds.). *Progress in physiological psychology* (Vol. 4). New York: Academic Press.

Vanderwolf, C. H., Kolb, B., & Cooley, R. K. (1978). Behavior of the rat after removal of the neocortex and hippocampal formation. *Journal of Comparative and Physiological Psychology, 92*, 156–175.

Walsh, R. (1981). *Towards an ecology of brain.* New York: SP Medical and Scientific Books.

Whishaw, I. Q., & Kolb, B. (1983a). "Stick out your tongue": Tongue protrusion in neocortex and hypothalamic damaged rats. *Physiology & Behavior. 30*, 471–480.

Whishaw, I. Q., & Kolb, B. (1983b). Can male decorticate rats copulate? *Behavioral Neuroscience, 97*, 270–297.

Whishaw, I. Q., & Kolb, B. (1984). Neuropsychological assessment of children and adults with developmental dyslexia. In: R. N. Malatesha & H. A. Whitaker (Eds.), *Dyslexia: A global issue.* Boston: Martinus Nijhoff.

Whishaw, I. Q., Kolb, B., & Sutherland, R. J. (1983). The analysis of behavior in the laboratory rat. In T. E. Robinson (Ed.), *Behavioral contributions to brain research.* London: Oxford University Press.

Whishaw, I. Q., Kolb, B., Sutherland, R. J., & Becker, J. (1983). Cortical control of claw cutting in the rat. *Behavioral Neuroscience, 97*, 370–380.

Whishaw, I. Q., Nonneman, A. J., & Kolb, B. (1981). Environmental constraints on motor abilities used in grooming, swimming, and eating by decorticate rats. *Journal of Comparative and Physiological Psychology, 95*, 792–804.

Whishaw, I. Q., Schallert, T., & Kolb, B. (1981). An analysis of feeding and sensorimotor abilities of rats after decortication. *Journal of Comparative and Physiological Psychology, 95,* 85–103.

Woods, B. T. (1980). The restricted effects of right-hemisphere lesions after age one; Weschler test data. *Neuropsychologia, 18,* 65–70.

Woods, B. T., & Teuber, H.-L. (1973). Early onset of complementary specialization of cerebral hemispheres in man. *Transections of the American Neurological Association, 98,* 113–117.

8

Functional Development of the Prefrontal System*

Arthur J. Nonneman,
James V. Corwin, Christie L. Sahley,
and John P. Vicedomini

Introduction

Early Lesion Effects

Because the brain of the infant differs in many important ways from that of the adult, the effects of focal brain lesions often are age-dependent in animals and in humans (Schneider, 1979). In many cases, brain damage sustained early in life produces less debility or greater recovery of function than comparable damage in adulthood. A dramatic example is the sparing of language function following left hemisphere removal in humans and children (e.g., Basser, 1962). However, some functions are even more seriously impaired by brain damage in children than in adults (e.g., Teuber & Rudel, 1962). Any attempt to predict the outcome of early brain damage is complicated by at least three factors: the nature of the behavioral test employed (Kolb & Whishaw, 1981; Nonneman & Isaacson, 1973), the age of the subject at the time of testing (Goldman, 1976), and the specific locus

*The rat research reported here was supported in part by Biomedical Research Support Grant 5S07RR07114-10, NIMH Grant MH 27345, NIH Grant NS 13516, NIH postdoctoral fellowship F 32 NS06402-01, and the University of Kentucky Research Fund.

and extent of the brain injury (Goldman, 1972; Johnson & Almli, 1978; Nonneman & Corwin, 1981).

FUNCTIONAL DEVELOPMENT AND SPARING OF FUNCTION

Even when two brain areas are closely related both anatomically and functionally, the severity of the effects of early lesions can differ dramatically. Differences in recovery potential may reflect the fact that different brain areas mature at different rates (Goldman, 1976). Thus, perinatal damage to a given structure may have little immediate effect on behavior if it has not yet developed a mature pattern of connections with functionally related brain regions (Corwin, Leonard, Schoenfeld, & Crandall, 1983). Behavioral deficits may emerge at a later age, when the damaged area would normally begin to exert an influence on the behavior of the developing individual (Goldman, 1976). In other cases, the functional sparing may be permanent, especially if new connections form between functionally related areas (Schneider, 1979).

THE PREFRONTAL SYSTEM AND THE STUDY OF EARLY LESION EFFECTS

The prefrontal systems of rhesus monkeys and laboratory rats provide convenient models for studying the relationship between functional development (at the time of injury) and behavioral effects of damage to closely related structures. In both species there are three major components of the prefrontal system: the prefrontal cortex, the head of the caudate nucleus (CN), and the mediodorsal thalamus (MD). Damage to any of these components in adults of either species produces serious deficits on spatial reversal and spatial delayed-response tasks. However, the effects of perinatal lesions in either species depend on the specific component of the system that is damaged.

These results lead to the major thesis of this chapter. Different components of the prefrontal system mature at different rates: subcortical before cortical, and orbital (sulcal) cortex before dorsal convexity (medial) cortex. This conclusion is supported by converging evidence from several sources: the age at which lesions first produce immediate effects, the age at which lesions first produce long-term effects, and the age at which long-lasting degeneration products (from degenerating projections) are first evident following early lesions of the MD.

The Prefrontal System: Anatomical Relationships

MONKEYS

The major interconnections between the various components of the prefrontal system are presented in Figure 1 for both rhesus monkey and rat. In the monkey, three cortical zones are connected reciprocally with three subdivisions of the MD: the arcuate cortex with the extreme lateral paralamellar subdivision, the convexity cortex with the midlateral parvocellular subdivision, and the orbital cortex with the medial magnocellular subdivision (Akert, 1964). In addition, both cortex and the MD project to the head of the CN.

RATS

In the rat, Leonard (1969) has described two cortical zones that receive primary projections from the MD. A strip of sulcal cortex lies dorsal to the rhinal sulcus on the rostral one-third of each hemisphere, and another strip of medial cortex lies on the medial wall of each hemisphere extending rostrally from the genu of the corpus callosum to the olfactory bulbs. These projections course through the caudate–putamen (CP), giving off collateral projections on the way. In addition, both zones of the prefrontal cortex project to the CP, the MD, and to each other (Beckstead, 1979; Divac, Kosmal, Bjorklund, & Lindvall, 1978; Krettek & Price, 1977). Because of the similarity of thalamocortical and corticothalamic projections, Leonard (1969) suggested that the sulcal cortex of the rat is analogous to the orbital cortex of the monkey, and that the medial cortex of the rat is analogous to the dorsolateral cortex of the monkey.

This pattern of anatomical connections between prefrontal cortex, MD, and CP, as well as the similarity of behavioral effects produced by lesions to these three areas, suggests that they normally function as integrated components of a prefrontal system in rats and monkeys. The immediate and long-term behavioral effects of damage to different components of this system at various ages are summarized in Table 1.

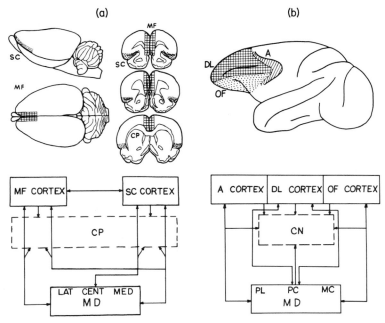

Figure 1. Anatomical locus (upper panel) and major connections (lower panel) of rat (a) and rhesus monkey (b) prefrontal systems. (A) arcuate cortex, (CENT) central segment of MD, (CN) caudate nucleus, (CP) caudate–putamen, (DL) dorsolateral prefrontal cortex, (LAT) lateral segment of MD, (MC) magnocellular portion of MD, (MD) mediodorsal thalamic nucleus, (MED) medial segment of MD, (MF) medial prefrontal cortex, (OF) orbital prefrontal cortex, (PC) parvocellular portion of MD, (PL) paralamellar portion of MD, (SC) sulcal prefrontal cortex. Rat SC and monkey OF cortices indicated by stippling. Rat MF and monkey DL cortices indicated by crosshatching. Monkey arcuate cortex indicated by slashes. Rat cortical terminology after Leonard (1969). Rat thalamic terminology after Krettek and Price (1977). Monkey terminology after Akert (1964). In the rat, the caudate nucleus and putamen comprise one fused nucleus, and the fibers interconnecting the cortex and MD course through this nucleus in a series of scattered fascicles. In the monkey, CN is separated from the putamen by the internal capsule.

Immediate Effects of Early Damage

CORTICAL

   The behavioral effects of early damage to the monkey prefrontal cortex suggest that the orbital subfield matures before the dorsolateral subfield. When year-old monkeys are tested on spatial de-

TABLE 1

Immediate and Long-Term Behavioral Effects
of Lesions to the Prefrontal System at Various Ages[a]

Subject and lesion[b]	Immediate	Long-term
Monkey		
Prenatal		
DL	−	−
Infant		
DL	−	+
OF	+	−
CN	+	+
MD	+	+
Juvenile		
DL	+	+
OF	+	+
CN	+	?
MD	+	?
Adult		
DL	+	+
OF	+	+
CN	+	+
MD	+	+
Rat		
Infant		
MF	−	−
SC	+	−
CP	+	−
MD	?	−
Juvenile		
MF	?	−
SC	?	+
CP	?	+
MD	?	+
Adult		
MF	+	+
SC	+	+
CP	+	+
MD	+	+

[a]+ = behavioral deficit; − = no deficit; ? = not studied.
[b]DL = dorsolateral cortex,   OF = orbital cortex, CN = caudate nucleus, MD = mediodorsal thalamus, MF = medial cortex,   SC = sulcal cortex,   CP = caudate–putamen.

layed-response tasks, those that received lesions of the orbital cortex at 2 months of age are seriously impaired, whereas monkeys receiving dorsolateral lesions at the same age perform as well as normal controls (Goldman, 1972). Lesions to either prefrontal subfield in juveniles (18–24 months old) produce serious deficits. Thus, the involvement of the orbital cortex in delayed-response performance seems to develop within the first few months after birth. In contrast, the involvement of the dorsolateral cortex continues to develop through the first 2 years of postnatal life.

Similar effects are obtained when local hypothermia is used to produce a reversible cryogenic "lesion" of the dorsolateral cortex. "Cryogenic depression of prefrontal cortex, at a temperature sufficient to induce 21–25% decrements in delayed-response performance in 34–36 month old monkeys, produced deficits of only 7–8% in 19–31 month olds and no detectable loss in younger monkeys, 9–16 months of age" (Alexander & Goldman, 1978, p. 233). Thus, functional depression of the dorsolateral cortex in the youngest age group had no effect. This suggests that the delayed-response performance of the infant monkey is mediated by (a) brain region(s) other than the dorsolateral cortex, but it becomes dependent on the dorsolateral cortex as the animal ages and this cortex matures.

In rats, the effects of early prefrontal cortex lesions on a spatial reversal task also suggest that the sulcal (orbital) cortex matures before the medial (dorsolateral) cortex. Sulcal lesions at 7 to 8 days of age produce (at 14 days) deficits that are similar to the effects of sulcal lesions in adults (Kolb, Nonneman, & Singh, 1974; Sahley & Nonneman, 1979). In contrast, lesions of the medial prefrontal cortex at 7 to 8 days of age produce no deficit, whereas similar lesions in adult rats produce serious deficits on this task.

SUBCORTICAL

Just as the effects of early cortical lesions lead to the suggestion that the orbital (sulcal) cortex matures before the dorsolateral (medial) cortex, the effects of early subcortical lesions to the CN and the MD suggest that these areas mature before the cortical components of the prefrontal system.

The behavioral effects of lesions to the CN or the MD of infant rhesus monkeys are indistinguishable from those of comparable lesions in juvenile monkeys (Goldman, 1974; Goldman & Rosvold, 1972). In rats, lesions of CP at 7 to 8 days of age produce a dramatic spatial reversal deficit when the animals are tested at 14 days of age (Sahley & Nonneman, 1979).

Long-Term Effects of Early Damage

Four patterns of long-term behavioral effects of early brain damage have been identified: (1) continued sparing of function throughout the subject's life, (2) initial sparing of function followed by the emergence of deficits as the subject matures, (3) recovery of function, in which an initial deficit disappears as the subject matures, and (4) continuous deficit throughout the subject's life. Each of these patterns is seen after early damage to various components of the prefrontal system.

CORTICAL

A pattern of functional recovery is seen after early lesions of the orbital cortex in monkeys or the sulcal cortex in rats. Although monkeys with orbital cortex lesions induced at 2 months of age are impaired on spatial delayed-response tasks when first tested at 12 months, they show dramatic improvement when retested at 24 months on the same task (Goldman, 1972, 1974). Also, rats with early sulcal cortex lesions show spatial reversal deficits when they are tested at 14 days of age (Sahley & Nonneman, 1979), but no deficit can be detected when spatial reversal testing is conducted at 120 days of age (Kolb & Nonneman, 1978).

In contrast with this recovery of function after neonatal orbital cortex destruction, infant monkeys with dorsolateral cortex lesions or with frontal lobectomies show initial sparing of function followed by later emergence of severe delayed-response deficits, whereas the performance of control subjects improves with age (Goldman, 1972; Tucker & Kling, 1967). This late emerging deficit was not seen, however, in a monkey with prenatal removal of the dorsolateral cortex. This animal showed complete sparing of delayed-response and delayed-alternation performance even at 24 months (Goldman & Galkin, 1978).

The long-term effects of medial cortex lesions or of frontal lobectomies in rats contrast with the recovery of function observed after neonatal sulcal lesions and also with the late-emerging deficits of monkeys with infant dorsolateral lesions or lobectomies. Lobectomies or medial prefrontal lesions induced at or before 25 days allow continued sparing on spatial reversal, delayed-response, or delayed-alternation tasks (Kolb & Nonneman, 1978; Kolb & Whishaw, 1981; Nonneman & Corwin, 1981; Vicedomini, Corwin, & Nonneman, 1982a). Thus the effects of early medial prefrontal lesions in rats are very much like those of the monkey that received a dorsolateral lesion before birth (Goldman & Galkin, 1978). Since the rhesus monkey is generally more mature at birth than the rat, it is not surprising that prenatal lesions in monkeys produce effects comparable to those of neonatal lesions in rats.

SUBCORTICAL

In monkeys, the initial sparing of delayed-response performance observed after neonatal dorsolateral cortex lesions is eliminated if damage to the head of the CN is added to the dorsolateral cortex lesion (Kling & Tucker, 1967). In like manner, rats receiving combined lesions of the medial cortex and the CP as infants show no sparing of spatial reversal or delayed-alternation performance when they are later tested as adults (Vicedomini, Isaac & Nonneman, 1984). However, neonatal lesions restricted to the CP or the MD produce no deficit on these same tasks when the rats are tested as adults. They perform as well as controls or subjects with neonatal lesions restricted to the medial prefrontal cortex (Vicedomini, Corwin, & Nonneman, 1982b).

The results are much different with juvenile subjects. In contrast with the long-term sparing of function allowed by neonatal MD, CP, or medial prefrontal lesions or by medial prefrontal lesions in juveniles, rats with CP or MD lesions as juveniles (25 days) or adults show severe long-term behavioral deficits (Kolb, 1977; Vicedomini et al., 1982b). These effects are consistent with the idea that subcortical components mature before cortical components of the rat prefrontal system.

Maturation of Prefrontal Connections

MONKEYS

The essential projections from the magnocellular portion of the MD to the orbital cortex apparently exist at birth in the rhesus monkey. The location and severity of retrograde degeneration in the MD following neonatal orbital or dorsolateral cortex removal is essentially the same as that produced by comparable lesions in adult monkeys. However, no retrograde degeneration is evident in the MD after prenatal removal of the dorsolateral cortex 2 months before birth. This may indicate that the projections from the MD to the dorsolateral cortex have not developed by the time of the lesion, at 106 days of gestation (Goldman & Galkin, 1978). There are no similar reports on the effects of prenatal orbital cortex lesions.

The major corticothalamic and corticocaudate projections also are present at birth in the monkey (Goldman & Nauta, 1977; Johnson, Rosvold, Galkin, & Goldman, 1976), but the corticocaudate projections may continue to mature for the first several postnatal months (Johnson et al., 1976).

RATS

In the rat, restricted lesions of the medial or sulcal prefrontal cortex within the first 10 days of life produce no detectable retrograde degeneration in the MD (Kolb & Nonneman, 1978; Nonneman & Corwin, 1981). In this respect, the neonatal rat is similar to the prenatally lesioned monkey described by Goldman and Galkin (1978). However, even in the adult rat the projections to the prefrontal cortex from the MD are more diffuse than the thalamocortical projections in the monkey; as a result, restricted cortical lesions do not produce the crisp, restricted MD degeneration characteristic of the monkey. The thalamocortical projections of the infant rat may be even more diffuse than in the adult. In any event, combined lesions of the medial and sulcal cortex in the neonatal rat do produce extensive retrograde degeneration in the MD, and this degeneration is even more severe after a complete frontal lobectomy (Kolb & Whishaw, 1981; Vicedomini et al., 1982a). These results are consistent with the suggestion that thalamic projections to the prefrontal cortex exist in the newborn rat and that they are distributed even more diffusely than in the adult (Divac et al., 1978; Krettek & Price, 1977).

Leonard (1974) has argued that the presence of stable degeneration argyrophilia provides a histological marker of the maturation of neural connections, because immature neurons degenerate more rapidly than mature neurons. Using this approach to study the development of thalamo–prefrontal connections of the rat, Corwin et al. (1983) have confirmed the presence of thalamic projections from the MD to both the medial and the sulcal prefrontal cortices and to the CP of the neonatal rat. But the CP and sulcal projections apparently mature before the medial projection, because stable anterograde degeneration develops several days earlier to the CP and the sulcal cortex (Day 13) than to the medial cortex (Day 20). Prior to these ages, degeneration products are cleared very quickly (< 72 hours), and the existence of the thalamocortical projections can be demonstrated only with very short survival times. Figure 2 illustrates the presence of stable degeneration to the sulcal cortex and the CP after an MD lesion at 13 days of age; Figure 3 shows the presence of stable degeneration in the CP, the medial cortex, and the sulcal cortex after a similar MD lesion at 20 days. These results are entirely consistent with the lesion–behavior data reported earlier that suggest that the CP and the sulcal cortex mature before the medial cortex of the rat.

Summary and Conclusions

Early brain damage can be either more or less debilitating than comparable damage suffered later in life. Both the immediate and the long-term behavioral effects of early brain damage depend on the maturational status both of the region destroyed and of the other brain areas with which it is anatomically and functionally interrelated. Within the prefrontal systems of the monkey and the rat, these interrelated components are the prefrontal cortex, the MD, and the head of the CN of the monkey or the CP of the rat.

In both species, the subcortical components are functionally mature (i.e., play an important role in behavior) before the cortical components: Subcortical lesions produce behavioral effects earlier than cortical lesions. Furthermore, the orbital cortex of the monkey seems to mature before the dorsolateral cortex, and the sulcal cortex of the rat matures before the medial cortex: Orbital or sulcal lesions produce deficits at an earlier age than dorsolateral or medial lesions in monkey and rat, respectively. In addition, the prognosis for functional recovery is typically poorer (i.e., behavioral deficits are still seen in adulthood) for subjects receiving early subcortical lesions (MD, CP, or CN) than for subjects receiving early cortical lesions. (See Table 1 for a summary of behavioral effects.) Finally, the projections from the MD to the sulcal cortex mature before those from the MD to the medial cortex of the rat, which is demonstrated by the presence of long-lasting, stable degeneration following early MD lesions.

In general, the rhesus monkey is more mature at birth than the rat, and the effects of either subcortical or cortical lesions in the infant

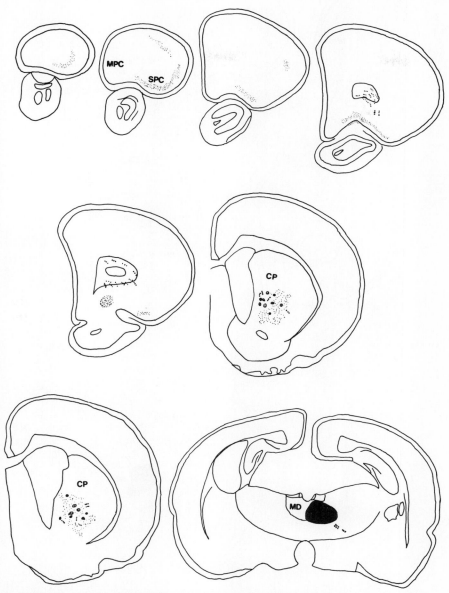

Figure 2. Serial reconstruction of long-lasting anterograde degeneration (72-hour survival) after unilateral lesion of the mediodorsal thalamic nucleus (MD) in a 13-day-old rat. Degeneration is visible in the caudate–putamen (CP) and the sulcal prefrontal cortex (SPC) but not in the medial prefrontal cortex (MPC). (Reprinted with permission from Corwin, Leonard, Schoenfeld, and Crandall, 1983, *Developmental Brain Research 8*, 89–100).

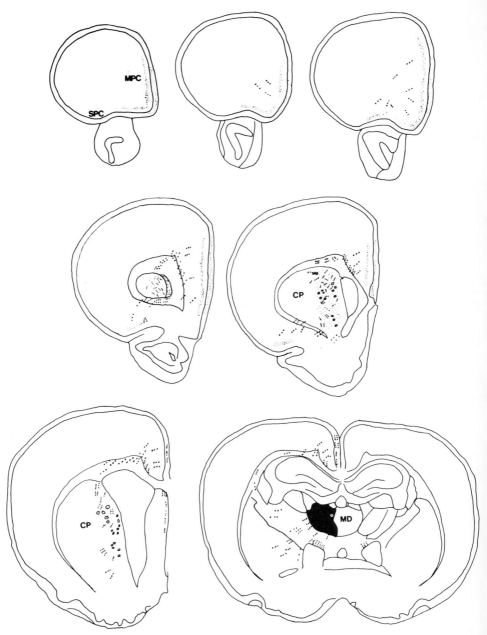

Figure 3. Serial reconstructions of long-lasting anterograde degeneration (72-hour survival) after unilateral lesion of mediodorsal thalamic nucleus (MD) in a 20-day-old rat. Degeneration is visible in the caudate–putamen (CP), the sulcal prefrontal cortex (SPC) and the medial prefrontal cortex (MPC). (Reprinted with permission from Corwin, Leonard, Schoenfeld, and Crandall, 1983, *Developmental Brain Research 8*, 89–100).

monkey are more serious than those of the corresponding lesions of the neonatal rat. However, prenatal destruction of the dorsolateral cortex of the monkey 2 months before birth allows the same degree of anatomical and behavioral sparing as neonatal removal of the medial prefrontal cortex in the rat. This similarity in the pattern of behavioral (Table 1) and anatomical results in monkeys and rats is remarkable if one considers the diverse ecology and evolutionary history of these species. It leads us to speculate that the same general relationships may be found in all mammals, including humans.

However, it should be noted that this review and these conclusions are based on the effects of early prefrontal system damage on learning and performance in a restricted group of tasks: spatial reversal, spatial delayed-response, and spatial alternation. Within these related structures and comparing these related tasks, the results of early damage are remarkably consistent. However, there are important species differences in the nature and variety of other tasks that are affected by prefrontal system damage. It was not appropriate or possible to review these in this chapter. Equally important is the well-established fact that all functions of a given structure do not mature at the same time or at the same rate. Therefore, there is probably no single time at which a brain region reaches functional maturity, and there is no time at which the outcome of brain damage becomes inexorably fixed. Rather, the degree of maturity and therefore the prognosis for recovery from early damage must be considered relative to each specific function of interest.

References

Akert, K. (1964). Comparative anatomy of the frontal cortex and thalamocortical connections. In J. M. Warren & K. Akert (Eds.), *The frontal granular cortex and behavior* (pp. 372–396). New York: McGraw-Hill.

Alexander, G. E., & Goldman, P. S. (1978). Functional development of the dorsolateral prefrontal cortex: An analysis utilizing reversible cryogenic depression. *Brain Research, 143,* 233–249.

Basser, L. S. (1962). Hemiplegia of early onset and the faculty of speech with special reference to the effects of hemispherectomy. *Brain, 85,* 427–460.

Beckstead, R. M. (1979). An autoradiographic examination of the corticocortical and subcortical projections of the mediodorsal-projection (prefrontal) cortex in the rat. *Journal of Comparative Neurology, 184,* 43–62.

Corwin, J. V., Leonard, C. M., Schoenfeld, T. A., & Crandall, J. E. (1983). Anatomical evidence for differential rates of maturation of the medial dorsal nucleus projections to prefrontal cortex in rats. *Developmental Brain Research, 8,* 89–100.

Divac, I., Kosmal, A., Bjorklund, A., & Lindvall, O. (1978). Subcortical projections to the prefrontal cortex in the rat as revealed by the horseradish peroxidase technique. *Neuroscience, 3,* 785–796.

Goldman, P. S. (1972). Developmental determinants of cortical plasticity. *Acta Neurobiologiae Experimentalis, 32,* 495–511.

Goldman, P. S. (1974) An alternative to developmental plasticity: Heterology of CNS structures in infants and adults. In D. Stein, J. Rosen, & N. Butters (Eds.), *Plasticity and Recovery of Function in the Central Nervous System* (pp. 149–174). New York: Academic Press.

Goldman, P. S. (1976). Maturation of the mammalian nervous system and the ontogeny of behavior. In J. Rosenblatt, R. Hinde, E. Shaw, & C. Beer (Eds.), *Advances in the Study of Behavior* (Vol. 7) New York: Academic Press.

Goldman, P. S., & Galkin, T. W. (1978). Prenatal removal of frontal association cortex in the fetal rhesus monkey: Anatomical and functional consequences in postnatal life. *Brain Research, 152,* 451–485.

Goldman, P. S., & Nauta, W. J. H. (1977). An intricately patterned prefrontocaudate projection in the rhesus monkey. *Journal of Comparative Neurology, 171,* 369–386.

Goldman, P. S., & Rosvold, H. E. (1972). The effects of selective caudate lesions in infant and juvenile rhesus monkeys. *Brain Research, 43,* 53–66.

Johnson, D. A., & Almli, C. R. (1978). Age, brain damage, and performance. In S. Finger (Ed.), *Recovery from brain damage: Research and theory* (pp. 115–134). New York: Plenum.

Johnson, T. N., Rosvold, H. E., Galkin, T. W., & Goldman, P. S. (1976). Postnatal maturation of subcortical projections from the prefrontal cortex in the rhesus monkey. *Journal of Comparative Neurology, 166,* 427–444.

Kling, A., & Tucker, T. J. (1967). Effects of combined lesions of frontal granular cortex and caudate nucleus in the neonatal monkey. *Brain Research, 6,* 428–439.

Kolb, B. (1977). Studies on the caudate–putamen and the dorsomedial thalamic nucleus of the rat: Implications for mammalian frontal ·ɔbe functions. *Physiology and Behavior, 18,* 237–244.

Kolb, B., & Nonneman, A. J. (1978). Sparing of function in rats with early prefrontal cortex lesions. *Brain Research, 151,* 135–148.

Kolb, B., Nonneman, A. J., & Singh, R. K. (1974). Double dissociation of spatial and perseverative impairments following prefrontal lesions in rats. *Journal of Comparative and Physiological Psychology, 87,* 772–780.

Kolb, B., & Whishaw, I. Q. (1981). Neonatal frontal lesions in the rat: Sparing of learned but not species-typical behavior in the presence of reduced brain weight and cortical thickness. *Journal of Comparative and Physiological Psychology, 95,* 863–879.

Krettek, J. E., & Price, J. L. (1977). The cortical projections of the mediodorsal nucleus and adjacent thalamic nuclei in the rat. *Journal of Comparative Neurology, 171,* 157–192.

Leonard, C. M. (1969). The prefrontal cortex of the rat. I. Cortical projection of the mediodorsal nucleus. II. Efferent connections. *Brain Research, 12,* 321–343.

Leonard, C. M. (1974). Degeneration argyrophilia as an index of neural maturation: Studies on the optic tract of the golden hamster. *Journal of Comparative Neurology, 156,* 435–458.

Nonneman, A. J., & Corwin, J. V. (1981). Differential effects of prefrontal cortex ablation in neonatal, juvenile, and young adult rats. *Journal of Comparative and Physiological Psychology, 95,* 588–602.

Nonneman, A. J., & Isaacson, R. L. (1973). Task dependent recovery after early brain damage. *Behavioral Biology, 8,* 143–172.

Sahley, C. L., & Nonneman, A. J. (1979). Sparing and recovery of function within the prefrontal system of the infant rat. *Society for Neuroscience Abstracts, 5,* 635.

Schneider, G. E. (1979). Is it really better to have your brain lesion early? A revision of the "Kennard principle." *Neuropsychologia, 17,* 557–583.

Teuber, H. L., & Rudel, R. G. (1962). Behavior after cerebral lesions in children and adults. *Developmental Medicine and Child Neurology, 4,* 3–20.

Tucker, T. J., & Kling, A. (1967). Differential effects of early and late lesions of frontal granular cortex in the monkey. *Brain Research, 5,* 377–389.

Vicedomini, J. P., Corwin, J. V., & Nonneman, A. J. (1982a). Role of residual anterior cortex in recovery from neonatal prefrontal lesions in the rat. *Physiology and Behavior, 28,* 797–806.

Vicedomini, J. P., Corwin, J. V., & Nonneman, A. J. (1982b). Behavioral effects of lesions to the caudate nucleus or mediodorsal thalamus in neonatal, juvenile, and adult rats. *Physiological Psychology, 10,* 246–250.

Vicedomini, J. P., Isaac, W. L., & Nonneman, A. J. (1984). Role of the caudate nucleus in recovery from neonatal mediofrontal cortex lesions in the rat. *Developmental Psychobiology, 17,* 51–65.

9

The Effects of Early Cerebellar Hemispherectomy in the Rat: Behavioral, Neuroanatomical, and Electrophysiological Sequelae

Albert Gramsbergen
and Jos IJkema-Paassen

Introduction

The so-called Kennard principle was derived from early animal experiments that suggested that brain lesions at early stages of maturation have less severe effects on later behavior than similar lesions in adult animals. Simply stated this principle states that the immature brain has a greater capacity for functional compensation after brain trauma than the mature brain. Further research has shown that early brain lesions lead to extensive neuronal rearrangement. For instance, Hicks and d'Amato (1970) demonstrated that cerebral hemispherectomy in the rat during the first days of life did not result in apparent impairment. However, lesioning at adult age led to severe handicaps. In the neonatally lesioned animals a strong ipsilateral corticospinal tract was found, and it was suggested that this aberrant projection effected the undisturbed locomotor development. Such findings have been regarded as a possible explanation for the Kennard principle. Still later investigations, especially those involving a meticulous analysis of behavioral sequelae, often indicate a complicated relationship between the maturational stage at lesioning and its effects on brain function.

Prendergast and co-workers (Prendergast & Shusterman, 1982; Prendergast, Shusterman, & Phillips, 1982), in studying the effects of spinal hemisection in rats, made lesions either before the 3rd day of life or at adult age. The neonatally lesioned rats appeared to perform well in the hopping reaction, whereas a considerable percentage of adult-lesioned rats failed. On the other hand, adult-lesioned rats recovered their ability to cross a narrow runway swiftly, whereas neonatally lesioned rats were clumsy and needed more time. Thus it would appear that no consistent behavioral outcomes necessarily result from early or late lesions. Bregman and Goldberger (1982) compared the effects of partial hemisection of the spinal cord in neonatal and adult cats. They applied kinematographic techniques and made computer reconstructions of limb movements. The most obvious difference in the comparison was the partial sparing of the tactile placing reaction in the neonatally lesioned cats and its abolition in the adult-lesioned cats. Anatomical evidence in the neonatally lesioned animals revealed that the corticospinal projection formed an aberrant pathway that bypassed the lesion. Furthermore, the authors demonstrated that the preserved tactile placing reaction was dependent on these fibers. However, a massive loss of neurons was observed in the red nucleus and Deiters' nucleus (contralateral and ipsilateral to the lesion, respectively) of the neonatally lesioned animals, which might explain the clumsy limb movements in these kittens. Schneider and Jhaveri (1974) showed that aberrant fiber projections occurring after early brain lesions may even produce abnormal behavioral patterns. They made unilateral tectal ablations in Syrian hamsters at birth, and on testing, these animals made abnormal head movements away from certain visual stimuli. Anatomically there were considerable numbers of retinotectal axons terminating in the medial zone of the remaining colliculus at the "wrong", ipsilateral side, whereas no such aberrant fiber projections were found after similar lesions at adult age. These few examples illustrate the intricate effects that may occur after such crude interferences—as surgical lesions—with highly complex and finely tuned neurodevelopmental processes. The evidence they contain acts as strong counterweight to the assumption of any simple relationship between early brain lesions and increased capacity for functional compensation.

The effects of cerebellar hemispherectomy at early and later ages in the rat on the development of locomotor behavior is unknown. However, early experiments in newborn puppies, rabbits, and cats suggested that early cerebellar lesions are better compensated for than lesions at adult age (Asratian, 1938; DeRenzi & Pompeiano, 1956; Di Giorgio, 1944). A common drawback of these experiments is that only decerebrated animals were involved, and consequently results are based on a relatively short survival period. In later experiments, several investigators have demonstrated the occurrence of extensive neuronal remodeling after hemicerebellectomy at early ages in the rat (e.g., Castro & Smith, 1979; Leong, 1978; Lim & Leong, 1975). It is against this background of previous research that we decided to study the development of locomotor behavior in the rat following cerebellar hemispherectomy at early and later ages. We choose the rat as the experimental animal because these animals were born at an early stage of maturation (Altman & Anderson, 1971). This permits experimental interference at early stages of brain development, which has apparent methodological advantages.

The first section of this chapter deals with the effects of cerebellar hemispherectomy on locomotor development, the second section deals with certain aspects of neuronal rearrangement, and in the third section, neurophysiological functioning of aberrant fiber connections are considered.

The Effects of Cerebellar Hemispherectomy at Early and Later Ages on Locomotor Behavior

METHODS

Rats of the white and black hooded Lister strain were studied. Inspection for litters occurred once daily. Unilateral cerebellar hemispherectomy was performed by aspiration under ether anaesthesia at the 5th, 10th, 20th, and 30th days. All rats of a litter were lesioned. Individual rats were marked in the first 10 days of life by spots of nontoxic ink on their back, and thereafter by recording the black and white patterning that emerges by that age. After completion of behavioral testing, the extent of the cerebellar lesion was verified microscopically. Only material of the experimental rats in which the roof of the metencephalic brainstem was intact and the vermis and one hemisphere and its nuclei were preserved was considered. For the numbers of rats in each of the age groups meeting these criteria see Table 1. Rats lesioned at the 5th, 10th or 20th day were tested daily after the operation until their 30th day and with 30-day intervals thereafter. The rats lesioned at the 30th day were tested at the 34th day for the first time, then at the 60th day and with 30-day intervals thereafter until the 360th day. Testing, lasting 15–20 min-

ALBERT GRAMSBERGEN AND JOS IJKEMA-PAASSEN

TABLE 1

Numbers of Rats per Age Group Used in the Different Experiments

	Experiments		
Test group	Locomotor behavior[a]	Neuronal remodeling	Neurophysiological functioning
2nd day	—	4	2
5th day	24	4	4
10th day	19	4	1
20th day	14	4	2
30th day	29	4	—
Control rats	—	4	4

[a]Behavioral categories based on pilot study in 30 control rats and 110 rats with cerebellar lesions.

utes per animal, occurred between 1400 and 1700 hours (lighting schedule of the animal room: from 800 until 1800 hours light). Rats were weighed until the age of 30 days. Reflexes listed in Table 2 were elicited while the animals were awake. Only the presence or absence of reflexes was noted. In rats of all ages, locomotion was tested on a table with a smooth surface. The developmental stage of locomotor abilities for rats until the age of 14 days was evaluated by applying a scale comprising four categories, a scale slightly modified from that of Almli and Fisher (1977).

A: Ventral body surface in contact with the testing platform; head motion and uncoordinated swimming movements and pivoting.
B: Ventral body surface in contact with the testing platform; coordinated and directive crawling with the forelimbs only.
C: Ventral body surface in contact with the testing platform; coordinated and directive crawling with all four limbs.
D: Walking on all four limbs with the ventral body surface off the testing platform.

Control data for weight increase, reflex ontogeny, and locomotor development were derived from normative data collected in rats of the same strain over several years (Gramsbergen, 1976, 1982; Gramsbergen, Schwartze, & Prechtl, 1970).

For rats aged 14 days and older, a scale of six locomotion categories was applied. This scale is designed to classify locomotor abilities of

TABLE 2

Description of Reflexes

Reflex	Stimulus	Positive response	Remarks
Righting	Rats placed on their back on a flat surface	Turns over	Elicitable until 20th day
Negative geotaxis	Rat placed on a 20° slope, head downward	Turns around to face upward	Elicitable until 20th day
Free-fall righting	Rat dropped, back downward, from 20 cm onto wood wool nesting material	Lands on all four limbs	
Palmar grasp; plantar grasp	Palm of forepaw or backpaw stimulated gently with paper clip	Digits flex to grasp clip	
Forelimb hopping, hindlimb hopping	Rat held at the flanks, slightly elevated; moving forward with limbs in contact with floor	Rhythmic walking movements with limbs	Elicitable until 20th day

rats with a cerebellar hemispherectomy relative to normal rats (Gramsbergen, 1981).

1: Ventral body surface in contact with ground; no effective movements.
2: Ventral body surface in contact with ground; locomotive movements in forelimbs.
3: Ventral body surface in contact with ground; locomotive movements in all four limbs.
4: Ventral body surface off the ground; locomotion on all four limbs; lateral sways exceeding half of body diameter.
5: Locomotion on all four limbs; slight swaying—less than one-half body diameter; clumsy locomotion.
6: Undisturbed locomotion.

Locomotion was scored according to the category predominating during testing.

Finally, an inventory of specific locomotor handicaps was made.

None of these handicaps was specifically associated with any of the locomotion categories.

Corkscrew movement:	Fall and turn over with a corkscrew-like distortion of the body axis.
Falling:	Falling on the lateral body flank.
Ataxia:	Marked swaying with large amplitude and low frequency.
Postural tremor:	Low amplitude and high frequency tremor of the trunk.
Increased gait width:	Abduction of one or both hindlimbs during locomotion.
Waddling gait:	Unstabilized pelvis during locomotion.
Hypermetria of paws:	Clearly audible locomotion due to hard slapping.

Data from behavioral testing were subjected to statistical treatment with nonparametric tests.

RESULTS AND DISCUSSION

The weight curves of the groups of rats lesioned at the 5th or 10th day in comparison to control rats are given in Figure 1. The weight gain of lesioned rats showed a decrease compared to the control curve 2–3 days after the operation. This is undoubtedly a symptom of the postoperative recovery period. What is striking, though, is that there is no catch-up in weight. Unpublished observations of our own in litters, of which a few were hemicerebellectomized, a few sham-lesioned, and the other littermates left undisturbed, have demonstrated that the mother rat does not show a preference in her maternal care either for normal or lesioned rats. The present results may imply, therefore, that the decreased weight gain of lesioned rats is the result of their handicap in reaching their food supply—their mother before weaning, and thereafter the solid-food container in the wire lid of the cage.

Reflex responses in rats lesioned at the 5th or 10th day are given in Table 3. Most of the reflexes listed have developed by the 5th day in normal rats, and these particular reflexes remain positive after lesioning at this age or at the 10th day. The plantar grasp reflex, which in normal rats can be elicited from the 6th or 7th day onward, devel-

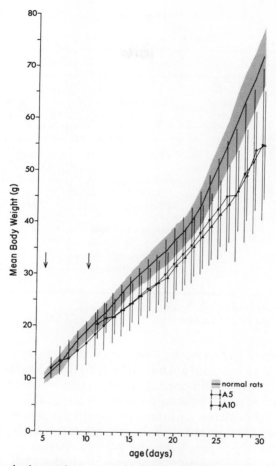

Figure 1. Mean body weight and standard deviations of rats lesioned at the 5th day and at the 10th day compared to control rats.

ops normally despite cerebellar hemispherectomy at the 5th day. However, free-fall righting, which normally becomes positive around the 16th–18th day, appears to be retarded in both groups of rats. In rats lesioned at the 5th day, the median age at which this motor pattern develops is 19.2 days (range, 16–24 days; in 1 rat out of 24 this reflex did not become positive at all), whereas for 50% of the rats lesioned at the 10th day, it does not appear until 22.0 days (range, 17–26 days; in 3 rats out of 19 no positive response developed). Hindlimb hopping, which can be elicited in normal rats from the 4th–6th day,

TABLE 3

Results from Reflex Testing

Reflex	Control rats	Postnatal days to positive reflex	
		Cerebellar hemispherectomy at 5th day	Cerebellar hemispherectomy at 10th day
Righting	1–3	Remains positive	Remains positive
Negative geo-taxis	4–5	Remains positive	Remains positive
Free-fall righting	16–18	Median, 19.2 days range, 16–24 days[a]	Median, 22.0 days range, 17–26 days[b]
Palmar grasp	2–3	Remains positive	Remains positive
Plantar grasp	6–7	6–7	Remains positive
Forelimb hopping	3–4	Remains positive	Remains positive
Hindlimb hopping	4–6	5–6; abnormal from 13th–14th day	Remains positive; abnormal from 13th–14th day

[a]Negative in one rat until last testing day (30th day).
[b]Negative in three rats until 30th day.

appears to be positive in both groups from the 1st day of testing. But in most of the rats lesioned at the 5th or 10th day a marked abduction that hampers the normal hopping reaction can be observed from the 13th–14th day onward. In rats lesioned at the 20th day, all reflexes tested remained positive without any symptom of a developmental drawback. Abnormal hopping of the hindlimb caused by limb abduction occurred in these rats from the 1st day of testing.

Development of locomotion is normal until the 12th day of life in rats lesioned at the 5th or 10th day. Until that day, both lesioned and normal rats show locomotion with the ventral body surface in contact with the ground. In the following days, normal rats start walking with their ventral body surface free from the ground (type "D" locomotion). A few rats with cerebellar hemispherectomy follow this development. However, in the groups of rats lesioned at the 5th and 10th days, some animals are retarded by 2 to 4 days in the onset of this type of locomotion. Some other rats are never able to walk freely on all four limbs for longer uninterrupted periods during their whole lifetime.

From the 14th day onward, locomotion of experimental rats was compared to that in normal rats by applying the scale of six locomotion categories. The median scores attained by both groups at the 14th day are between 4.3 and 4.5. A slight improvement can be observed until the 28th–30th day (median scores for rats lesioned at the 5th day, 5.1; at the 10th day, 4.9). Rats lesioned at the 20th day and tested at the 21st day show handicapped locomotion from that day onward. The median score attained at the age (4.7) is comparable to that of the group of rats lesioned at the 5th or 10th day and tested at the same age. It then increases slightly up to the 30th day. All rats lesioned at the 30th day show abnormal locomotion when tested at the 34th day, but they perform clearly better than rats of the other age groups. However, neither of the experimental groups attains normal levels. From the 60th day onward, locomotion becomes increasingly hampered with age in all experimental groups.

Both the improvement until the 30th day and the decline thereafter are statistically significant ($p < .01$; rank test for independent samples). When comparing the results of the different experimental groups, it appears that rats lesioned at the 30th day consistently attain the highest median scores. Scores of rats lesioned at the 5th or 20th day range in between, and scores of rats lesioned at the 10th day are lowest when compared at the respective ages (for further details see Gramsbergen, 1981, 1982).

Essentially the same trends can be observed when comparing the incidence of locomotor handicaps in the different groups of rats. Handicaps become apparent from the 14th day onward in the rats lesioned at the 5th and 10th day. The incidence of most handicaps increases with age. However, the incidence of corkscrew movements and falling remains stable over age, and that of postural tremor decreases in all groups. The incidence of ataxia decreases in the groups of rats lesioned at the 20th and 30th day but remains the same in rats lesioned at the 5th or 10th day (Figure 2). For the groups of rats lesioned at the 20th or 30th day, it is remarkable that the more disabling handicaps (such as corkscrew movements and falling) either do not occur (in rats lesioned at the 30th day) or occur only infrequently (in rats lesioned at the 20th day). These severe handicaps occur more frequently in rats lesioned at the 5th or 10 day.

To summarize, we begin with the following point. During the first 14 days of life, no major neurological abnormalities occur despite a cerebellar hemispherectomy at the 5th or 10th day. The first signs of major handicaps become apparent at a stage in neuroontogeny at which rats normally start the adult-type locomotion: with their ventral body surface off the ground. Although this outcome might be a chronological coincidence, it suggests that cerebellar functioning

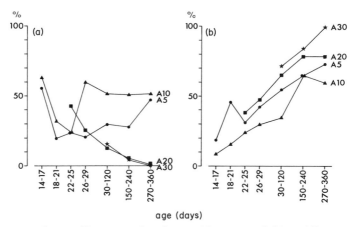

Figure 2. Incidence of locomotor handicaps, (a) *ataxia* and (b) *waddling gait*, in rats lesioned at the 5th, 10th, 20th, or 30th day. Because data appeared to be stable over time, the plots are based on four consecutive test sessions until the 29th day and on three sessions thereafter.

does not play a major role in the regulation of locomotor movements in the preceding life span. As far as the long-term effects of cerebellar hemispherectomy are concerned, two conclusions may be drawn. First, complete improvement does not occur in any of the experimental groups. Second, locomotion of rats lesioned at the 30th day remains less impaired than that of rats lesioned at earlier ages. Earlier reports about the effects of hemicerebellectomy or total cerebellectomy in puppies, young rabbits, and kittens suggested that a lesion in the newborn period jeopardizes locomotor behavior less than a similar lesion at a later age (Asratian, 1938; DeRenzi & Pompeiano, 1956; Di Giorgio, 1944). However, apart from differences in the species studied, it should be remembered that in these experiments, decerebrated animals with relatively short survival periods (of only a few weeks) were involved.

Might the more severe effects of cerebellar hemispherectomy at early ages be explained by the development of aberrant fiber connections? Aberrant projections in the rat after early hemicerebellectomy have been reported to emanate from the deep nuclei of the remaining cerebellar hemisphere onto the *ipsilateral* red nucleus and *ipsilateral* thalamic nuclei (Castro, 1978; Leong, 1978, 1980; Lim & Leong, 1975; Yamamoto, Kawaguchi, & Samejima, 1981). In normal rats, only contralateral projections onto these nuclei occur (Chan-Palay, 1977). Preliminary findings of our own have demonstrated aberrant rubrocerebellar fibers onto the ipsilateral anterior interpositus nucleus in the remaining hemishere. Normally, these fibers, which are collaterals of the rubrospinal tract, project onto the contralateral side (Huisman, Kuypers, & Verbrugh, 1981). In addition, aberrant fibers from the cerebral cortex—contralateral to the cerebellar lesion—project onto pontine nuclei (Leong, 1980). Castro and Smith (1979) reported a spinal projection onto the lateral vestibular nucleus—ipsilateral to the lesion—that is increased after neonatal hemicerebellectomy. They claim that these fibers are rerouted from what would have been their normal trajectory if the cerebellar hemisphere had not been removed. There are two findings common to the authors cited. First, the earlier the lesion is performed, the more pronounced the neuronal remodeling appears to be. Second, lesions after the 10th day produce hardly any aberrant fiber projections.

In rats with early hemicerebellectomy there is a striking impairment in locomotor behavior that is associated with extensive neuronal rearrangement. This finding raises the possibility that the neuronal remodeling adversely affects locomotor behavior. If so, an important problem to be solved is the quantitative relation of aberrant and normal fibers in rats lesioned at different ages. The double-labeling technique allows investigation of this problem. With this technique, two retrogradely transported fluorescent tracers are applied that label different features of the parent cells in different colors. Injection of one tracer in the normal and the other in the aberrant projection area enables quantification of the cells projecting onto the normal and "wrong" projection area. Because marked neuronal remodeling has been demonstrated in the cerebellorubral projection and because the red nuclei are important in the regulation and maintenance of tone in limbs (Kuypers, 1982), we decided to study this projection.

Quantitative Relations between Aberrant and Normal Cerebellorubal Connections

METHODS

In the following experiments, the strain of rats and the housing conditions were identical to those described in the first experiment. Animals lesioned at the 5th, 10th, 20th, and 30th days were studied, as well as a group lesioned at the 2nd day. A group of control rats was included. At adult age, true blue (0.3 μl, 2%) and nuclear yellow (0.15 μl, 1%) were injected stereotaxically into the red nuclei under general anaesthesia. After appropriate survival periods the animals were perfused, and the brains were removed and cut transversely (30-μm sections). Only material from experimental rats with appropriate cerebellar lesions was investigated (see preceding section). From these animals 1 out of 3 sections was studied with a fluorescence microscope at an excitation wavelength of 360 nm (Leitz Ploemopack; filter mirror system A). The injection sites from the experimental rats as well as from control rats were inspected for proper localization. Collection of material continued until there were 4 rats meeting all the criteria in each of the five experimental age groups and the control group (Table 1). (For further technical details, see Gramsbergen & IJkema-Paassen, 1982.)

RESULTS AND DISCUSSION

In control rats nearly 99% of labeled cells in the lateral nucleus and the interpositus nuclei are labeled from the contralateral red nucleus, with only about 1% labeled from the ipsilateral red nucleus. Less than 0.4% of the cells are double labled, indicating that these cells project bilaterally. These results, showing the projection from the lateral nucleus and the interpositus nuclei to be predominantly contralateral, confirm earlier reports in the literature (Chan-Palay, 1977).

In rats with a cerebellar hemispherectomy performed at the 2nd day, 70–80% of cells are still labeled by the tracer injected into the contralateral side, but 1 out of 3 to 4 cells are labeled from the ipsilateral side (Figure 3). In rats lesioned at the 5th day, the numbers of cells labeled from the ipsilateral side via aberrantly projecting fibers has decreased, and there are even fewer lesions at the 10th day. However, even in these rats 5% of cells in the lateral nucleus and about 10% in the interpositus nuclei are labeled from the abnormal projection area. In rats lesioned at the 20th or 30th day, the numbers of axons to the abnormal, ipsilateral red nucleus are comparable to the numbers found in control rats. Values obtained on the 2nd, 5th, and 10th days differ significantly from those found on the 20th and 30th days, whereas values from the 20th and 30th days do not differ significantly from those of the control rats.

Another striking result from this investigation is that more than

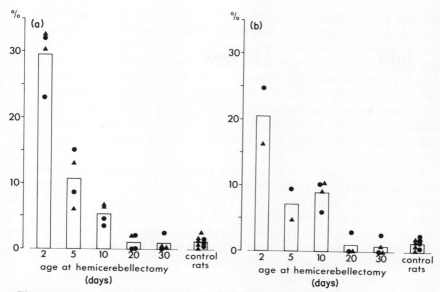

Figure 3. Percentages of retrograde-labeled cells in (a) lateral nucleus and (b) interpositus nuclei due to aberrant axons directed to the abnormal, ipsilateral red nucleus in the deep cerebellar nuclei. Circles represent values per rat by true blue injections; triangles values by nuclear yellow; columns show average values. (From Gramsbergen & IJkema-Paassen, 1982; by courtesy of Elsevier Biomedical Press.)

99% of the cells in the remaining deep cerebellar nuclei are labeled singly: either from the contralateral or from the ipsilateral side. This means that cells projecting via aberrant fibers onto the ipsilateral red nucleus stem from separate parent cells and are not collaterals from normally projecting fibers.

Our findings concerning the aberrantly projecting cerebellorubral fibers onto the ipsilateral side after early cerebellar hemispherectomy are in agreement with the literature (Castro, 1978; Leong, 1978, 1980; Lim & Leong, 1975). However, they extend this knowledge by demonstrating a clear-cut relationship between the age of lesioning and the proportion of rerouted axons. It appears that even in rats lesioned at the 10th day, considerable numbers of fibers still project onto the abnormal, ipsilateral red nucleus. One possible explanation for the presence of aberrantly projecting fibers is that they are remnants of an uncrossed projection that would normally be present at very early stages of brain maturation. In order to test this hypothesis, we injected a minute amount of [^{3}H]leucine into rats on their 1st day of life at one side in the lateral cerebellar nucleus. This radioactively labeled amino acid is transported orthogradely and can be made visible by means of autoradiography. The projection patterns in both red nuclei were studied after a survival period of 7 days. Results from this pilot experiment in 6 rats clearly show that there is a predominantly contralateral projection even at this early stage of brain maturation. Having excluded this possibility, the most plausible explanation seems to be that the aberrant projection is the result of a directional change of outgrowing fibers. This outcome might possibly be induced by an abundance of predilectional synaptic sites in the ipsilateral red nucleus.

The present data relate extremely well with results from our behavioral investigation in which rats lesioned at the 5th or 10th day show distinctly more impaired locomotion than animals lesioned at a later age. It should be kept in mind, however, that the present data refer only to cerebellorubral projections. The possibility cannot be ruled out that the occurrence of other aberrant projections after early cerebellar hemispherectomy has a different relation to the age at lesioning. Apart from this point, data obtained seem to point toward a causal relationship between neuronal remodeling and impaired locomotor behavior. However, the feasibility of this hypothesis depends heavily on a crucial unsolved problem: Are aberrant fibers functional, and what are the effects of neuronal remodeling on neurophysiological functioning? In order to elucidate this problem we decided to investigate electrical activity in the red nuclei in relation to locomotor behavior.

Electrical Activity in the Red Nuclei after Early Cerebellar Hemispherectomy

METHODS

In these experiments the strain of rats, housing conditions, and operation procedures were identical to those described in the previous sections. At adult age (180–360 days), insulated tungsten microelectrodes for chronic recording of extracellular activity were implanted under general anaesthesia. Pairs of electrodes (with an intertip distance of 1 mm) were implanted stereotaxically in the left and right red nucleus and in the remaining lateral cerebellar nucleus (in both lateral nuclei in control rats). Furthermore, triplets of electrodes were implanted in the left and right motor cortices. Only red nuclei recordings are considered here. A small, brass screw (diameter 1 mm) fastened into the skull served for both securing the electrodes and connecting the rat to the preamplifier common. Electrodes were connected to a miniature socket and fixed to the skull by dental acrylic. After the rats recovered from the implantation, the socket was connected to the amplifier system by a flexible cable. Electrical activity and the rat's movements were recorded on paper and on magnetic tape (Bell and Howell system 80). In addition, the rat's behavioral state and its movements were monitored by means of a TV camera so that they could be assessed and documented on the paper read-out. The behavioral-state definitions, based on behavioral criteria were

Quiet sleep: Eyes closed, regular respiration, no body movements.

Active sleep: Eyes closed, irregular respiration, eye movements, twitches in extremities.

Wakefulness: Eyes opened, movements may occur.

Neurophysiological signals were analyzed automatically (Perkin Elmer system 3220) for computation of power spectra and coherence functions.[1] Several recordings lasting several hours each were made per animal. After the last recording, electrode positions were marked by small electrolytic lesions, and positions of the electrodes as well as the cerebellar lesion in the experimental animals were verified histologically. For numbers of rats in the different age groups meeting all criteria, see Table 1.

RESULTS AND DISCUSSION

RED NUCLEI ACTIVITY IN NORMAL RATS

When rats are in quiet sleep, the red nuclei electrical activity shows high amplitudes (up to 300 μV) and predominantly low frequencies. Amplitudes decrease (90–120 μV) and higher frequencies occur when the rats awaken (but remain still), or when they enter active sleep.

---

[1]Power spectra give the power of the signal as a function of the frequency with a spectral resolution of 0.1 Hz; coherence functions are a measure of the probability that the electrical activities recorded from two areas are linearly related as a function of frequency.

During particular movements, a distinct pattern can be observed that is characterized by a regular 7.5–8.0 Hz-rhythm with amplitudes of about 40 μV (Figure 4). Movements that co-occur with this pattern include gross body movements and locomotion when rats are awake and movements for readjustment of body posture in periods of quiet sleep. However, other movements such as shortlasting isolated movements of extremities or head movements appear not to be accompanied by this particular pattern. Computation of 3-minute epochs of the recordings confirm these results. During quiet sleep, power is concentrated in the lower frequencies—from 0.1 to 3 Hz. During active sleep or quiet wakefulness, the power content of the signal has decreased and moreover has shifted toward the higher frequencies (higher than 5.0 Hz). When rats are active, or when they walk around, power spectra show a prominent peak at 7.5 to 8.0 Hz. A consistent finding in control rats is that power spectra from right and

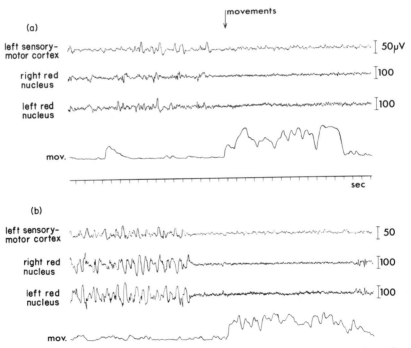

Figure 4. In (a) wakefulness and (b) quiet sleep, electrical activity in the right and left red nucleus (recorded unipolarly) and the electrocorticogram (at a depth of 1200 μm; recorded bipolarly) of a control rat, age 200 days (time constant = 0.3 sec). Movements are indicated by the traces (mov.).

left red nuclei are remarkably similar in all behavioral states. Co-herence functions are high at frequencies up to 3 Hz during quiet sleep, but this shifts toward a higher frequency range when rats are in active sleep or awake. (For further details, see Gramsbergen, Schuling, & Vos, in press.)

In order to study the electrical activity pattern during movements in more detail, spectra and coherence functions were computed from the signals just before and after the occurrence of these movements. The recording was divided into 10-sec epochs: two epochs in the 20 sec preceding the movement followed by 8 epochs during the move-ment and often the quiescence after the movement. Power spectra of the 10-sec epochs preceding the movement show the characteristics described earlier, depending on which behavioral state the animal is in. With the appearance of the rhythm, a peak occurs in the power spectra of the left and right red nucleus at the specific pattern fre-quency (Figure 5).

RED NUCLEI ACTIVITY IN LESIONED RATS

When lesioned rats are in quiet sleep, active sleep, or awake but quiescent, red nuclei signals do not show clear-cut differences from recordings in normal rats. This holds true for both red nuclei and for rats of all age groups. Power spectra demonstrate the behavioral-state-related patterns that have been described for control rats. How-ever, when comparing power spectra from left and right red nuclei, differences between sides become apparent. Humps occur in one spectrum with a dip in the other, and vice versa. These differences, which are neither consistent nor related to the side of the lesion, indicate that electrical activity in the two red nuclei is unrelated. This finding is confirmed by the computation of coherence functions, which have decreased considerably.

When movements occur in rats lesioned at the 20th day, recordings from both red nuclei show a pattern that is identical to that found in control rats. Power spectra of both red nuclei signals show a peak within the normal range (7.5–8.0 Hz) and coherence functions are high at these frequencies. In rats lesioned at the 5th or 10th day, a patterning in the electrical activity occurs, but the peak in the power spectra has shifted toward a distinctly lower frequency (i.e., 5.6–6.4 Hz). Coherence functions are high at these frequencies. In rats le-sioned at the 2nd day, no change in patterning in relation to move-ments occurs. This striking finding is supported by the computation

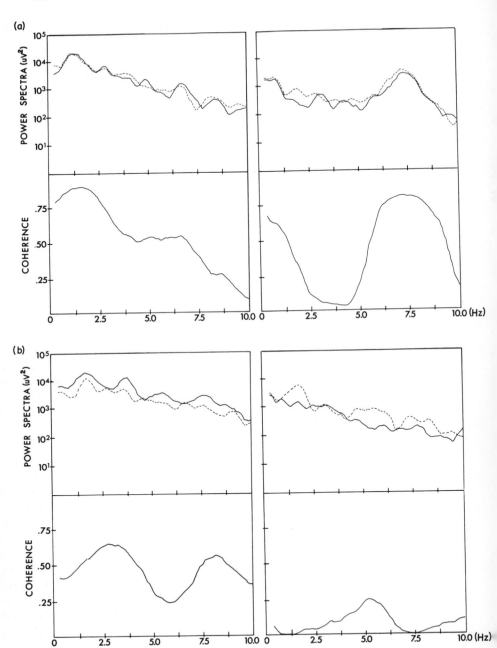

of power spectra (Figure 5). Spectra do not show a consistent profile during movements, and left–right differences are remarkable. Coherence functions remain low at all frequencies.

COHERENCE FUNCTIONS OVER ABERRANT PROJECTIONS

The electrical activity in both lateral nuclei in control rats is characterized by high amplitudes and low frequencies during quiet sleep and low amplitudes and higher frequencies during active sleep and wakefulness. A striking difference with the red nuclei electrical activity pattern described earlier is that no specific patterning during movements occurs. Coherence functions between left lateral nucleus and right red nucleus, and between the other contralaterally connected pair, show high coherences in the lower frequencies during quiet sleep. During active sleep and wakefulness, high coherences have shifted toward the higher frequencies. In control rats, coherences between the ipsilaterally connected nuclei remain low and do not surpass chance level.

In rats with a cerebellar hemispherectomy performed at the 2nd or 5th day, coherence functions between the remaining lateral nucleus and its *ipsilateral* red nucleus are increased and in general well above chance level: during quiet sleep in the low frequency range and during active sleep and wakefulness in the higher frequency range. In rats lesioned at the 10th or 20th day, coherences between these activities remain low, as in control rats. In rats with a cerebellar hemispherectomy at the 2nd or 5th day, 30 and 11%, respectively, of the fibers from the lateral nucleus are rerouted toward the ipsilateral red nucleus (see previous section). Our electrophysiological data demonstrate that these aberrant fibers induce correlated electrical activity. This indicates, therefore, that aberrant fiber projections are indeed functioning. However, in rats lesioned at the 10th day, coherence functions of activity in the remaining lateral nucleus and its ipsilateral red nucleus remain low, although they are connected via 6%

Figure 5. Power spectra and coherence functions of the red nuclei electrical activity. (a) plots from a control rat; (b) plots from a rat lesioned at the 2nd day. In both cases the left plots are computed during quiet sleep, the right plots during movements thereafter. Power in μV^2; broken line, spectrum from the right red nucleus; continuous line, spectrum from the left red nucleus.

of aberrant cerebellorubral fibers. These data further indicate that a certain critical number of fibers is required for inducing coherent electrical activity.

Power spectra of activity from both red nuclei during the rat's quiescence are markedly different in lesioned rats of all age groups. It can be concluded that these differences are due to the loss of one cerebellar hemisphere and its nuclei. However, in early lesioned rats, both red nuclei are connected via the remaining lateral nucleus through normally and aberrantly projecting fibers. Despite the fact that these fibers are functioning, no coherent activity in the red nuclei is observed. Only one conclusion is possible here: namely, that the neurons in the deep cerebellar nuclei that make aberrant connections to the ipsilateral red nucleus are unrelated in their activity to those neurons with normally projecting fibers. This conclusion is further supported by our finding that fibers projecting normally onto the contralateral side and fibers projecting aberrantly onto the ipsilateral side stem from separate parent cells.

The main finding from the electrophysiological experiments relates to the age specificity of the lesion effects.

1. In rats lesioned at the 2nd day, specific patterning in red nuclei electrical activity during movement is absent.
2. In rats lesioned at the 5th or 10th day, patterning occurs, but with a lower frequency.
3. In rats lesioned at the 20th day, patterning occurs that is closely similar to that in control rats.

These findings correspond closely to the degree of neuronal rearrangement and to the degree of locomotor impairment.

Conclusion

Behavioral investigations into the effects of cerebellar hemispherectomy have revealed that lesioning at the 5th or 10th day leads to more impairment in locomotor behavior than similar lesions at a later age. Hemicerebellectomy at early ages leads to extensive neuronal remodeling, and we have demonstrated a clear-cut relationship between the age at lesioning and the degree of neuronal remodeling. In addition, we have demonstrated these fiber connections to be functional and neurophysiological phenomena related to locomotor behavior to be distinctly abnormal. We conclude that neuronal remodeling after early hemispherectomy is a causal factor in locomotor impairment.

Our results contribute to the accumulating evidence that age-related neuronal rearrangement leads to deleterious effects on later functioning. Neuronal remodeling in the central nervous system is not restricted to early stages of brain maturation; it may also occur after lesions at adult age (for review see, Cotman & Nieto-Sampedro, 1982). However, collateral sprouting at this stage has been observed only within a restricted area. The effect of this collateral sprouting on behavior seems limited compared with the dramatic effects after lesions in the neonate. There have been a few examples showing that aberrant fiber systems following neonatal lesions in the rat have positive effects on later functioning (e.g., Hicks & d'Amato, 1970; Prendergast & Shusterman, 1982). Our data, however, stress once more (see also, Schneider, 1979) that the dogma of the young brain having a greater compensational capacity is not generally valid.

Acknowledgments

The advice, criticism, and comments of H. F. R. Prechtl, J. B. Hopkins, and M. J. O'Brien are greatfully acknowledged.

This research is supported by Programme Grant 13-51-91 from the Foundation for Medical Research (FUNGO), which is subsidized by the Organization for the Advancement of Pure Research (ZWO).

References

Almli, C. R., & Fisher, R. S. (1977). Infant rats: sensorimotor ontogeny and effects of substantia nigra destruction. *Brain Research Bulletin, 2*, 425–459.

Altman, J., & Anderson, W. J. (1971). Irradiation of the cerebellum in infant rats with low-level X-ray: histological and cytological effects during infancy and adulthood. *Experimental Neurology, 30*, 492–509.

Asratian, E. A. (1938). Beitrage zur Alterscharakteristik des Kleinhirns. *Fiziolohichnyi Zhurnal (Kiev), 19*, 448–453.

Bregman, B. S., & Goldberger, M. E. (1982). Anatomical plasticity and sparing of function after spinal cord damage in neonatal cats. *Science, 217*, 553–554.

Castro, A. J. (1978). Projections of the superior cerebellar peduncle in rats and the development of new connections in response to neonatal hemicerebellectomy. *Journal of Comparative Neurology, 178*, 611–628.

Castro, A. J., & Smith, D. E. (1979). Plasticity of spinovestibular projections in response to hemicerebellectomy in newborn rats. *Neuroscience Letters, 12*, 69–74.

Chan Palay, V. (1977). *Cerebellar dentate nucleus*. New York: Springer.

Cotman, C. W., & Nieto-Sampedro, M. (1982). Brain function, synapse renewal, and plasticity. *Annual Review of Psychology, 33*, 371–401.

DeRenzi, C., & Pompeiano, O. (1956). La comparsa dell'attivita tonica della corteccia e dei nuclei del cerbeletto nel gatto neonato. *Archives of Biological Science, 40*, 523–534.

Di Giorgio, A. M. (1944). Sulla organizzazione della attivita cerebellari nei mammiferi neonati. *Archivio di Fisiologia, 43*, 47–63.

Gramsbergen, A. (1976). EEG development in normal and undernourished rats. *Brain Research, 105*, 287–308.

Gramsbergen, A. (1981). Locomotor behaviour after cerebellar lesions in the young rat. In: H. Flohr and W. Precht (Eds.), *Neuronal plasticity in sensorimotor systems: Mechanisms of recovery from lesions* (pp. 324–336). Berlin: Springer.

Gramsbergen, A. (1982). The effects of cerebellar hemispherectomy in the young rat. I. Behavioural sequelae. *Behavior and Brain Research, 6*, 85–92.

Gramsbergen, A., & IJkema-Paassen J. (1982). CNS plasticity after hemicerebellectomy in the young rat. Quantitative relations between aberrant and normal cerebello-rubral projections. *Neuroscience Letters, 33*, 129–134.

Gramsbergen, A., Schuling, F. H., & Vos, J. E. (in press). Electrical activity in the red nuclei of rats and the effects of hemicerebellectomy at young ages.

Gramsbergen, A., Schwartze, P., & Prechtl, H. F. R. (1970). The postnatal development of behavioral states in the rat. *Developmental Psychobiology, 3*, 267–280.

Hicks, S. P., & d'Amato, C. J. (1970). Motor-sensory and visual behavior after hemispherectomy in newborn and mature rats. *Experimental Neurology, 29*, 416–438.

Huisman, A. M., Kuypers, H. G. J. M., & Verbrugh, C. A. (1981). Quantitative differences in collateralization of the descending spinal pathways from red nucleus and other brainstem cell groups in rat as demonstrated with the multiple fluorescent retrograde tracer technique. *Brain Research, 209*, 271–286.

Kuypers, H. G. J. M. (1982). A new look at the organization of the motor system. In H. G. J. M. Kuypers, & G. F. Martin (Eds.), *Descending pathways to the spinal cord* (pp. 381–403). Amsterdam: Elsevier.

Leong, S. K. (1978). Plasticity of cerebellar efferents after neonatal lesions in albino rats. *Neuroscience Letters, 7*, 281–289.

Leong, S. K. (1980). A qualitative electron microscopic study of the cortico-pontine projections after neonatal cerebellar hemispherectomy. *Brain Research, 194*, 299–310.

Lim, K. H., & Leong, S. K. (1975). Aberrant bilateral projections from the dentate and interposed nucleus in albino rats after neonatal lesions. *Brain Research, 96*, 133–154.

Prendergast, J., & Shusterman, R. (1982). Normal development of motor behavior in the rat and effect of midthoracic spinal hemisection at birth on that development. *Experimental Neurology, 78*, 176–189.

Prendergast, J., Shusterman, R., & Phillips, T. (1982). Comparison of the effect of midthoracic spinal hemisection at birth or in adulthood on motor behavior in the adult rat. *Experimental Neurology, 78*, 190–204.

Schneider, G. E. (1979). Is it really better to have your brain lesion early? Revision of the Kennard Principle. *Neuropsychologia, 17*, 557–584.

Schneider, G. E., & Jhaveri, S. R. (1974). Neuroanatomical correlates of spared or altered function after brain lesions in the newborn hamster. In D. G. Stein, J. J.

Rosen, & N. Butters (Eds.), *Plasticity and recovery of function in the central nervous system* (pp. 65–109). London: Academic Press.
Yamamoto, T., Kawaguchi, S., & Samejima, A. (1981). Electrophysiological studies on plasticity of cerebellothalamic neurons in rats following neonatal hemicerebellectomy. *Japanese Journal of Physiology, 31,* 217–224.

10

Neonatal Cerebral Hemispherectomy: A Model for Postlesion Reorganization of the Brain

Jaime R. Villablanca,
J. Wesley Burgess,
and Bobby Jo Sonnier

Introduction

Following the pioneer experiments in dogs by Goltz (1888) and the first therapeutic ablations by Dandy (1933), it has been widely recognized that removal of one cerebral hemisphere results in outstanding recovery of neurological functions in all species studied, including man (Ueki, 1966; Zulch & Micheler, 1978), monkey (White, Shreiner, Hughes, MacCarty, & Grindlay, 1959), cat (Bogen, 1974; Villablanca, Marcus, & Olmstead, 1976a), dog (Goltz, 1888), and rat (Hicks & D'Amato, 1970). Unfortunately, few investigators have attempted quantification; therefore, their results are difficult to compare and their observations are often only ancedotal. Terminology also complicates the interpretation of the reports, because removals have been performed to different degrees of completeness. In this chapter, the term *hemispherectomy* exclusively denotes the removal of the neocortex, neostriatum, and most of the limbic system on one side (hemitelencephalon), but excludes any parts of the diencephalon.

The extensive recoveries seen in even a cursory inspection of hemispherectomized subjects have fascinated us from the very beginning

(Teasdall, Villablanca, & Magladery, 1965), and this feeling appears to be shared by most investigators. However, efforts to shed light on the basic neural processes that may account for the amelioration have not been proportional to that sense of perplexity. In a first attempt to understand the functional and anatomical consequences of hemispherectomy, we demonstrated heightened discharges and lower thresholds for monosynaptic components of the stretch reflex on the side contralateral to a long-standing ablation in cats (Teasdall et al., 1965). Although this pattern persisted after spinal cord transection, and therefore was firmly imprinted on segmental organization, we could not demonstrate sprouting of dorsal roots, a possible basis for the electrophysiological changes (Liu & Chambers, 1958), in our material using the protargol stain (Nathanson, 1965).

Persistent changes at the level of the brainstem were suggested later by our studies in diencephalic cats (Norman, Villablanca, Brown, Schwafel, & Buchwald, 1974; Villablanca & Marcus, 1972). In some of these animals, a two-stage removal of the telencephalon was performed; that is, following recovery from a first hemispherectomy, the remaining hemisphere was removed. To our surprise, the side contralateral to the second ablation was now clearly more neurologically impaired, and this functional asymmetry did not disappear during the ensuing few months of survival. This observation directed our attention to the brainstem as a site for possible anatomical remodeling.

In our ongoing research, we use neonatal and adult hemispherectomy in the cat as a model to understand the neuroanatomical and neurophysiological basis for the self-healing properties of the mammalian brain. The rationale for this approach is that extensive brain lesions followed by an unequivocal recovery, as seen in hemispherectomy, should render the basic processes involved in the repair much easier to identify, localize, and quantify. This key feature of the design should also facilitate study of the influence of interventions (e.g., motor training) upon the hypothetical central nervous system remodeling, as well as provide a firm framework for the demonstration of the seemingly elusive structure–function correlations.

In the first part of this chapter, we report the results of comparing the neurological and behavioral recovery of both hemispherectomized adult cats and neonatal kittens. In the second part, we summarize the current status of our research that demonstrates reorganization in the brain of these animals.

Neurological and Behavioral Studies

GENERAL METHODS

SUBJECTS, SURGERY, MAINTENANCE

We used 12 kittens (HEMI K) that received hemispherectomy at a median age of 8 days (range, 5–25) and 14 adult cats (HEMI C). In all cases, the left hemisphere was removed.

Hemispherectomy is a standard technique in our laboratory and results in practically no mortality or morbidity. Under deep anesthesia and hypothermia, the calvarium over the hemisphere is removed and the underlying dura mater is cut. Using blunt dissection with a suction pipette and under a fiber-optics headlight, the hemisphere is separated from the thalamus at the level of the internal capsule and caudate nucleus. After the pedicle of the middle cerebral artery is ligated and sectioned, the entire hemisphere is removed in a block. The ablation (Figure 1) includes the neocortex and medial walls of the hemisphere, the neostriatum and the hippocampus, except for its ventromedial portion, as well as variable ventromedial portions of the rhinencephalon. The diencephalon and mesencephalon are spared and only occasionally does the dorsal thalamus sustain accidental injury.

For the night after surgery, HEMI K are maintained in a thermostatically controlled incubator. Supplementary or intragastric feeding may be occasionally required for a day. The animals are reared with the littermates until weaning (2 months of age), when they are transferred to larger colony cages, and at about 5–6 months of age they are moved to standard individual cages. Only routine postoperative care is necessary for the HEMI C.

GENERAL HISTOLOGICAL PROCEDURES

At the end of experiments, each animal is deeply anesthetized with barbiturate and sacrificed by pressure-controlled cardiac perfusion of saline followed by 10% neutral buffered formalin. Brains are immediately removed, carefully inspected, and photographed from several angles. After 2 to 4 weeks postfixation in formalin, each brain is appropriately blocked, immersed in 20% ethanol overnight, frozen, and serially sectioned in the coronal or sagittal planes at a thickness

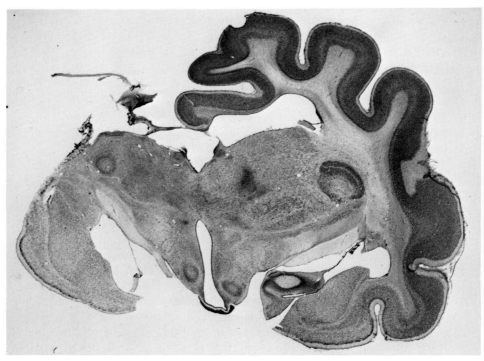

Figure 1. Frontal section at approximately A 8.0 (Jasper & Ajmone-Marsan, 1954) of the brain of an adult cat with removal of the left cerebral hemisphere at 8 days of age to show extent of a typical ablation. Note considerable atrophy of the left thalamus. Thionine stain.

of 50 μm. Alternate sections are used for autoradiographic (*vide infra*) and thionine staining.

To verify the extent and gross topography of the hemispherectomy, the lesions in each brain are reconstructed on at least eight coronal plates from the atlas of Reinoso-Suarez (1961) at regularly spaced rostro-caudal planes. For this purpose, sections corresponding to these planes are projected on copies of plates of the atlas and the lesion is drawn. In general, the lesions were well-placed as described in the previous section. In only 5 HEMI K and 6 HEMI C was there some accidental damage to the dorsal thalamus. In all animals, the left hemithalamus was considerably reduced in size due to atrophy consecutive to extensive degeneration of the projection cells, as has been repeatedly described following extensive cortical ablations (Macchi, Quattrini, Chinzari, & Capocchi, 1975). Whether there is a differential atrophy in the two age groups has not been assessed. For additional technical details see Villablanca and Marcus (1972), Villablanca, Marcus, Olmstead, and Avery (1976b), and Villablanca, Olmstead, Levine, and Marcus (1978).

STATISTICAL ANALYSIS

Continuous numerical data were processed using analyses of variance (ANOVAs) with repeated measures and unweighted mean models where applicable (Winer, 1972). Ordinal and frequency data were analyzed using nonparametric tests (Siegel, 1972) including χ^2.

TESTING METHODS AND RESULTS

All animals were studied starting immediately after surgery and continuing into adulthood (HEMI K), or for at least 6 months postsurgery (HEMI C) (Burgess, Villablanca, Olmstead, & Levine, 1982). Due to limitations in space, only the results collected during the late, stable state are described in detail, and only a brief statement about early recovery is included. Except as indicated, the results of long-term recovery were derived from 10 HEMI K, kept for over 1 year and hence adults, and 14 HEMI C, studied for at least 6 months after surgery (4 for over a year). During this period, all animals were given the neurological test battery every 1–3 months and other tests as described in the following. Additional details about our testing methods are in Villablanca *et al.* (1976a) and in Villablanca and Olmstead (1979).

All HEMI K showed normal growth; that is, their adult weight was similar to that of their littermates. Few changes in test scores were seen either in HEMI Ks or Cs after the 6th month postsurgery, and therefore the scores for all tests from that date onward were used for statistical comparisons. In Table 1 the mean scores and ranges are shown for comparison of relative group differences, with statistical probability values shown in the right column.

MOVEMENT AND POSTURE

1. As seen in Table 1, HEMI C showed more right-sided paresis than HEMI K as follows. The limb's attitude and strength were evaluated while the animals walked spontaneously in an open field, and the following scores were given: 0 = no impairment; 1 = minor or irregular slipoff and/or dragging of the right limbs; 2 = clear and reliable right limb weakness. The latter was not seen in HEMI K.

TABLE 1

Neurobehavioral Impairments after Hemispherectomy

Test	Kitten-lesioned			Cat-lesioned			Probability: kitten vs. cat
	Score[a]	n	Range	Score[a]	n	Range	
Movement—posture tests							
R. limb paresis	0.4	10	0–1	1.8	14	1–2	.0005
R. limb abduction	1.0	10	1–2	2.2	14	2–3	.0002
Eyelid asymmetry	0.2	10	0–1	1.8	14	1–3	.0007
R. limb tonus	−1.2	10	0–(−2)	1.6	14	1–3	.008
R. limb posture	−0.1	10	0–(−2)	1.8	14	1–3	.025
Spontaneous l. turning	1.0	10	0–3	2.9	14	2–3	.0009
Limb placing reactions							
Visual placing	1.1	10	1–2	1.9	14	1–2	.0002
Chin placing	1.1	10	1–2	2.0	14	1–2	.0001
Proprioceptive placing	1.6	10	1–3	2.4	14	2–3	.007
Plank walking	1.3	10	0–3	4.4	14	2–5	.0015
Sensory tests							
Tactile facial response	0.1	10	0–1	0.8	6	1–2	.004
R. paw withdrawal (water test) (sec to withdraw: 38°)	4.8	7	0.2–16.7	27.5	5	17.5–30.0	<.0001
Intact:	0.2	6	0.2–0.2				
Pupil asymmetry	0.2	10	0–1	1.0	12	0–2	.02
Neurobehavioral tests							
%R. Paw use (string test)	44.4	9	42.5–50.2	36.1	7	23.3–40.6	.0003
Intact:	47.9	17	43.5–53.2				
Food retrieval (# sessions to criterion)	1.0	4	1–1	7.6	7	2–13	.001
T maze reversal (reversals/10 trials)	5.0	4	0.7–8.7	2.9	11	0.5–5.8	<.0001
Intact:	7.6	8	3.7–9.5				

[a]Unless specified under the test description, these indicate mean scores.

Right forelimb weakness was further evaluated by estimating the angle of abduction of the extended forelimb in relation to the body while the animal was held by the scruff of the neck and pushed forward across a textured tile floor. Under these conditions the left (normal) limb hops while resisting the forward displacement. Scoring: 0 = no abduction; 1 = less than 45° abduction angle; 2 = 45–90° angle; 3 = more than 90° abduction angle. HEMI K had few 2 and no 3 scores.

Right facial weakness was shown in HEMI C by a larger (lagging) eyelid opening and a brisker, more marked closure of the left eyelids after any facial stimuli: Scoring: 0 = no right–left asymmetry on eyelid opening; 1 = opening 0–2 mm larger at right; 2 = eyelid opening 2–3 mm larger at right; 3 = opening at right is 3 mm or more larger than at left. Only 1 scores were seen in HEMI Ks.

2. The muscle tone of the limbs was tested by passive mobilization with the animal held by the scruff of the neck. Compared to the left limbs, in the HEMI K the tone of the right limbs was either normal or decreased, whereas in the HEMI C it was increased. With the animal in the same testing position, the posture of the forelimbs tended to be adducted and extended in HEMI C and adducted and flexed in HEMI K. Therefore, the scores ranged from +3 = markedly extended to −3 = markedly flexed.

3. Turning bias: During spontaneous walking in an open field, all HEMI animals tended to make more left than right turns, and this bias clearly predominated in HEMI C. After at least 10 spontaneous turns, the scoring was: 0 = about same number of turns to each side; 1 = 50–70% turns to left; 2 = 79–90% turns to the left; 3 = about 100% turns to the left.

4. Usage of the forepaws: Initially, for the young kittens, we counted the spontaneous, directed movements of the forepaws. Later we used a string test, which markedly increased the number of movements elicited; statistically the left versus right limb counts obtained by either method were equivalent ($p = .54$), and therefore we continued using only this more efficient test. For the string test, we used a 10–30-cm string manipulandum, which was presented in the visual field, alternating between left and right to avoid bias, with the animals in their home cages. In Table 1, the number of responses with the right paw is expressed as mean percentage of the total number of responses counted (HEMI K age, 9–65 weeks). Compared to intact animals, both lesioned groups showed a significantly lower percentage of responses with the right paw, but, as seen in Table 1, the bias

to use the left, unimpaired paw was significantly stronger for the HEMI C.

Limb placing reactions were tested according to our described methods (Villablanca & Olmstead, 1979; Villablanca *et al.*, 1976b). None of the animals recovered *contact*-placing reactions of the right limbs. Clear cat–kitten differences were found in other components of the reactions. Visual and chin placing were almost invariably absent for the right forepaw of HEMI C (score = 1). Proprioceptive placing was either absent (score = 3) in the HEMI C or required a limb extension angle of 90° or more (score = 2). In contrast, HEMI K frequently placed with a limb extension angle between 45° and 90° (score = 1) or less (score = 0). As a consequence, the ability to walk on a narrow plank was markedly impaired in HEMI C such that they either fell as soon as they started to move or were barely able to traverse the plank, whereas HEMI K could traverse the plank easily and even do turns without falling.

1. To assess cutaneous sensation we used a Rowan model RA 100 aesthesiometer calibrated to provide a 2-g contact pressure. When applied to the right side of the face of the HEMI K, usually both the forehead and the cheek areas responded, although the response was weaker and with longer latency than in normals (score = 1). In contrast, in the HEMI C only the lower portion of the face responded regularly (score = 2). The same method was used to study the withdrawal response of the limbs on food pad stimulation. In both groups, although more reliably in the HEMI C, the right limbs did not react to a stimulus that was constantly effective on the left limbs.

A more sensitive water test to evaluate cutaneous sensation was also developed (Feeney & Wir, 1979). The right forepaw was immersed in water to wrist level, and time to withdrawal (to a maximum of 30 sec) at each of 10 different temperatures was measured for at least three trials. Intact cats withdrew the paw almost immediately at all temperatures but, in contrast, the time for withdrawal was prolonged for both HEMI groups. As seen in Figure 2, the delay was maximal for temperatures ranging between 30 and 50°C, and

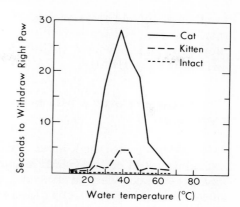

Figure 2. Time to withdrawal of the paw (ordinate) from water at temperatures indicated on the abscissa.

within that range the time to withdrawal by HEMI C was 4–6 times longer than by HEMI K, with a peak differential effect at the thermoneutral level of 38°C.

2. Our standard tests for vision (Villablanca *et al.*, 1976a) suggested that none of our HEMI animals could see with the right eye. The visual palpebral reflex was regularly absent at the right. Visual tracking of objects moving horizontally in the visual field from the left stopped at midline, and visual placing was absent when the left eye was blindfolded. However, anecdotal observations of left-eye blindfolded HEMI animals walking on counters or tables suggested that they had some perception of visual cliff and that this might be better in the HEMI K. Anisocoria was noted in HEMI subjects, with the right pupil clearly (score = 2) or marginally (score = 1) larger than the left. This difference was more marked in HEMI C and was not correlated with accidental damage to the left lateral geniculate.

SPATIAL REVERSAL LEARNING

The ability for spatial reversal learning was evaluated (HEMI K, n = 4; HEMI C, n = 11) in a walk-through T maze by an investigator blind to the surgical intervention. Each cat's preferred turning direction was ascertained during five daily sessions of 10 trials, in which responses to the left or the right side of the maze were reinforced with food. All HEMI animals were strongly biased to turn to the left side of the maze. Thereafter, each cat was trained for an additional 50 reversal trials, during which the animal was reinforced for responses to the side opposite its initial preference. Table 1 shows the mean number of correct responses in all five reversal sessions. Intact cats readily switched direction, whereas HEMI animals were significantly more resistant; however, HEMI K were significantly less resistant to switching than HEMI C.

DEVELOPMENT OF PAW PREFERENCES IN INTACT
AND HEMI K

The ability to use the forepaws was measured by the string test (see above) was studied in 4 HEMI K and in 5 littermate controls in which paw preferences were measured 2–4 times weekly between 5 and 2 weeks of age. Intact kittens did not show any left–right bias during the 6-month period. The same was true for HEMI K, but only until about 9 weeks of age. Thereafter, there was a significant, increasing bias against use of the paw contralateral to the ablation. Age, therefore, was significantly correlated with the development of asymmetric usage of the paws in HEMI Ks ($p < .001$).

EFFECT OF TRAINING ON PAW USAGE

Once again, due to space limitations, we here only report that: (1) we have preliminary data demonstrating that the bias to preferentially use the left paw on the string test can be easily reversed in HEMI cats and kittens, and (2) in a more discrete task for paw usage consisting of food retrieval from a selectively positioned narrow feeder, HEMI C show a marked impairment such that in order to perform directed movements with the right paw they require restriction (but not immobilization) of the left paw, a mean of 7.6 training sessions (30 minutes each), extensive food deprivation, and at least 1 month recovery postsurgery. In contrast, HEMI Ks are easily trainable in the food-getting paradigm (Table 1; Burgess & Villablanca, 1983).

The early postsurgical recovery also is more marked for a HEMI K. For example, all kittens are active and nursing the day after surgery. They show a strong bias to turn and circle to the left, and to arch the body and neck toward that side when held by the scruff of the neck. However, these postural biases quickly attenuate such that by the 5th–10th days postsurgery they are either weak or not apparent at all. Indeed, by the end of the 1st postsurgical month, nothing obvious permits differentiating the HEMI K from their intact littermates. HEMI Cs, in contrast, are unable to stand steadily for about 2–4 days and they often fall to the right. They also show clear right paresis as well as tonus–posture changes such that by the end of the 1st month they appear distinctly neurologically abnormal and demonstrate the highest scores in most of the tests described.

Anatomical Studies

METHODS

For analysis of brain reorganization, we selected the autoradiographic method for tracing of anterograde axonal transport of tritiated amino acids. The advantages of this technique are reviewed in Edwards and Hendrickson (1981) and in Jones (1978). The pericruciate motor area of the cortex and the nucleus interpositus of the cerebellum were targets for injection of the radioactive material. Pathways originating in these sites are unilateral in the cat and provide the opportunity of examining any "new" projections that cross the midline to reinnervate areas partially denervated by lesions. In addition, these pathways overlap in some of their terminal target areas, for example, the red nucleus (RN) and the thalamus, which is convenient for examination of possible interactive remodeling.

SURGICAL AND INJECTION PROCEDURES

Under thiopental sodium anesthesia and with aseptic techniques, all cats received injections of a 1:1 mixture of [³H]leucine–proline at 50 µCi/µl. Injections were placed stereotaxically using a 1.0-µl Hamilton syringe equipped with a 26-gauge needle mounted in a microinjector (Kopf model 5000) attached to the stereotaxic carrier.

1. Cortical injections:The animal was positioned in the stereotaxic frame in such a way that the surface of the pericruciate cortex was in the horizontal plane, and an ample craniotomy was performed over the right frontal pole. Starting 2–3 mm from the midline to avoid the medial supplementary cortical areas, which have sparse contralateral projections (Rinvik, 1968), 4–6 injections (depending on the length of the sulcus) were made 2 mm apart, 1.0–1.5 mm in front of and behind the cruciate sulcus, respectively, at a 3-mm depth (Figure 3). The volume of each injection ranged from 0.3 to 0.6 µl, depending on the estimated thickness of cortical lamina V at each of the injection

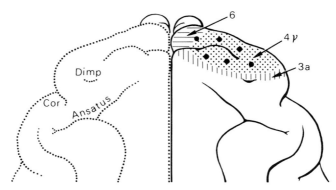

Figure 3. Dorsal view of the frontal areas of the cat brain to show the location of the injection sites (black dots) of tritiated amino acids in relation to the Hassler and Muhs-Clement (1964) cytoarchitectural fields. (Cor) coronal sulcus; (dimp) postcruciate dimple.

sites, and proceeded at the rate of 0.1 μl/5 minutes, allowing 10 minutes of equilibration at the beginning and end of each injection.

2. Cerebellar injections: Using the same surgical procedures, the syringe was mounted at a 30° posterior angle and the tip of the needle was aimed at either the anterior or posterior divisions of the right nucleus interpositus at the following stereotaxic coordinates (Snider & Niemer, 1969): for anterior nucleus interpositus, A 8.0, L 4.0, and H + 1.0; for posterior nucleus interpositus, A 9.5, L 4.0 and H + 1.0. The total volume of the injections was 0.2 μl and it was deposited in 0.05-μl increments with 3-minute intervals.

HISTOLOGY AND DATA ANALYSIS

The animals were sacrificed 5 days after the injections and, following the procedures described earlier, every fourth 50-μm brain section was mounted on a gelatinized slide and processed for autoradiography (methods of Cowan, Gottlieb, Hendrickson, Price & Woolsey, 1972). After a 6-week exposure period, the sections were developed, stained with thionine, and cover-slipped. Adjacent control sections were prepared without emulsion coating and stained with thionine. Using both light- and dark-field illumination, injection sites and terminal fields were reconstructed from appropriate sections by making serial drawings with the aid of a drawing tube attached to a Wild M5A stereomicroscope. Specific nuclear groups were identified by using the atlases of Snider and Niemer (1961) and Berman (1968). Illustrative sections of the terminal fields were photographed at a higher magnification with a Leitz Dialux 20 microscope.

For quantitative analysis of the terminal fields in the RN, we used the following methods. Eight frontal sections at 0.5-mm intervals through the RN from A 3.0 to A 6.5 were selected from each brain. Each of the sections was projected, at constant magnification and distance, over a 5-mm-square grid paper under dark-field illumination. The contour of the RN was reconstructed, and for the assessment of terminal distribution, each square inside the RN was visually scored for terminal-field density on a 4-point scale: 0 = no terminal fields, that is, equal to background; 1 = minimal; 2 = medium; 3 = maximal relative density. The RN on each section was divided into four quadrants: dorsolateral, dorsomedial, ventrolateral, and ventromedial. The total number of grid squares overlying the RN as well as the number of squares containing each of the four estimated density scores (or "type of observation") were counted per quadrant of the RN in each of the eight anterior to posterior (A–P) sections across both groups of animals and entered on a computer.

The graphic display SAS graphic G-Plot computer program provided three-dimensional blocks (Figure 4), each showing, at the bottom, the mean number of grid squares that overlay the surface of the RN in each of the quadrants, with the proportion of the mean number of grid squares for each of the terminal density scores indicated by the different shadings within each block. For example, if a larger proportion of Observation Type 3 is seen for a block in a given quadrant, this indicates a larger terminal density for that particular quadrant.

With this approach to statistical analysis, the grid squares may be treated (1) homogeneously, as areas of the RN showing or not showing terminal fields, or (2) heterogeneously, as proportions of the RN exhibiting different terminal densities; that is, different density scores. The computer statistics used for area comparisons were from BMDPO 2V and BMDP 3S.3 programs (Kruskal–Wallis and Mann–Whitney), and those for the density-score comparisons were from the BMDP 3S.1 program (Wilcoxon). Both are available from the computer facilities of our Mental Retardation Research Center at UCLA (D. Guthrie, director).

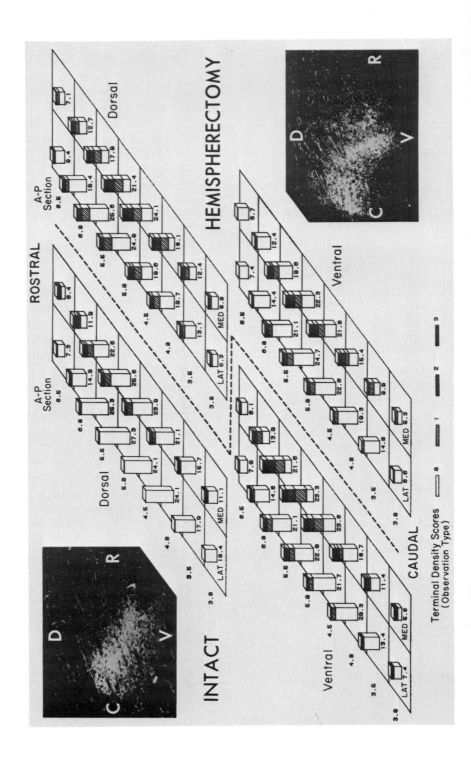

RESULTS

PROJECTIONS FROM THE RIGHT
PERICRUCIATE CORTEX

For these studies we used 6 *kittens*, which received left hemi-spherectomy at a median age of 8.5 days (range, 8–25) and were sacrificed when all were over 14 months of age. The control group was 10 intact adult cats.

At the injection sites, the radioactive material typically filled most of the dorsal pericruciate areas 4 and 3a of Hassler and Muhs-Clement (1964) but excluded, in most cases, approximately the medial quarter of the anterior (area 6) and posterior sigmoid gyri (Figure 3). In 4 intact control cats and 2 HEMI K, the latter areas were partially labeled, including deep layers of small portions of gyri located in the medial surface of the hemisphere. The labeling in the lateral sigmoid gyrus extended into parts of the upper bank of the coronal sulcus (area 3a) in the majority of the brains, but never into the lower bank of that sulcus.

1. Corticorubral projections: In intact cats we found terminal fields only in the RN ipsilateral to the cortical injection site (Figure 5[a]). In all brains there was some terminal labeling along the entire rostro-caudal extent of the nucleus, without any gross clustering at any particular frontal section, but with a clearly greater density of terminals in the entire ventral half (Figure 5) of the nucleus (McAllister, Villablanca, Olmstead, Gómez, & Sonnier, 1982b). The existence of ipsilateral projections from the pericruciate cortex to the RN in

---

Figure 4. Computer graphics display showing an statistical summary of the distribution of terminal fields in the red nucleus in intact (left of dotted line) and hemispherectomized (right of dotted line) animals. For the eight coronal sections throughout the nucleus (A–P Section) (stereotaxic planes A 6.5 through A 3.0), the mean total area for each quadrant of the nucleus is shown by the number under each of the blocks and the mean proportions of the estimated terminal densities is shown in each of the blocks by the different shadings within each block. The photomicrographs, oriented as the graphic displays, show a representative sagittal section at about L 2.0 of the left red nucleus of an intact (upper left) and of an hemispherectomized (lower right) cat as examples of the distribution of terminal fields as seen with autoradiography and under dark-field illumination. Magnification: 12×. Note that in the hemispherectomized animals, the terminals now occupy a larger area (expansion) of the dorsal quadrants. (R) Rostral; (C) caudal; (D) dorsal; (V) ventral. (Taken from Olmstead, Villablanca, Sonnier, McAllister & Gómez, 1983 with permission from Elsevier Scientific Publishers.)

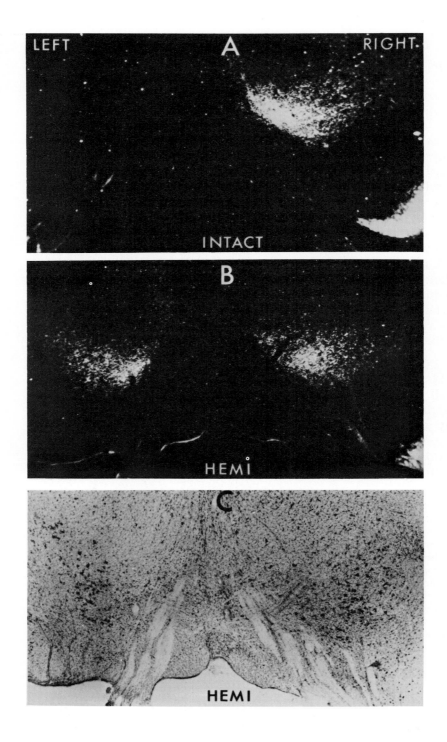

intact cats has been well documented using silver-impregnation methods (Massion, 1967; Padel, Smith, & Armand, 1973; Rinvik & Walberg, 1963; Sadun, 1975), but we know of only a single, brief note using autoradiography (Flindt-Egebak, 1979).

In all HEMI animals the outstanding finding was the presence of terminal fields in the RN of both sides (Figure 5[b]). The terminals in the RN contralateral (left) to the cortical injection originated from labeled fibers that ran medially in the mesencephalon from the right cerebral peduncle and coursed toward the midline either through or under the ipsilateral RN (Villablanca, Olmstead, Sonnier, McAllister, & Gómez, 1982). Inspection of all frontal sections throughout the RN showed that fibers reached the nuclei at all A–P levels in all cats and suggested that there were no marked differences in topography of the distribution of terminals between HEMI K (both RN) and intact animals. This important finding of a normal pattern of new innervation for the RN partially deafferented by the hemispherectomy was clearly documented by the computer statistics and graphic display.

Further quantification showed the following additional features of the RN and its terminal fields in intact and HEMI animals: (1) Area measurements of the RN for all eight frontal sections demonstrated no differences between intact and HEMI K or between the two RN of HEMI K, thus indicating no changes in size of the nuclei consecutive to the ablation. (2) Proportions of the area of the RN with terminal fields showed a slight decrease for the two nuclei of the HEMI K. In the RN of intact animals, the mean proportional area with terminal fields across all eight frontal sections was 0.57 (range, 0.41–0.68), whereas in the right and left RN of the HEMI K the values were 0.48 (range, 0.40–0.60), and 0.44 (range, 0.28–0.59), respectively. However, these reductions in terminal field areas occurred rather evenly

---

Figure 5. Autoradiographic labeling of right pericruciate cortical projections to the red nucleus. (A) Dark-field view of a frontal section at about A 5.0 (Berman, 1968) through the red nucleus of an intact adult cat. Note that the terminal label is restricted to the red nucleus of only the side ipsilateral to the injection site, as is shown by the intensely labeled mesencephalic peduncle at the lower right. (B and C) Dark- and bright-field photomicrographs, respectively, of a frontal section at about the same level through the red nucleus of an adult cat with neonatal removal of the left cerebral hemisphere and right-pericruciate injection of leucine–proline. Although the injection site was identical to that of the intact cat in (A), terminal label is now present (B) in both right and left red nuclei, with terminal field density and topography similar to that in the intact cat. (C) thionine-stained section showing large cells outlining the red nuclei. Magnification: 12× for all pictures (Taken from Villablanca, Olmstead, Sonnier, McAllister & Gómez, 1982, with permission from Elsevier Scientific Publishers.)

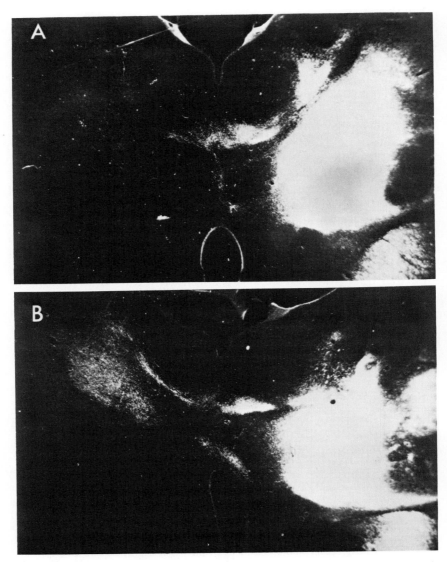

Figure 6. Autoradiographic labeling of right pericruciate cortical projections to the thalamus under dark-field illumination. (A) Frontal section at about A 10.0 (Jasper & Ajmone-Marsan, 1954) of the brain of an adult intact cat. (B) Section at about same level as in (A) of the brain of an adult cat with removal of the left cerebral hemisphere at 8 days of age (same shown in Figure 1). In the intact brain (A), most terminal labeling stops at the midline except for sparse terminal fields continuing for about 2 mm into the left side at the level of the nucleus centralis medialis. In the hemispherec-

along the rostral–caudal extent of the nuclei, with no overall significant difference between the nuclei. (3) We also found a tendency for
decreases in the proportions of areas with Type 2 and Type 3 scores in
both RN of HEMI K (which are practically identical) compared to the
RN of intact animals. But once again, these differences were usually
too small to reach significance. In addition, these also occurred
rather evenly across all eight frontal sections of the nuclei. Although
not statistically significant, the decreases in areas showing terminals
and in the density of these terminals in both RN of the lesioned
animals may have some meaning relative to processes underlying
reorganization in the RN, as is discussed later.

2. Corticothalamic projections: In intact cats there were cortical
projections along the entire A–P extent of the thalamus. From anterior to posterior, projections were found in the following main nuclei:
ventralis anterior, reticularis, ventralis lateralis, centralis lateralis–
paracentralis, ventralis medialis, lateral portions of medialis dorsalis, centralis medialis, ventralis posteromedialis, and centrum me-
dianum. Many of these can be seen in Figure 6(a). All projections were
ipsilateral except for sparse terminals that continued 1–3 mm into
the left side at two dorsoventral levels: dorsally at the level of the
centralis medialis, and ventrally and more posteriorly at the level of
the nucleus subparafascicularis and at dorsal aspects of zona incerta.

There is only one autoradiographic study that we know of (Jones &
Burton, 1974) that examines the projections of the motor cortex to
the thalamus in the cat. Although the authors did not describe any
crossing fibers (admittedly minimal in our material), our results generally agree with their findings. The results of Rinvik (1968), who
used fiber-degeneration methods, also agree in that there are only a
minimal number of cortical fibers that cross to the opposite side of
the thalamus.

In all 6 HEMI K, we observed that the distribution of corticothalamic fibers on the intact side was quite similar to that just described
for intact animals. Once again, the outstanding difference was the
presence of fibers crossing the midline and terminating in most of the
atrophic left thalamus (Figure 6[b]). As in intact animals, the cross-

---

tomized brain, cortical projections continue into the left side after crossing at two
dorsoventral levels, and they terminate sparsely in the area of the left centralis lateralis–parafascicularis complex (under the nonlabeled nucleus medialis dorsalis) and
diffusely at the level of most of the left atrophic ventrolateral thalamus (see Figure 1).
Magnification: 6×.

ing was in two dorsoventral contingents, but both were denser, so that caudal to A 10.0 they tended to coalesce and to fill most of the ventral half of the midline. In the left thalamus, the dorsal pathway terminated along the entire extent of the intralaminary nuclei, whereas the ventral contingent filled whatever was left of the ventral thalamus. These crossed terminal fields were relatively sparse and diffuse (Figure 6[b]), never reaching the degree of density seen for the terminals in the intact side.

3. Projections to the area of the n.III nucleus complex: In all HEMI K, we found terminal fields bilaterally in an area located dorsolateral to the rostral end of the n.III nucleus, which included the insterstitial nucleus of Cajal and Darkschewitsch's nucleus. In intact cats this projection was seen only unilaterally, ispilateral to the injection site, and appeared to originate from fibers ascending through the RN of that side. The origin and distribution of the new contralateral projection seen in the HEMI K appeared to be identical to that in intact cats (or to the corresponding ipsilateral terminals in the HEMI K).

PROJECTIONS FROM THE RIGHT NUCLEUS
INTERPOSITUS

For these studies, we used 7 intact and 7 left-hemispherectomized adult cats lesioned at least 4 months earlier. At the injection sites, although the injections were aimed independently at the anterior and posterior nucleus interpositus subdivisions, the label was confined to the posterior nucleus interpositus in only 1 of the intact brains. In 4 intact brains and 4 HEMI cases it filled mainly the anterior nucleus interpositus, and in the remaining 2 intact and 3 HEMIs, both divisions were labeled almost equally. Therefore, the injection sites of the two age groups were comparable.

1. Cerebellorubral projections: Inspection of all sections throughout the RN showed that terminal distributions were similar in all cats of both groups in that they were found exclusively in the RN contralateral to the injection site and along the entire rostral–caudal extent of the nucleus. These findings agree with all previous literature for *intact* cats (Courville, 1966; Dekker, 1981), but in this species ours is the first study using autoradiographic tracing methods (Olmstead, Villablanca, Sonnier, McAllister & Gómez, 1983).

Comparisons of the total area of the nucleus in each of the eight A–P sections showed that there were no significant differences between animal groups in the actual size of the nucleus. However, comparison of the proportion of the RN areas showing terminal fields at each of the A–P sections demonstrated an uneven distribution between groups. In intact cats, the area containing terminal fields increased gradually toward the center of the nucleus, such that at A 5.0 and through A 6.0 the proportion of the overall nucleus area that contained terminals was equal to or greater than 0.33, with significant tapering at A 6.5 ($p = .028$). In the HEMIs, increases surpassed 0.33 from A 3.5 to A 6.0 ($p = .028$), where decreases started. Therefore, in the HEMIs a larger proportion of the RN area contained terminal fields.

Inspection of the graphic displays (Figure 6) suggested that the greater area covered by terminal fields in the HEMIs might be accounted for by increases in the dorsal quadrants. This was documented by comparisons between proportions of quadrant areas containing terminal fields in the two groups. The proportion of the dorsolateral quadrant exhibiting terminal fields was significantly larger in the HEMIs between A 5.5 and 3.5 (encompassing most of the A–P extent of the nucleus). There were also larger terminal-field areas for the dorsomedial quadrant in these animals, but the increases were significant only at A 4.5 and A 4.0 levels. A similar analysis for the ventral quadrants showed no significant differences between groups except for a decrease in proportional area in the HEMI at A 6.0 ($p = .0128–.008$ for these differences).

Because these analyses suggested a slight decrease in terminal-field areas for the ventral quadrants of the HEMIs, and because the graphic display suggested that there might be reduction of terminal densities in that region, the possibility of displacement of terminals from ventral to dorsal quadrants received a closer scrutiny. Statistical analysis showed no significant decrease in proportions of Observation Type 2 or 3 for the ventral quadrants in these animals. This indicated that a possible displacement of terminals from ventral to dorsal areas was not the main factor responsible for the increase in terminal areas in the dorsal aspects of the partially deafferented RN, and that expansion of the terminals was, therefore, the main mechanism involved (Olmstead et al., 1983).

2. Cerebellothalamic terminal fields: Projections from the nucleus interpositus to the ventralis lateralis–ventralis anterior nuclei of the contralateral thalamus have been shown in the cat by both degeneration and autoradiographic methods (Angaut, 1979; Sugimoto, Mizuno, & Itoh, 1981). In our intact animals, the projections were

present only to the contralateral side and were distributed as reported in the cited literature. The interesting new results were in the hemithalamus ipsilateral to the hemispherectomy in the HEMI C. Cytoarchitecturally, that thalamus was conspicuously gliotic and, to a great extent, devoid of large thalamocortical relay neurons (Macchi *et al.*, 1975). In spite of this atrophy, we found abundant terminal fields. Terminal fields in the contralateral ventralis lateralis were seen in 5 HEMI C. The terminals were patchy and appeared qualitatively identical to those in intact animals. Additional terminals in areas of the parafascicularis, centralis lateralis, and anterior pretectal thalamic nuclei were seen in 2 animals. The density of the labeling appeared greater in the HEMI than in the intact cats, but this could be due to a passive contraction of the original terminals into denser aggregations consecutive to the atrophy. In 2 animals, in which injections were mostly confined to the anterior nucleus interpositus, we did not see any thalamic labeling. This persistence of dense cerebellar terminal fields in the partially degenerated thalamus may represent an attempt at reorganization (McAllister, Olmstead, Villablanca, & Gómez, 1982a).

Discussion

Neurology and Behavior

Overall, the neonatally lesioned kittens studied into adulthood performed significantly better than the cats lesioned as adults on the great majority of our tests. For the tests that explored vision, we did not detect age-related differences, but based on anecdotal observations, we suspected that we would have done so had we used more sensitive assessment methods. These age-related differences in recovery included the trainability of the impaired paw. Here, an impressive degree of functional plasticity was common to all animals. However, although in both groups the bias not to use the impaired paw in a simple action (string test) could easily be reversed, only the HEMI K could be easily trained to perform with their right paw in a more complex, purposeful task (food retrieval from the narrow box).

Some of the objections leveled at studies comparing results of early and late brain injury (Isaacson, 1976; Villablanca & Olmstead, 1981) are not applicable to the present experiments. First, the larger sparing in the HEMI K was a general finding; it was not limited to a few of the functions tested (Nonneman & Isaacson, 1973). Second, the larger recovery seen in the HEMI K persisted into adulthood, and recovery was not limited to a relevative brief time period in the HEMI C (Lawrence & Stein, 1978). Third, throughout the years our ablation technique has become so standardized that lesions were not different in the two age groups (Isaacson, 1976).

The present results unambiguously support the Kennard principle (Teuber, 1973; Villablanca & Olmstead, 1981), holding that the earlier in life a brain lesion is sustained, the better is the overall chance for recovery (Kennard, 1936). This conclusion surprised us initially in view of our previous experience with other brain lesions. In a series of experiments in cats and kittens with frontal or caudate nuclei ablations, we found that a number of other factors, in addition to the age at surgery, could influence the long-term effects of the lesion (Villablanca & Olmstead, 1981). Quite often those influences were dominant to the extent of rendering the Kennard principle irrelevant. For example, caudate-lesioned kittens performed worse in the paw-usage task (Olmstead & Villablanca, 1979b) and showed longer lasting impairment of contact placing reactions than similarly lesioned adult cats (Villablanca et al., 1978; Villablanca & Olmstead, 1982). In other tasks, including a bar-pressing battery (Olmstead & Villablanca, 1979a) and a passive avoidance test (Olmstead & Villablanca, 1980), there were practically no age-related differences. Similarly, our findings in cats and kittens with a mesencephalic transection (Olmstead & Villablanca, 1982) were even less supportive of the Kennard principle. Here, young kittens showed crippling postural and motor control defects of an extent that we have not seen following comparable decerebration in adult cats (Villablanca, 1966) or after any other central nervous system lesions in cats of any age.

Why then was the HEMI K performance so uniformly better than that of the adult counterparts? At this stage of our ongoing work we can only offer reasonable clues. It is possible that the pathways that we have discovered crossing from the intact hemisphere to partially deafferented areas of the remaining left brain were not formed after the lesion, but were naturally present in the neonatal kitten at the time of ablation. Since those pathways are absent in the intact brain of adult cats, we may be lesioning brains of different structures depending on the age at surgery: that is, that of the kitten, with bilateral innervation of some subcortical areas, or that of the adult, with pathways descending only unilaterally. If that were the case, the role of early hemispherectomy would essentially be to sustain preexisting crossing pathways, thereby allowing bilateral control by the remaining hemisphere.

This hypothesis seems reasonable on the basis of two considerations. From the anatomical standpoint, there are several reports in the literature demonstrating that pathways that cross the midline early in life disappear during the course of development (Innocenti, 1981; Ivy, Akers, & Killackey, 1979; Nah, Ong, & Leong, 1980). From the functional standpoint, early presence of bilateral cortical projections would be a good explanation for the relatively few immediate effects of hemispherectomy in the neonatal kitten. However, other processes may contribute to this remarkable early recovery, for example, the apparent absence of neurological shock in the neonatal kitten (Bradley, Smith & Villablanca, 1983).

Either because the earlier lesion is instrumental in maintaining crossing pathways that would otherwise disappear, or because it promotes the growth of new axon terminals (to be discussed subsequently), the present results document the fact that unilaterality of brain damage is a powerful factor in favor of recovery and reorganization. Indeed, in the examples quoted above from our past work, the animals with unilateral ablation of the caudate nucleus showed less abnormal paw usage than the bilaterally acaudate cats, and that deficit clearly improved with training (Olmstead & Villablanca, 1979b).

Finally, we are greatly impressed with the role that training appears to play in the recovery of motor functions. This is illustrated by the contrast between decerebrate kittens, which remain helpless and inactive after the lesion and show minimal recovery (Olmstead & Villablanca, 1982), and the HEMI K, which are active the morning following surgery and show extensive recovery. Furthermore, in the present studies, the remaining motor impairment of both HEMI groups also showed considerably plasticity in response to motor training. For the food-retrieval task, in particular, it was impressive to discover that the HEMI C could be literally coerced into using the seemingly useless right paw for this task, and this subsequently resulted in a regular performance of food retrieval with that paw. Will timely exercise and training cancel the developmental bias against use of the impaired paw in our HEMI Ks? Will it also enhance the recovery of usage of that paw in adult cats? Will we find an enhanced anatomical remodeling as a counterpart to activity-induced recovery? These all are tantalizing questions that we are eager to answer using the present animal model.

ANATOMY

In the anatomical portion of our studies, the reorganization that we have discovered is certainly widespread in scope. Admittedly, we have not fully ascertained the exact differences between cat and kitten reorganization; however, assuming, as it seems reasonable to do, that the changes we have demonstrated for HEMI C should occur at least to a similar extent in HEMI K, it is quite clear at this point that the total rearrangement we expect to finally disclose in the neonates will certainly be massive.

In addition to being extensive, none of the new terminal fields that we have found could be described as abnormal (Schneider, 1981). For example, the pattern of distribution of the terminals in the newly innervated RN of the HEMI K was remarkably similar to that in our intact cats. This seemingly normal reorganization, together with the suggestion that the larger reorganization appears to accompany the larger recovery of function, as in the HEMI K, might indicate that anatomical remodeling is in this case directly related to recovery.

We do not know of any such widespread anatomical remodeling previously reported in the literature. However, fragments of similar changes have been communicated, as illustrated by the following examples.

1. In a Finck–Heimer study, Nah (1976) demonstrated that a new contralateral projection to the RN developed from corresponding regions in the intact hemisphere following a unilateral neonatal sensory–motor cortex ablation in rats. The crossing axons were not seen in adult rats with a similar lesion. In the brain of the only HEMI C that we have studied, we have not seen any crossing corticorubral fibers, either.

2. Using the horseradish peroxidase tracing method, Pritzel and Huston (1981) and Neumann, Pritzel, and Huston (1982) demonstrated, in hemispherectomized adult *and* infant rats, the appearance of a crossed pathway to the thalamus on the side of the ablation originating from the corresponding projection area in the cortex of the remaining hemisphere. There were no systematic behavioral studies on these animals, but the authors stated that the appearance of the crossed connection coincided in time with the cessation of the turning behavior induced by the unilateral lesion. Since the crossing pathway was seen in the animals studied 7 days postlesion, but not in those injected with the peroxidase immediately after the lesion, it is probable that the terminals in the thalamus ipsilateral to the abla-

tion did not exist before the lesion. Similarly, in a preliminary study of the brain of 2 intact kittens (ages 2 and 28 days) after cortical injections of labeled amino acids, we failed to see any crossed corticothalamic pathway.

3. Several studies indicate that there is anatomical remodeling following both neonatal and adult lesions of the cerebellar input to the RN. For example, electron microscopic studies after lesion of cerebellar afferents to the RN in adult cats suggested that the corticorubral terminals moved from distal segments of the dendrites of RN neurons to the cell soma or to proximal parts of the dendrites (Murakami, Katsumaru, Sato, & Tsukahara, 1982). It is known that the dendrites of the large rubral neurons are extremely long (Dekker, 1981), and that in the intact cat, cortical terminals selectively contact distal dendrites, whereas cerebellar terminals synapse proximally or are axosomatic (Nakamura, 1975). In view of this, we tentatively propose that in our HEMI C the cerebellar terminals might have sprouted to contact the distal site of the rubral dendrites vacated by cortical afferents after hemispherectomy. This proposed cerebellorubral reorganization would therefore be similar but opposite in direction to the corticorubral response following cerebellar lesions described by Nakamura and his colleagues (1974). Tsukahara (1979) and Tsukahara and Fujito (1981) have provided electrophysiological evidence from cats and kittens for the anatomical changes summarized in (1) and (3).

For the basic processes underlying the reorganization that we have seen, the following possibilities may be offered: (1) collateral sprouting of new axon terminals (Raisman & Field, 1973), also called *reactive synaptogenesis* (Cotman & Nadler, 1978); (2) displacement of terminals from existing synapses with subsequent elongation, or growth, in order to occupy new sites now vacated by degenerated afferents; (3) persistance of neonatal pathways.

Our available evidence suggests that sprouting might be the principal mechanism involved in our results. This is because expansion (i.e., increases in size of terminal-field areas) is the main phenomenon that we have seen, particularly in fibers crossing past the midline into the left thalamus and into the normally non-cross-innervated RN, and because this process occurred with little depopulation of terminals in areas that normally received innervation.

The nonsignificant but clear displacement of terminals that we observed, particularly in the cerebellorubral projections, might represent a tendency of the system to comply with the principle of conservation of the total axon terminal arborization (Schneider, 1973). However, it also might be that only (or mainly) those terminals that move are the ones that sprout, and in such a case this seemingly small change would be much more relevant to the reorganization.

Whether the persistence into adulthood of neonatal pathways that would normally disappear during development has any relevance to our findings (see preceding discussion) will depend on the results of our ongoing search for crossed thalamic and rubral projections in intact young kittens and in HEMI Cs.

As might have been gleaned from our citation of the literature, there are very few studies of hemispherectomy that can be compared to ours. The experiments in rats by Hicks and D'Amato (1970) come closer than others, because both adult and neonatal subjects were included, and because attention was paid to both functional recovery and anatomical reorganization. However, in that study the extent of the lesions was more variable than in our ablation, and the battery of tests used was smaller and less systematically applied. The authors found practically no differences between age groups except for more impairment of the forelimb stride component of running in adult animals. Using Finck–Heimer–Nauta stains, they demonstrated that infant but not adult rats developed a small, uncrossed corticospinal tract after hemispherectomy. Other studies in animals with hemi-decortication (Ramirez De Arellano, 1961; Wenzel, Tschirgi, & Taylor, 1962) have provided additional pieces of evidence in favor of larger recovery in younger subjects. Finally there are numerous reports of hemispherectomy in children (Arnott, Guieu, Blond, Charlier, Vanceloo, Lejeune, Clarisse, Delandsheer, & Laine, 1982; Austin & Grant, 1955; Cairns & Davidson, 1951), and most agree on remarkable neurological and behavioral recoveries, some of which are not seen after hemispherectomy in adult patients.

Conclusions

Following hemispherectomy in cats and kittens there is a remarkable, quantifiable recovery that encompasses a wide neurobehavioral range. This recovery is significantly more pronounced following neonatal lesion and persists indefinitely into adulthood. Remaining motor impairments are modifiable, and this functional plasticity also appears to be more pronounced in kittens.

Parallel to the functional recovery there is an extensive anatomical remodeling that consists essentially of the presence of axon terminals in brainstem areas devoid of such endings in intact adult cats. These new terminals, which presumably originate from intact sprouting axons, follow a normal distribution pattern, and the overall reorganization also appears to be more pronounced after the neonatal lesion. All this evidence suggests that the structural reorganization does serve a functional purpose, although further research is needed for direct proof of this statement.

We propose neonatal hemispherectomy as an excellent animal model in which to continue analysis of the processes involved in self-healing of the brain after injury and particularly to test the possible ameliorative role of intervention factors such as motor training.

Acknowledgments

Ch. E. Olmstead participated in stages of both the behavioral and the anatomical work reported here. J. P. McAllister and F. Gomez collaborated in the autoradiographic studies. The authors wish to thank A. F. Koithan, A. Seraydarian, and S. Belkin for their assistance with the histological, computer, and art work, respectively supported by USPHS grants HD-05958, HD-04612, and BR-05750-04.

References

Angaut, P. (1979). The cerebello-thalamic projections in the cat. In J. Massion & K. Sasaki (Eds.), *Cerebro-cerebellar interactions* (pp. 19–43). Amsterdam: Elsevier/North Holland Biomedical Press.

Arnott, G., Guieu, J. D., Blond, S., Charlier, J., Vanceloo, F. M., Lejeune, E., Clarisse, J., Delandsheer, E., & Laine, E. (1982). Hémisphérectomie droite totale. Etude neurophysiologique après vingt-six ans. *Revue Neurologique, 1384*, 305–316.

Austin, G. M., & Grant, F. C. (1955). Physiologic observations following total hemispherectomy in man. *Surgery, 38*, 239–257.

Berman, A. L. (1968). *The brain stem of the cat: A cytoarchitectonic atlas with sterotaxic coordinates*. Madison: University of Wisconsin Press.

Bogen, J. E. (1974). Hemispherectomy and the placing reaction in cats. In M. Kinsbourne & W. L. Smith (Eds.), *Hemisphereic disconnection and cerebral function.* (pp. 48–94). Springfield, IL: Thomas.

Bradley, N. S., Smith, J. L., & Villablanca, J. R. (1983). Absence of handlimb tactile placing in spinalized cats and kittens. *Experimental Neurology, 82*, 73–88.

Burgess, J. W., & Villablanca, J. R. (1983). Paw preference and motor training in cats with adult or neonatal removal of one cerebral hemisphere. *Society for Neuroscience Abstracts, 9*, 695.

Burgess, J. W., Villablanca, J. R., Olmstead, C. E., & Levine, M. S. (1982). Differential recovery from hemispherectomy in kittens and cats. *Society for Neuroscience Abstracts, 8,* 746.

Cairns, H., & Davidson, M. A. (1951). Hemispherectomy in the treatment of infantile hemiplegia. *The Lancet, September 8,* 411–415.

Cotman, C. W., & Nadler, J. V. (1978). Reactive synaptogenesis in hippocampus. In C. W. Cotman (Ed.), *Neuronal plasticity* (pp. 227–271). New York: Raven Press.

Courville, J. (1966). Somatotopical organization of the projection from the nucleus interpositus anterior of the cerebellum to the red nucleus. An experimental study in the cat with silver impregnation methods. *Experimental Brain Research, 2,* 191–215.

Cowan, W. M., Gottlieb, D. I., Hendrickson, A. E., Price, J. L., & Woolsey, T. A. (1972). The autoradiographic demonstration of axonal connections in the central nervous system. *Brain Research, 37,* 21–51.

Dandy, W. E. (1933). Physiological studies following extirpation of the right cerebral hemisphere in man. *Bulletin of the Johns Hopkins Hospital, 53,* 31–51.

Dekker, J. J. (1981). Anatomical evidence for direct fiber projections from the cerebellar nucleus interpositus to rubrospinal neurons. A quantitative EM study in the rat combining anterograde and retrograde intra-axonal tracing methods. *Brain Research, 205,* 229–244.

Edwards S. B., & Hendrickson, A. (1981). The autoradiographic tracing of axonal connections in the central nervous system. In L. Heimer & M. J. Robards (Eds.), *Neuroanatomical tract-tracing methods* (pp. 171–204). New York: Plenum.

Feeney, D. M., & Wir, C. S. (1979). Sensory neglect after lesions of substantia nigra or lateral hypothalamus: Differential severity and recovery of function. *Brain Research, 178,* 329–346.

Flindt-Egebak, P. (1979). An autoradiographical study of the projections from the feline sensorimotor cortex to the brain stem. *Journal für Hirnforschung, 20,* 375–390.

Goltz, F. (1888). Uber die Verrichtungen des Grosshirns. *Pflugers Archive, 42,* 419–467.

Hassler, R., & Muhs-Clement, K. (1964). Architektonischer Aufbau des sensomotorischen und parietalen Cortex der Katze. *Journal für Hirnforschung, 6,* 377–420.

Hicks, S. P., & D'Amato, C. J. (1970). Motor-sensory and visual behavior after hemispherectomy in newborn and mature rat. *Experimental Neurology, 29,* 416–438.

Innocenti, G. M. (1981). Growth and reshaping of axons in the establishment of visual callosal connections. *Science, 212,* 824–827.

Isaacson, R. L. (1976). Recovery (?) from early brain damage. In T. D. Tjossem (Ed.), *Intervention strategies for high risk infants and young children* (pp. 37–62). London: University Park Press.

Ivy, G. O., Akers, R. M., & Killackey, H. P. (1979). Differential distribution of callosal projection neurons in the neonatal and adult rat. *Brain Research, 173,* 532–537.

Jasper, H. H., & Ajmone-Marsan, C. (1954). *A stereotaxic atlas of the diencephalon of the cat.* Ottawa: The National Research Council of Canada.

Jones, E. G. (1978). Recent advances in neuroanatomical methodology. *Annual Review of Neuroscience, 1,* 215–296.

Jones, E. G., & Burton H. (1974). Cytoarchitecture and somatic sensory connectivity of thalamic nuclei other than the ventrobasal complex in the cat. *Journal of Comparative Neurology, 154,* 395–432.

Kennard, M. A. (1936). Age and other factors in motor recovery from precentral lesions in monkey. *American Journal of Physiology, 115,* 138–146.

Lawrence S., & Stein, D. G. (1978). Recovery after brain damage and the concept of localization of function. In S. Finger (Ed.), *Recovery from brain damage* (pp. 369–407). New York: Plenum.

Liu, C. N., & Chambers, W. W. (1958). Intraspinal sprouting of dorsal root axons. *Archives of Neurology & Psychiatry, 79*, 46–61.

McAllister, J. P., Olmstead, C. E., Villablanca, J. R., & Gómez, F. (1982a). Residual cerebellothalamic terminal fields following hemispherectomy in the cat. *Neuroscience Letters, 29*, 25–29.

McAllister, J. P., Villablanca, J. R., Olmstead, C. E., Gomez, F., & Sonnier, B. J. (1982b). Autoradiographic tracing of the cortico-rubral terminal fields in cats. *Society for Neuroscience Abstracts, 8*, 746.

Macchi, G., Quattrini, A., Chinzari, P., & Capocchi, G. (1975). Quantitative data on cell loss and cellular atrophy of intralaminar nuclei following cortical and subcortical lesions. *Brain Research, 89*, 43–59.

Massion, J. (1967). The mammalian red nucleus. *Physiological Reviews, 47*, 383–436.

Murakami, F., Katsumaru, H., Saito, K., & Tsukahara, N. (1982). A quantitative study of synaptic reorganization in red nucleus neurons after lesions of the nucleus interpositus of the cat: An electron microscopic study involving intracellular injection of horseradish peroxidase. *Brain Research, 242*, 41–53.

Nah, S. H. (1976). Bilateral corticofugal projection to the red nucleus after neonatal SNC lesions in the albino rat. *Brain Research, 107*, 433–436.

Nah, S. H., Ong, L. S., & Leong, S. K. (1980). Is sprouting the result of a persistent neonatal connection? *Neuroscience Letters, 19*, 39–44.

Nakamura, Y. (1975). An electron microscopic study of the red nucleus in the cat, with special reference to the quantitative analysis of the axosomatic synapses. *Brain Research, 94*, 1–17.

Nakamura, Y., Mizuno, N., Konishi, A., & Sato, M. (1974). Synaptic reorganization of the red nucleus after chronic deafferentation from cerebellorubral fibers. An electron microscope study in the cat. *Brain Research, 82*, 298–301.

Nathanson, N. (1965). Failure to demonstrate dorsal root sprouting using the protargol stain following spinal cord hemisection or hemispherectomy in the cat. *Bulletin of the Johns Hopkins Hospital, 116*, 116–243.

Neumann, S., Pritzel, M., & Huston, J. P. (1982). Plasticity of cortico-thalamic projections and functional recovery in the unilateral detelencephalized infant rat. *Behavioral Brain Research, 4*, 377–388.

Nonneman, A. J., & Isaacson, L. (1973). Task dependent recovery after early brain damage. *Behavioral Biology, 8*, 143–172.

Norman, R. J., Villablanca, J. R., Brown, K. A., Schwafel, J. A., & 8uchwald, J. S. (1974). Classical eyeblink conditioning in the bilaterally hemispherectomized cat. *Experimental Neurology, 44*, 363–380.

Olmstead, C. E., & Villablanca, J. R. (1979a). Effects of caudate nuclei or frontal cortical ablations in kittens. Bar pressing performance. *Experimental Neurology, 63*, 257–265.

Olmstead, C. E., & Villablanca, J. R. (1979b). Effects of caudate nuclei or frontal cortical ablations in kittens: Paw usage. *Experimental Neurology, 63*, 559–572.

Olmstead, C. E., & Villablanca, J. R. (1980). Effects of caudate or frontal cortex ablation in cats and kittens: Passive avoidance. *Experimental Neurology, 68*, 335–345.

Olmstead, C. E., & Villablanca, J. R. (1982). The development of decerebrate kittens, *Neuroscience, 7*, 162.

Olmstead, C. E., Villablanca, J. R., Sonnier, B. J., McAllister, J. P., and Gómez F. (1983). Reorganization of Cerebellorubral terminal fields following hemispherectomy in adult cats. *Brain Research, 274*, 336–340.

Padel, Y., Smith, A. M., & Armand, J. (1973). Topography of projections from the motor cortex to rubrospinal units in the cat. *Experimental Brain Research, 17,* 315–332.

Pritzel, M., & Huston, J. P. (1981). Unilateral ablation of telencephalon induces appearance of contralateral cortical and subcortical projections to thalamic nuclei. *Behavioral Brain Research, 3,* 43–54.

Raisman, G., & Field, P. M. (1973). A quantitative investigation of the development of collateral reinnervation of the septal nuclei. *Brain Research, 50,* 241–264.

Ramírez De Arellano, M. (1961). Hemidecortication in monkeys. Comparison of rate and degree of recovery of neurological deficit as related to age at time of operation. *Seventh International Congress of Neurology, Abstracts, 38,* 150–151.

Reinoso-Suárez, F. (1961). *Topographischer Hirnatlas der Katze.* Darmstadt: Merk AG.

Rinvik, E. (1968). The corticothalamic projection from the pericruciate and cornal gyri in the cat. An experimental study with silver-impregnation methods. *Brain Research, 10,* 79–119.

Rinvik, E., & Walberg, F. (1963). Demonstration of a somatotopically arranged corticorubral projection in the cat. *Journal of Comparative Neurology, 120,* 393–407.

Sadun, A. (1975). Differential distribution of cortical terminations in the cat red nucleus. *Brain Research, 99,* 145–151.

Schneider, G. E. (1973). Early lesions of superior colliculus: Factors affecting the formation of abnormal retinal projections. *Brain, Behavior and Evolution, 8,* 73–109.

Schneider, G. E. (1981). Early lesions and abnormal neuronal connections. *Trends in Neuroscience, 4,* 187–192.

Siegel, S. (1972). *Nonparametric statistics for the behavioral sciences.* New York: McGraw Hill.

Snider, R. S., & Niemer, W. T. (1961). *A stereotaxic atlas of the cat brain.* Chicago: University of Chicago Press.

Sugimoto, T., Mizuno, N., & Itoh, K. (1981). An autoradiographic study on the terminal distribution of cerebellothalamic fibers in the cat. *Brain Research, 215,* 29–47.

Teasdall, R. D., Villablanca, J., & Magladery, J. W. (1965). Reflex responses to muscle stretch in cats with chronic suprasegmental lesions. *Bulletin of the Johns Hopkins Hospital, 116,* 229–242.

Teuber, H. L. (1973). Recovery of function after lesions of the central nervous system: History and prospects. *Neurosciences Research Program Bulletin, 11,* 1–12.

Tsukahara, N. (1979). Plastic and dynamic properties of red nucleus neurons: A physiological study. In M. A. B. Brazier (Ed.), *Brain mechanisms in memory and learning: From single neuron to man* (pp. 65–70). New York: Raven.

Tsukahara, N., & Fujito, Y. (1981). Neuronal plasticity in the newborn and adult feline red nucleus. In H. Flohr & W. Precht (Eds.), *Lesion-induced neuronal plasticity in sensorimotor systems* (pp. 67–74). New York: Springer-Verlag.

Ueki, K. (1966). Hemispherectomy in the human with special reference to the preservation of function. *Progress in Brain Research, 21b,* 285–338.

Villablanca, J. R. (1966). Behavioral and polygraphic study of "sleep" and "wakefulness" in chronic decerebrate cats. *Electroencephalography and Clinical Neurophysiology, 21,* 562–577.

Villablanca, J. R., & Marcus, R. J. (1972). Sleep–wakefulness, EEG and behavioral studies of chronic cats without neocortex and striatum: The "diencephalic" cat. *Archives Italiennes de Biologie, 110,* 348–382.

Villablanca, J. R., Marcus, R. J., & Olmstead, C. E. (1976a). Effects of caudate nuclei or frontal cortical ablations in cats. I. Neurology and gross behavior. *Experimental Neurology, 1976, 52,* 389–420.

Villablanca, J. R., Marcus, R. J., Olmstead, C. E., & Avery, D. L. (1976b). Effects of caudate nuclei or frontal cortex ablations in cats. III. Recovery of limb placing reactions including observations in hemispherectomized animals. *Experimental Neurology, 53,* 289–303.

Villablanca, J. R., & Olmstead, C. E. (1979). Neurological development of kittens. *Developmental Psychobiology, 12,* 101–127.

Villablanca, J. R., & Olmstead, C. E. (1981). Conditions which may influence the effects of neonatal brain lesions. In P. Mittler (Ed.), *Frontiers of knowledge in mental retardation* (pp. 197–209). Baltimore: University Park Press.

Villablanca, J. R., & Olmstead, C. E. (1982). The striatum: A fine tuner of the brain. *Acta Neurobiologiae Experimentalis, 42,* 225–297.

Villablanca, J. R., Olmstead, C. E., Levine, M. S., & Marcus, R. J. (1978). Effects of caudate nuclei or frontal cortical ablations in kittens: Neurology and gross behavior. *Experimental Neurology, 61,* 615–634.

Villablanca, J. R., Olmstead, C. E. Sonnier, B. J., McAllister, J. P., & Gómez, F. (1982). Evidence for a crossed corticorubral projection in cats with one cerebral hemisphere removed neonatally. *Neuroscience Letters, 33,* 241–246.

Wenzel, B. M., Tschirgi, R. D., & Taylor, J. L. (1962). Effects of early postnatal hemidecortication on spatial discrimination in cats. *Experimental Neurology, 6,* 332–339.

White, R. J., Schreiner, L. H., Hughes, R. A., MacCarty, C. S., & Grindlay, J. H. (1959). Physiologic consequences of total hemispherectomy in the monkey. *Neurology, 9,* 149–159.

Winer, B. J. (1972). *Statistical principles in experimental design.* New York: McGraw-Hill.

Zulch, K. J., & Micheler, E. (1978). Hemispherectomy—25 years later—findings and concepts. *Neurosurgical Review, 1/2,* 69–78.

11

Bases of Recoveries from Perinatal Injuries to the Cerebral Cortex*

*Donald R. Meyer
and Patricia Morgan Meyer*

Introduction

We think it fair to say that in the early 1960s, when the contemporary era of studies of perinatal injuries to the brain was just beginning, the very great majority of workers in the field expected to observe that such injuries would have lesser effects upon behaviors than would comparable injuries in adulthood. We suspected that there might be exceptions to the rule but thought that there would not be many. The overall attitude was nicely summarized by a still-remembered quip of Lukas Teuber, who said that if he had to have a cerebral injury, he would rather have it sooner than later.

This presumptive rule is often termed Kennard's principle. The honor is accorded because, in the 1930s and 1940s, Kennard and her associates had studied the effects of perinatal injuries to the motor cortex of monkeys (e.g., Kennard, 1936, 1938, 1940, 1942). They observed two phenomena that have been pursued in a number of experimental contexts. The first was that animals with early injuries seemed at first to be completely normal, but as they grew up they had increasingly apparent impairments. The second was that the impairments, when apparent, were for Kennard's particular conditions less severe than the deficits of subjects with comparable injuries in

*This review was prepared with support from the Donald Jansen Fund of The Ohio State University.

211

adulthood. The latter phenomenon has been the most thoroughly explored. In part this has been for a practical reason: It is much the easier to study. However, it is also by far the more important of the two for the question of in what respects the organization of the young brain is relatively plastic will only be answered through empirical assessments of functions that are spared after early damage to the organ.

The universal version of Kennard's principle fared very well at the beginning. Thus, for example, Benjamin and Thompson (1959) reported that somatosensory cortex-damaged cats could discriminate differences in roughness if, and only if, the damage was inflicted very soon after birth. Next, Doty (1961) found that cats with perinatal lesions of the posterior cortex could learn to discriminate between certain kinds of visual patterns. Kling (1962) amygdalectomized kittens and failed to observe symptoms that appear after comparable injuries in adulthood such as increased oral activity and changes in sexual or emotional behaviors. And in what seemed an apparent contradiction to the findings of a study of Jacobsen, Taylor, and Haslerud (1936) of monkeys with early prefrontal injuries, Akert, Orth, Harlow, and Schiltz (1960) and Harlow, Akert, and Schiltz (1964) found that such subjects were able to perform the classical delayed-response problem (see Harlow, Blumquist, Thompson, Schiltz, & Harlow, 1968, for review).

The trend continued with Raisler and Harlow's (1965) finding that posterior associative injuries, if inflicted in very young monkeys, have minimal effects on performances of object-discrimination problems. Also, Kling (1965) extended his observations of kittens with amygdalectomies and found that there was only a transient increase in sexual and aggressive behaviors by the subjects when they reached the age of puberty. And Tucker and Kling (1967), in a study of monkeys with perinatal prefrontal injuries, confirmed the observation of Harlow and his colleagues that the animals could solve the classic delayed-response problem.

However, there was one difficulty. Although Tucker and Kling (1967) had observed that their monkeys with early ablations of the prefrontal cortex were proficient at delayed responding, they also observed that their perinatal subjects were as poor as monkeys with adult prefrontal lesions in performance of delayed alternation. The finding was disturbing because at that time it was thought by some workers that delayed alternation and delayed responding were different measures of the same function (e.g., Mishkin, 1964). However, although it challenged that idea and also the "general rule" concern-

ing the effects of early versus late brain damage, the observation was
not taken very seriously.

But the crack in the dam began to grow with a report of Isaacson,
Nonneman, and Schmaltz (1968). They had studied the behaviors of
cats with early hippocampal injuries and found, as had Tucker and
Kling (1967), that the animals exhibited sparing of functions when
given certain tasks but not others (see also Nonneman and Isaacson,
1973). However, that message also was stonily received and indeed
was not effectively transmitted until, in a much later paper, Isaacson
(1975) proclaimed that infant sparing was a myth.

Our First Approaches to the Problem

Our own investigations of perinatal subjects began with an experiment by Wetzel, Thompson, Horel, and Meyer (1965). We had previously observed that cats with large ablations of the neocortex in
adulthood fail a visual pattern-discrimination problem in which an
array of black and white checks is presented in conjunction with
arrays of horizontal or vertical black and white stripes (Meyer, 1963).
The particular problem was employed because the cats had performed a visual cliff discrimination and then, when given treatments
with d-amphetamine, had exhibited the visual placing reflex (Meyer,
Horel, & Meyer, 1963). Hence it was already clear that such animals
still have some form of spatial vision but, for some reason that was
not apparent to us, have great difficulty with two-dimensional visuo-
spatial tests.

In Wetzel et al. (1965), we found that cats prepared with injuries to
areas 17, 18, 19, and the suprasylvian gyrus in adulthood only very
rarely exhibit a capacity to learn the checks–stripes discrimination.
In contrast, kittens that had suffered the same kinds of injuries at 7
days of age not only learned the problem but were somewhat faster to
learn it than were normal controls. Although we viewed the latter
finding as disturbing, we considered the overall results to be consistent with Doty's (1961) previous observations.

Next, because we knew of no reason to doubt the "general rule" for
early injuries, the just-mentioned finding encouraged us to study the
effects of perinatal frontal injuries. Our approach to the problem was
conditioned by the fact that we had a breeding colony of cats, and by
the further fact that even normal cats usually fail the classic delayed-

response problem. Happily, Lawicka and Konorski (1961) had devised a useful alternative procedure—a test that they had shown to be a sentitive detector of perseverative tendencies in animals with prefrontal injuries in adulthood.

The test was employed in a study by Thompson (1968), who expected to find that early prefrontal injuries would have lesser effects on performance of the task than injuries sustained at 6 weeks of age or when the brain was fully mature. However, the subjects of all three groups exhibited perseverative behaviors. Hence the outcomes were seemingly at variance with findings for perinatal prefrontal monkeys except for the result of Tucker and Kling (1967) with respect to delayed alternation. But like the latter outcome, the findings were largely ignored, and most investigators continued to believe in the validity of the "general rule."

While the study of Thompson (1968) was in progress, we were also heavily engaged in studies of the functions of limbic mechanisms. Our most dramatic finding was that rats with injuries to the septum of the forebrain are socially cohesive, in that such subjects spend nearly all of their time in a free field within a body length of one another. We also observed that amygdalar subjects exhibit a converse effect: In free-field encounters, they pay no attention to other rats as social objects (Jonason and Enloe, 1971).

We also observed that the cohesiveness effect disappears if septal rats are also prepared with injuries to the amygdala (Jonason, Enloe, Contrucci, and Meyer, 1973). Moreover, we found that although such rats much prefer to be with other rats, they would rather be with cats than by themselves in empty enclosures (see Meyer, Ruth, & Lavond, 1978, for review). We concluded from the findings that amygdalar systems are involved in mother–infant separations, and that the septal cohesiveness effect is due to a release of the Harlows' contact-comfort motive (Harlow & Harlow, 1965).

Johnson (1972), who was working in our laboratory at the time that the effect was discovered, decided to employ it as one of several measures in a systematic study of the consequences of perinatal injuries to the septum. The expectation from both the "general rule" and from Kling's (1962, 1965) observations of cats was that the effect, if detectable at all, would be less pronounced than it is in adult preparations. However, Johnson found that it did not matter when the septal injury was inflicted: The same effect appeared in perinatal subjects, in subjects that were lesioned in their young adulthood, and in subjects that were lesioned after they were many months old.

Nature of the Spatial Vision of Decorticated
Mammals

The findings of Thompson (1968) and Johnson (1972) had shown that at least some perinatal injuries to the brain have severe and enduring consequences. Hence, in three studies, the only support we had encountered for Kennard's principle was that cats with early injuries to the visual neocortex, but not cats with comparable injuries in adulthood, could learn to discriminate between checked and striped visual patterns (Wetzel *et al.*, 1965). Moreover, a question had developed as to whether the latter result was replicable, for Thompson (1970) had reported that it could not be confirmed through experiments conducted with rats.

Thompson had employed a two-choice task, the oblique-stripes (OB) discrimination problem, that we had also used in our own investigations of the substrates of visual-form perception (Horel, Bettinger, Royce, and Meyer, 1966). The task was a version of the horizontal–vertical (HV) discrimination problem (Lashley, 1939) in which the black-and-white stripes were oriented at 45 and 135° instead of at 0 and 90°. Initially, we thought that the OB problem was better than the HV problem because it excluded solutions on the basis of flicker cues that might be generated through a process of horizontal scanning of the patterns by the subjects.

In Horel *et al.*, we had found that rats prepared with bilateral ablations of the posterior cortex in adulthood were completely incapable of learning the OB problem. Thompson confirmed that result. However, he observed that the same thing was true for rats that were prepared with comparable ablations when they were 17 days old. The latter result was disappointing to us, but we found that we could wish it away by presuming that the outcome would surely have been different had Thompson's early injuries been inflicted when the animals were younger.

However, that surmise was incorrect. Thus we were to find that Thompson's negative result and the findings of Wetzel *et al.* were functions of the tasks that were employed in the studies, and not of such variables as species differences or age at the time of operation. The studies that led us to the latter conclusion were initially concerned with the nature of the spatial vision of decorticated mammals, and principally of mammals that had suffered injuries to the visual neocortex in adulthood.

In the 1960s, it was generally believed that decorticated mammals are form-blind, but that they retain a capacity to learn discriminations if two visual stimuli are different with respect to visual flux. The principal exception to the generalization was an under-quoted finding of Klüver (1941) that monkeys deprived of both occipital lobes could learn to discriminate between a single square and a grouping of four smaller squares. But as we have observed, we already knew that cats with huge cortical ablations have a latent capacity for visual placing and can see some difference between the shallow side and the deep side of a visual cliff. Also, an experiment of Braun (1966) with rats had confirmed our results for visual placing, and Braun, Lundy, and McCarthy (1970) had observed that posteriorly decorticated rats can readily be trained to discriminate between a shallow and a deep visual alley.

But it still remained a fact that the same kinds of subjects would usually fail a flux-equated task in which they were required to discriminate between a pair of two-dimensional patterns. Hence we were prompted to ask if cats prepared with injuries to the visual neocortex could learn to discriminate between perspective drawings of a deep and shallow visual alley. Wetzel (1969) demonstrated that the animals could solve such a problem, and the question then was whether they could also discriminate between other kinds of visual patterns. Wetzel approached the latter question by employing patterns with no perspective depth cues—specifically, arrays of black and white squares of high and low spatial frequencies. He found that his cats could also learn the latter coarse checks–fine checks problem, and despite variations in the cues that precluded detections of differences in flux.

We next addressed the question of whether the cats had learned the checks problem by responding to differences between the numbers of corners in the two discriminanda. We found that they had not, for decorticated cats can also discriminate between visual patterns that present flux-equated arrays of large and small black discs (Dalby, Meyer, and Meyer, 1970). Thereafter, we constructed pairs of visual patterns that were carefully equated with respect to flux and also with respect to the amounts of contour in the patterns, but that differed with respect to the numbers of enclosed visual spaces or figures in the patterns (Ritchie, Meyer & Meyer, 1976). We found that the latter problem was unlearnable by cats with injuries to the visual cortex, and hence we concluded that the spatial vision of decorticated cats is an ability to tell if two visual patterns are different with respect to edginess.

We found that the generalization was consistent with Klüver's (1941) anomalous result and also with a finding that the checks discrimination is learnable by rats with large lesions of the visual cortex (Mize, Wetzel, and Thompson, 1971). However, although we regarded the conclusion as of the first importance in its own right, we saw that it meant that the task we has used in the Wetzel *et al.* (1965) experiment with kittens was not a test of visual-form perception. Instead, it was a task in which the checkerboard cues contained more contour than the vertical and horizontal stripes. Hence it was a task that should have been learnable by both of the study's two groups, and not just the subjects whose injuries to the visual cortex were sustained in infancy.

We also believed that we had found the reason why the perinatal subjects had not only learned the checks–stripes problem, but had learned that problem at a faster rate than normal animals. In our efforts to control for solutions of the problem on the basis of flux differentials, we had varied the positions of the checks within the checkerboards and also the positions of the stripes. Also, the checkerboards had been presented with two varieties of stripes, which served to complicate the problem for a subject that could see a difference between them. Hence, despite their handicaps, the perinatal subjects were working with two advantages: For them, the striped patterns were the same kinds of cues, and they had learned to rely on contour differentials in finding their way in visual space.

We saw that one simple way to check our speculations would be to prepare a group of perinatal cats and test them for performance of the OB problem in adulthood. The task is a rigorous test of form perception because it is insoluble in terms of either local or overall flux differentials and also is insoluble in terms of either local or overall contour differentials. To pass it, the subject must be able to detect the spatial orientations of the contours. We view that as important because we find ourselves unable to imagine how a brain-injured animal could lack that capacity and yet be able to recognize the shapes of visual objects. We have yet to carry out such a study, and have no plans to do so in the future, and hence we invite our junior colleagues to try it for themselves. Should they choose to do so, our prediction would be that their posteriorly decorticated cats would fail the task no matter how long they were trained and no matter when their injuries were inflicted.

The prediction is explicitly for cats that would be tested with the OB discrimination problem. It would fail if the animals were tested, instead, with the HV discrimination problem. The reason is simply that the HV problem, like the task employed by Wetzel *et al.* (1965), is not a rigorous test of visual-form perception because it does not exclude solutions on the basis of local amounts of visual contour. Thus if rats with injuries to the posterior cortex are trained on one problem or the other, they can learn the HV discrimination problem but will fail to learn the OB problem (Lavond, Hata, Gray, Geckler, Meyer, & Meyer, 1978). Moreover, that result is independent of the fact that the OB problem is the harder of the two for a normal animal to learn (Lavond & Dewberry, 1980). Both of the problems are soluble by rats with injuries to area 17 (Hughes, 1977), but in our long experience we have yet to encounter a rat with a radical posterior ablation (and no matter how inflicted) that did any better than chance when it was trained on the OB discrimination problem.

Although, as we have said, we have no present plans to test the prediction for ourselves, an unpublished study by our student, Mary Hata, has yielded a result that has served to strengthen our convictions. Hata observed that if rats are prepared with bilateral ablations of the posterior half of the cortex at 7 days of age, they will fail to learn the OB discrimination problem if they are tested in adulthood. Hence, we believe that the evidence at hand is supportive of the notion that form recognition is a function that depends on the cortex, and that even very early injuries to the cortex will not permit recovery of the function.

The Equipotential Function of the Cerebral Cortex

Although we have found that it is not especially easy to show that perinatal injuries to the brain have lesser effects than later injuries, we have one set of findings that strongly suggest that the young brain is relatively plastic. The studies from which the findings have emerged were a part of a program that has mainly been directed toward the problem of the bases of recoveries from reversible amnesias (Meyer & Meyer, 1977). Therefore, we must first describe the salient results of that endeavor.

It has long been established that radical ablations of the posterior cortex not only affect a rat's performances of visual-form discriminations but also bring about impairments of remembering of a brightness discrimination problem (Lashley, 1935). Although, as we have noted, the impairment of form recognition is irreversible, a posterior subject will rapidly relearn the brightness discrimination problem. Moreover, if the posterior injuries are inflicted before the rat is trained on that problem, the rat will learn the problem at about the same rate that a trained rat will relearn the problem.

When we first began the program, we were interested in whether the extravisual or anterior cortex is critically involved in learning or relearning of the problem by posterior subjects (Horel *et al.*, 1966). We approached that question by first preparing rats with bilateral anterior injuries. Then we trained the rats on the problem, and then we prepared them with second-stage posterior ablations. Much to our suprise, we found that the subjects relearned the problem at exactly the same rate as rats that were trained when they were normal animals and then were prepared with first-stage posterior ablations. Hence, because it did not seem to matter in the slightest whether a recovering posterior preparation had its anterior cortex or not, we concluded that the process was mediated by a change in the functions of subisocortical systems.

We also observed that the converse was true for subjects that were tested for relearning of the problem after they had undergone first-stage or second-stage ablations of the anterior cortex. Some of the animals were trained while they were normal, and others were trained after having first sustained ablations of the posterior cortex. We found that first-stage and second-stage subjects relearned the problem at the same rate, even though the second-stage subjects had by then been deprived of the entire neocortex.

As the program continued, we began to discover that the rates at which partially decorticated subjects relearned the problem conformed to what we first termed the pseudomathematics of the cortex. For example, we found that animals with injuries to any one quadrant of the cortex would relearn the problem in 8 to 9 trials regardless of the locus of the injury. We also observed that if an anterior quadrant and the ipsilateral posterior quadrant were destroyed in one stage, the subjects would require about 17 trials to relearn the problem after surgery. We also observed that the same thing was true for subjects with crossed-quadrant injuries (that is, of injuries to one posterior quadrant and the contralateral anterior quadrant) and for subjects prepared with one-stage bilateral ablations of both anterior quadrants.

There was only one exception to the rule. Thus, although the scores for two-quadrant subjects were, in most instances, two times as high as the scores for one-quadrant subjects, animals with injuries to both posterior quadrants required 25 trials instead of 17 to relearn the problem after surgery. The question then was whether the extra 8 trials, the posterior-specific deficit, was due to an impairment that could be dissociated from the ones that are observed after any kind of injury to the cortex.

We approached the question by studying the effects of various combinations of injuries to quadrants of the cortex (Cloud, Meyer, & Meyer, 1982). Rats were first trained on the brightness problem, and then were prepared with first-stage ablations of one or two quadrants of the cortex. Then they were retrained on the problem and, as we had previously observed, two-quadrant subjects with injuries that had spared at least one quadrant of the posterior cortex took about twice as long to relearn the problem as subjects with one-quadrant injuries. The animals were then prepared with second-stage injuries in a manner such that after operation, the subjects had one remaining quadrant. That is, if the rat was a first-stage two-quadrant subject, its second operation destroyed one additional quadrant; but if it was a first-stage one-quadrant subject, its second operation destroyed two additional quadrants.

The animals were then re-retrained, and yielded a remarkable result. The subjects that still had a posterior quadrant required only 1 to 3 trials to re-reach criterion. The subjects that had lost both posterior quadrants, regardless of whether they had been one-quadrant or two-quadrant first-stage subjects, required about 8 trials to relearn the problem following their second operations. That was a most interesting number because it was almost exactly equal to the difference between the effects on performance of the problem of two-quadrant injuries that destroy the visual cortex and other kinds of two-quadrant injuries.

We were prompted by the findings to conclude that the cortex has functions that are regionally specific but also has a function that is shared by all sectors of the cortex. Thus we supposed that when both of the quadrants of the posterior cortex are destroyed, most of the impairment of performance of the problem is due to the injury of the equipotential mechanism. We presumed that the cost of such an injury, which is 17 trials, becomes 25 for posterior subjects because their perceptual impairments have an added cost of 8 trials. We also presumed that any kind of injury to the holistic system will permit compensations that will serve to protect performance of the problem after any further injuries to the system, but that injuries that destroy or complete the destruction of the visual neocortex will always have a cost of 8 trials.

We must stress that the foregoing findings were for subjects that were trained on the task prior to surgery. Thus, as we observed at the beginning of this section, serial anterior–posterior preparations that receive their first training between the operations require as many trials to relearn the problem as first-stage posterior preparations. If, instead, the subjects had been trained prior to surgery and then re-trained between the operations, their scores for eventual relearning of the problem would have been about 8 trials instead of the usual 25. The reason for the difference is that interoperative training conveys no protection of performance unless the subject already has a memory to remember (Bodart, Hata, Meyer, & Meyer, 1980). Moreover, interoperative training is required as well as preoperative training, for animals prepared with two-stage ablations that are trained prior to surgery but are not retrained in the interval between the operations have the same deficits as animals prepared with comparable one-stage ablations (Kircher, Braun, Meyer, & Meyer, 1970). The two constraints suggest that the holistic system is a memory-retrieval mechanism, and that compensations for injuries to the system involve alterations in the processes by which the brain uses information that is stored within its core.

Effects of Early Injuries to the Holistic System

What could be some possible effects of early injuries to the brain's holistic mechanism? First, the victim of a perinatal injury would have formed very few memories. However, if we knew what they were, and if we also thought that the rules for adults were predictive regardless of the age of the subject at the time that the injury was inflicted, our presumption would be that further injuries to the system would have no effect on recall of the memories, provided that the subject had employed them. But that did not appear to us to be a researchable idea: It is not an easy task to train a very young rat, and had we tried to do that we would certainly have found that the early operations would have had to be delayed until the animals were juveniles.

We therefore decided to study the effects of bilateral ablations of the posterior cortex of rats that were 7 days old (Howarth, Meyer, & Meyer, 1979). The subjects then were trained on the brightness problem after they had reached maturity, and then they were prepared with second-stage bilateral ablations of the anterior cortex. We thought that the outcomes would go in either one of two ways. The first was that the animals would relearn the problem in approximately 17 trials, for that was what would be expected if the early posterior injury had the same effect as a comparable injury in adulthood. The second was that inasmuch as the subjects had grown up with only half their cortex, it might matter less and perhaps not at all if the rest of the organ were destroyed.

But both of the hypotheses were wrong. When the subjects were given their initial training, they learned the problem very quickly, but after their decortications were completed, they learned the problem very slowly. Just how slowly? As slowly as subjects that are trained while they are normal adults and are then tested for performance of the problem after they have been prepared with one-stage bilateral ablations of the entire neocortex. Therefore, the results suggested that very early injuries to the holistic system enhance the importance of its still-intact components for remembering or recall of the problem.

We saw that the finding implied that if our theory that the cortex is equipotentially involved in retrieval of memories was correct, perinatal injuries to the anterior cortex should also increase a subject's dependence on its remaining posterior cortex for performance of the brightness problem. We checked that prediction by preparing animals with early anterior and late posterior injuries (Hata, Diaz, Gibson, Meyer, & Meyer, 1980). As we have observed, if both the operations are performed while the subjects are adults, and the animals receive their first training on the problem following their anterior injuries, they will relearn the problem as quickly as subjects that are trained while they are normal and then are prepared with bilateral posterior ablations. In contrast, we found that early anterior subjects that are trained on the problem in adulthood require about as many trials to relearn the problem after second-stage posterior ablations in adulthood as animals prepared with early posterior injuries and second-stage anterior injuries.

Among the many questions posed by the results was whether early injuries to the posterior cortex induce alterations of the visual innervations of the anterior quadrants of the cortex. Gray and LeVere (1980) examined that question by searching for atypical evoked potentials in the anterior cortex of perinatal posterior subjects. No such potentials were found. Their observations serve to confirm our belief that our findings with respect to the role of the cortex in remembering of memories are completely independent of the fact that the task that we have used in our studies is a visual discrimination problem.

Reflections, Suggestions, and Conclusions

As we have observed, we first began our studies of perinatal injuries to the brain with a general expectation that the injuries would have a lesser effect on behaviors in adulthood than comparable injuries in adulthood. We also believed that there would be some exceptions to the rule. But now we have a converse opinion. Thus, in our experience, the injuries tend to have the same effects as injuries in adulthood, and the only exception we have found to that rule is the one that we have just been discussing.

We have pondered for a long time whether that exception and the ones that our colleagues have discovered are governed by a law that would permit us to predict new exceptions. At one time, our interests in recoveries of functions after serial ablations in adulthood prompted us to think that there might be a parallel between such effects and recoveries after early injuries. However, that idea was unproductive. For example, although it fitted observations with respect to the effects of prefrontal injuries on performance of delayed alternation, it failed to account for the fact that serial injuries suppress delayed responding and early frontal injuries do not (Meyer, Hughes, Buchholtz, Dalhouse, Enloe, & Meyer, 1976).

We also considered the possibility that potentials for recoveries from perinatal injuries are largely a function of the evolutionary status of the injured mechanism. But that idea was also unproductive. Although it could readily account for the fact that early septal injuries have the same effects as comparable injuries in adulthood, it was inconsistent with the finding of Thompson (1968) that cats with early injuries to the prefrontal cortex exhibit the same perseverative impairments that are commonly observed in mammals prepared with prefrontal injuries in adulthood.

Perhaps resolution of the problem will come from the thoughts of some genius in our midst. However, we believe that our present difficulties will not go away until we have a much larger data base. Hence, instead of offering some further speculations that would be off the tops of our heads, we propose to address the rest of our comments to youngsters who are just now beginning explore the effects of perinatal injuries.

Our first piece of what we view as very good advice is that they should know, and should always keep in mind, the fact that the study of behavior is a complicated subject. Thus, in our own investigations we have found that the likeliest sources of differences between the outcomes of two experiments that seem to be asking the same kind of question are often—subtle differences between the tasks that the animals are asked to perform. We contrast that conclusion with traditional beliefs that most of the variance in neurobehavioral studies of perinatal subjects is due to variations in placements of the injuries or to the times of placements of the injuries.

We also have found that a single swallow does not make a summer. To illustrate, a rat that is prepared with a perinatal injury to its posterior cortex will learn the brightness problem in about as many trials as it takes a normal rat to learn the problem. Hence, by that criterion, the animal is just as good as new. However, such a subject is profoundly abnormal, as is shown by its reactions to a further injury to its cortex. We believe that our results with serial procedures have shown them to be a potent tool, both for the identification of impairments and of modes of compensation for them. Their main limitation is that they are not for use by a worker in a hurry, but we also have observed that workers who hurry usually do not achieve their goals.

We also have found that brain-injured animals are clever. Thus, if they are given an unintended cue, the odds are very high that they will use it, and then they will seem to have recovered a function when in fact they are unable to perform it. Hence, the first thing that we tell our own students is to watch their subjects very closely: Are they using some trick, or have the methods excluded every possibility of tricks? When that has settled in, we ask our students not to tell us what their tests are called, and we ask them: Do you understand your methods, and how do you know you understand them?

The last is of course the hardest question, regardless of the nature of the function one is trying to assess. But it is the question that defines the province of neuropsychological research. Unless it is attended to, no amount of skill with either a knife or a syringe will serve an individual who shares our own goal of trying to understand the brain. The functions of the organ are the things that it does in one situation or another, and hence close analyses of situations are fundamental to our knowledge of it. That has been our personal part of the action, and to us, at least, its fruits have been rewarding.

References

Akert, K., Orth, O. S., Harlow, H. F., & Schiltz, F. (1960). Learned behavior of rhesus monkeys following neonatal bilateral prefrontal lobotomy. *Science, 132,* 1944–1945.

Benjamin, R. M., & Thompson, R. F. (1959). Differential effects of cortical lesions in infant and adult cats on roughness discrimination. *Experimental Neurology, 1*, 305–321.

Bodart, D. J., Hata, M. G., Meyer, D. R., & Meyer, P. M. (1980). The Thompson effect is a function of the presence or absence of preoperative memories. *Physiological Psychology, 8*, 15–19.

Braun, J. J. (1966). The neocortex and visual placing in rats. *Brain Research, 1*, 381–394.

Braun, J. J., Lundy, E. G., & McCarthy, F. V. (1970). Depth discrimination in rats following removal of visual neocortex. *Brain Research, 20*, 283–291.

Cloud, M. D., Meyer, D. R., & Meyer, P. M. (1982). Inductions of recoveries from injuries to the cortex: Dissociation of equipotential and regionally specific mechanisms. *Physiological Psychology, 10*, 66–73.

Dalby, D. A., Meyer, D. R., & Meyer, P. M. (1970). Effects of occipital neocortical lesions upon visual discriminations in the cat. *Physiology & Behavior, 5*, 727–734.

Doty, R. W. (1961). Functional significance of the topographical aspects of the retino-cortical projection. In R. Jung & H. Kornhuber (Eds.), *The visual system: Neurophysiology and psychophysics.* (pp. 228–243). Berlin: Springer-Verlag.

Gray, T., & LeVere, T. E. (1980). Infant posterior neocortical lesions do not induce visual responses in spared anterior neocortex. *Physiological Psychology, 8*, 487–491.

Harlow, H. F., Akert, K., & Schiltz, K. A. (1964). The effects of bilateral prefrontal lesions on learned behavior of neonatal, infant, and preadolescent monkeys. In J. M. Warren & K. Akert (Eds.), *The frontal granular cortex and behavior* (pp. 126–148). New York: McGraw-Hill.

Harlow, H. F., Blumquist, A. J., Thompson, C. I., Schiltz, K. A., & Harlow, M. K. (1968). Effects of induction-age and size of frontal lobe lesions on learning in rhesus monkeys. In R. L. Isaacson (Ed.), *The neuropsychology of development* (pp. 79–120). New York: Wiley.

Harlow, H. F., & Harlow, M. K. (1965). The affectional system. In A. M. Schrier, H. F. Harlow, & F. Stollnitz (Eds.), *Behavior of nonhuman primates* (Vol. 1, pp. 287–334). New York: Academic Press.

Hata, M. G., Diaz, C. L., Gibson, C. F., Jacobs, C. E., Meyer, P. M., & Meyer, D. R. (1980). Perinatal injuries to extravisual cortex enhance the significance of visual cortex for performance of a visual habit. *Physiological Psychology, 8*, 9–14.

Horel, J. A., Bettinger, L. A., Royce, G. J., & Meyer, D. R. (1966). Role of neocortex in the learning of two visual habits by the rat. *Journal of Comparative & Physiological Psychology, 61*, 66–78.

Howarth, H., Meyer, D. R., & Meyer, P. M. (1979). Perinatal injuries to the visual cortex enhance the significance of extravisual cortex for performance of a visual habit. *Physiological Psychology, 7*, 163–166.

Hughes, H. C. (1977). Anatomical and neurobehavioral investigations concerning the thalamocortical organization of the rat's visual system. *Journal of Comparative Neurology, 175*, 311–335.

Isaacson, R. L. (1975). The myth of recovery from early brain damage. In N. R. Ellis (Ed.), *Aberrant development in infancy* (pp. 1–25). Potomac, MD: Erlbaum.

Isaacson, R., Nonneman, J., & Schmaltz, L. W. (1968). Behavioral and anatomical sequelae of damage to the infant limbic system. In R. L. Isaacson (Ed.), *The neuropsychology of development* (pp. 41–78). New York: Wiley.

Jacobsen, C. F., Taylor, F. V., & Haslerud, G. M. (1936). Restitution of function after cortical injury in monkeys. *American Journal of Physiology, 116*, 85–86.

Johnson, D. A. (1972). Developmental aspects of recovery of function following septal lesions in the infant rat. *Journal of Comparative & Physiological Psychology, 78*, 331–348.

Jonason, K. R., & Enloe, L. J. (1971). Alterations in social behavior following septal and amygdaloid lesions in the rat. *Journal of Comparative & Physiological Psychology, 75*, 286–301.

Jonason, K. R., Enloe, L. J., Contrucci, J., & Meyer, P. M. (1973). Effects of simultaneous and successive septal and amygdaloid lesions on social behavior of the rat. *Journal of Comparative & Physiological Psychology, 83*, 54–61.

Kennard, M. A. (1936). Age and other factors in motor recovery from precentral lesions in monkeys. *American Journal of Physiology, 115*, 138–146.

Kennard, M. A. (1938). Reorganization of motor function in the cerebral cortex of monkeys deprived of motor and premotor areas in infancy. *Journal of Neurophysiology, 1*, 477–497.

Kennard, M. A. (1940). Relation of age to motor impairment in man and sub-human primates. *Archives of Neurology & Psychiatry, 44*, 377–397.

Kennard, M. A. (1942). Cortical reorganization of motor function: Studies on a series of monkeys in various ages from infancy to maturity. *Archives of Neurology & Psychiatry, 48*, 227–240.

Kircher, K. A., Braun, J. J., Meyer, D. R., & Meyer, P. M. (1970). Equivalence of simultaneous and successive neocortical ablations in production of impairments of retention of black-white habits in rats. *Journal of Comparative & Physiological Psychology, 71*, 420–425.

Kling, A. (1962). Amydalectomy in the kitten. *Science, 137*, 429–430.

Kling, A. (1965). Behavioral and somatic development following lesions of the amygdala in the cat. *Journal of Psychiatric Research, 3*, 263–273.

Klüver, H. (1941). Visual functions after removal of the occipital lobes. *Journal of Psychology, 11*, 23–45.

Lashley, K. S. (1935). The mechanism of vision. XII. Nervous structures concerned in the acquisition and retention of habits based on reactions to light. *Comparative Psychology Monographs, 11*, 43–79.

Lashley, K. S. (1939). The mechanism of vision. XVI. The functioning of small remnants of the visual cortex. *Journal of Comparative Neurology, 70*, 45–67.

Lavond, D. G., & Dewberry, R. G. (1980). Visual form perception is a function of the visual cortex: II. The rotated horizontal–vertical and oblique-strips pattern problems. *Physiological Psychology, 8*, 1–8.

Lavond, D. G., Hata, M. G., Gray, T. S., Geckler, C. L., Meyer, P. M., & Meyer, D. R. (1978). Visual form perception is a function of the visual cortex. *Physiological Psychology, 6*, 471–477.

Lawicka, W., & Konorski, J. (1961). The effects of prefrontal lobectomies on the delayed responses in cats. *Acta Biologica Experimentalis Warsaw, 21*, 141–156.

Meyer, D. R., Hughes, H. C., Buchholz, D. J., Dalhouse, A. D., Enloe, L. J., & Meyer, P. M. (1976). Effects of successive unilateral ablations of principalis cortex upon performances of delayed alternation and delayed response by monkeys. *Brain Research, 108*, 397–412.

Meyer, D. R., & Meyer, P. M. (1977). Dynamics and bases of recoveries of functions after injuries to the cerebral cortex. *Physiological Psychology, 5*, 133–165.

Meyer, D. R., Ruth, R. A., & Lavond, D. G. (1978). The septal social cohesiveness effect: Its robustness and main determinants. *Physiology & Behavior, 21,* 1027–1029.

Meyer, P. M. (1963). Analysis of visual behavior in cats with extensive neocortical ablations. *Journal of Comparative & Physiological Psychology, 56,* 397–401.

Meyer, P. M., Horel, J. A., & Meyer, D. R. (1963). Effects of *dl*-amphetamine upon placing responses in neodecorticate cats. *Journal of Comparative & Physiological Psychology, 56,* 402–404.

Mishkin, M. (1964). Perseveration of central sets after frontal lesions in monkeys. In J. M. Warren & K. Akert (Eds.), *The frontal granular cortex and behavior* (pp. 219–241). New York: McGraw-Hill.

Mize, R. R., Wetzel, A. B., & Thompson, V. E. (1971). Contour discrimination in the rat following removal of posterior neocortex. *Physiology & Behavior, 6,* 861–867.

Nonneman, A. J., & Isaacson, R. L. (1973). Task dependent recovery after early brain damage. *Behavioral Biology, 8,* 143–172.

Raisler, R. L., & Harlow, H. F. (1965). Learned behavior following lesions of posterior association cortex in infant, immature, and preadolescent monkeys. *Journal of Comparative & Physiological Psychology, 60,* 167–174.

Ritchie, G. D., Meyer, P. M., & Meyer, D. R. (1976). The residual spatial vision of cats with lesions of the visual cortex. *Experimental Neurology, 53,* 227–253.

Thompson, V. E. (1968). Neonatal orbitofrontal lobectomies and delayed response behavior in cats. *Physiology & Behavior, 3,* 631–635.

Thompson, V. E. (1970). Visual decortication in infancy in rats. *Journal of Comparative & Physiological Psychology, 72,* 444–451.

Tucker, T. J., & Kling, A. (1967). Differential effects of early and late lesions of frontal granular cortex in the monkey. *Brain Research, 5,* 377–389.

Wetzel, A. B. (1969). Visual cortical lesions in the cat: A study of depth and pattern discrimination. *Journal of Comparative & Physiological Psychology, 3,* 580–588.

Wetzel, A. B., Thompson, V. E., Horel, J. A., & Meyer, P. M. (1965). Some consequences of perinatal lesions of the visual cortex of the cat. *Psychonomic Science, 3,* 381–382.

12

Consequences of Early Visual Cortex Damage in Cats

Peter D. Spear

Introduction

Studies of a variety of species indicate that the behavioral consequences of neonatal visual cortex damage often are less severe than
the consequences of similar damage in adults (Dineen, Vermeire, &
Boothe, 1982; Schneider, 1970; Stewart & Riesen, 1972; Teuber,
1961; and see following section). These behavioral observations imply that remaining regions of the visual system possess a greater
capacity for neural compensation in the neonatal brain than in the
adult brain. The purpose of this chapter is to consider the nature of
the neural changes that occur following early visual cortex damage
and to relate these changes to the behavior of the animal. Whenever
possible, the results following neonatal lesions are compared directly
with results in animals with lesions received as adults so that any
differences in the neural mechanisms of compensation for brain
damage in neonates and adults can be assessed. The discussion con-
centrates on work carried out in the cat because this species has been
the most intensively studied and it is the only species in which extensive behavioral, anatomical, and physiological data are available for
comparison. An attempt is made to provide an overview and synthesis of these data and to indicate both the implications of what is
known and some questions that remain. A more detailed review of
the relevant literature is presented elsewhere (Spear, in press).

The chapter begins with a brief review of the behavioral consequences of early visual cortex damage in cats and an evaluation of the extent to which visual abilities are spared in these animals. Then the neural consequences of visual cortex damage in newborn kittens is considered, followed by a discussion of the critical period (or periods) for these effects. The final section considers the relationships between the neural and behavioral consequences of early visual cortex damage.

Behavioral Consequences
of Visual Cortex Damage

The visual cortex in mammals actually consists of multiple regions with separate anatomical inputs and visuotopic maps (Kaas, 1980; Van Essen, 1979). In the cat, electrophysiological mapping studies indicate that there are at least 13 different visual areas of cortex (Palmer, Rosenquist, & Tusa, 1978; Tusa & Palmer, 1980; Tusa, Palmer, & Rosenquist, 1978; Tusa, Rosenquist, & Palmer, 1979), and additional areas also may be present (Heath & Jones, 1971; Kalia & Whitteridge, 1973; Olson, & Graybiel, 1981; Updyke, 1982). All of these cortical areas receive some thalamic input (Graybiel & Berson, 1981; Symonds, Rosenquist, Edwards, & Palmer, 1981). However, the major pathways from retina to thalamus (lateral geniculate nucleus) to cortex in the cat terminate in areas 17 (striate cortex) and 18, and to lesser extent in area 19 (Rodieck, 1979; Sherman & Spear, 1982; Stone, Dreher, & Leventhal, 1979). Perhaps because of this, virtually all studies of the effects of neonatal visual cortex lesions have involved cats with damage to these three cortical areas.

There is good agreement that cats that received damage to areas 17, 18, and 19 as infants can learn simple visual discrimination tasks more readily than cats that received similar damage as adults. For example, cats that received visual cortex lesions when they were 2–4 days old can easily learn brightness and photic frequency discriminations in a shuttle-box situation, whereas cats with adult damage are deficient (Tucker, Kling, & Scharlock, 1968). In addition, several studies have found that cats that received visual cortex damage from within a few hours of birth to 9 days of age are much better than cats with adult damage at learning two-choice form and pattern discriminations (Doty, 1961; Murphy, Mize, & Schechter, 1975; Wetzel, Thompson, Horel, & Meyer, 1965). Thus, there is greater sparing or recovery of performance on these tasks following neonatal lesions than following adult lesions.

There is disagreement, however, concerning whether animals with neonatal visual cortex lesions can learn visual discriminations as rapidly as can normal animals; that is, whether there is complete sparing of function for these tasks. Most studies have found that the learning rates of cats that received neonatal visual cortex damage are not significantly different than normal (Doty, 1961; Murphy et al., 1975; Tucker et al., 1968; Wetzel et al., 1965). However, two studies by Cornwell and his colleagues (Cornwell & Overman, 1981; Cornwell, Overman, & Ross, 1978) found that cats with neonatal visual cortex lesions (received at 3 to 4 days of age) learn both form and pattern discriminations significantly more slowly than normal cats (unfortunately, no comparisons were made with cats that received lesions as adults).

The reasons for this disagreement are not clear. It is unlikely that the different results are due to differences in lesion extent, age at which the lesion was made, or age at the time of testing (Cornwell & Overman, 1981; Spear, in press). However, differences between studies in stimulus size, salience (e.g., presence of distracting background stimuli), or luminance levels (scotopic vs. photopic) may contribute to whether or not complete sparing of form- and pattern-discrimination ability occurs (Cornwell & Overman, 1981). It is important to test these possibilities directly because a determination of the conditions under which cats with neonatal visual cortex damage show partial (or even no) sparing of discrimination learning ability rather than complete sparing will aid understanding of the mechanisms of the sparing that occurs.

The studies discussed so far were concerned with simple discrimination learning ability. Unfortunately, there is a paucity of information about the detailed psychophysical capacities of animals with neonatal visual cortex damage. Kaye and Mitchell (1983) have made a start in obtaining this information by testing the visual acuity of cats with damage to areas 17, 18, and part of 19 that was incurred between 12 and 26 days of age. In agreement with other investigators (Berkley & Sprague, 1979; Lehmkuhle, Kratz, & Sherman, 1982), they found that cats that received damage to these areas as adults have lower than normal visual acuity (2.3–3.1 cycles/degree). In contrast, cats with early lesions have acuities (5.2–7.5 cycles/degree) that are within the normal range.

Kaye, Mitchell, and Cynader (1981, 1982) have tested binocular depth perception in cats that received lesions of areas 17, 18, and part of 19 between 10 and 26 days of age or as adults. They found that cats with adult lesions have no stereopsis and are deficient at using monocular depth cues as well. Cats with neonatal visual cortex damage have a normal use of monocular depth cues, which is consistent with their normal visual acuity. However, there is no sparing of stereopsis in these animals.

These results indicate that at least some of the psychophysical capacities that are disturbed by visual cortex damage in adult cats are spared following damage early in life (visual acuity), whereas others are not (stereopsis). Other psychophysical functions, such as thresholds for orientation discrimination, vernier acuity, and spatial contrast sensitivity, also are known to be affected by removal of visual cortex in adult cats (Berkley & Sprague, 1979; Sprague, Hughes, & Berlucchi, 1981). It is important for future studies to determine the extent to which these abilities develop normally following neonatal visual cortex damage.

Neural Consequences of Visual Cortex Damage

Before considering the neural consequences of visual cortex damage in newborn kittens, it is necessary to outline the organization of the relevant visual pathways in normal adult cats. In addition, the changes that occur following visual cortex damage in adult cats are described briefly for comparison.

NORMAL VISUAL SYSTEM

Figure 1(a) is a schematic diagram that summarizes the major visual pathways that are relevant to a discussion of the effects of early visual cortex damage in cats. In normal cats, retinal ganglion cells from both eyes project to the lateral geniculate nucleus (LGN) of the thalamus. These projections arise from three functional classes of ganglion cells, called X, Y, and W cells (or brisk sustained, brisk transient, and sluggish cells, respectively) (Lennie, 1980; Rodieck, 1979; Sherman & Spear, 1982; Stone et al., 1979). These three classes of cells differ in a number of receptive-field characteristics and dynamic response properties. For example, X cells have the smallest

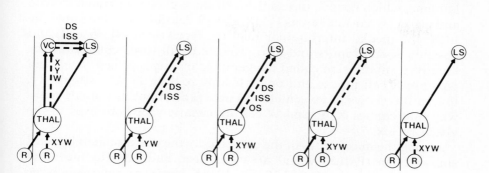

Figure 1. (a) Schematic representation of inputs from the two eyes (R) to the thalamus (THAL) and from there to ipsilateral visual cortical areas 17, 18, and 19 (VC) and the posteromedial lateral suprasylvian cortex (LS) in normal cats. The thin vertical line indicates the midline. (b–e) Schematic representation of the changes in these inputs following damage to cortical areas 17, 18, and 19 at different ages. These diagrams are intended to show only the functional information that is provided to LS cortex neurons by the primary retinogeniculocortical pathways and by the thalamic–LS cortex pathways independent of visual cortex. Details of the pathways and the thalamic nuclei involved have not been drawn for the sake of clarity. (DS) direction selectivity; (ISS) inhibits response to stationary flashing stimuli; (OS) orientation selectivity; (X,Y,W) X, Y, or W cell functional classes.

receptive fields and highest spatial resolution (visual acuity), and they generally give a sustained response to continuous stimulation of the receptive-field center. In contrast, Y cells have large receptive fields and lower spatial resolution and generally give a transient response to visual stimulation. W cells are a heterogeneous group that generally have large receptive fields and very low spatial resolution and give low peak discharges (respond sluggishly) to visual stimulation.

The LGN is divided into a number of subdivisions, each of which receives a somewhat different mix of X, Y, or W cell retinal inputs. Neurons in each of these subdivisions have response properties that correspond to their retinal inputs, and therefore each subdivision contains a different mix of X, Y, or W cells. In addition, each subdivision projects differently to cortical areas 17, 18, and 19 (Lennie, 1980; Rodieck, 1979; Sherman & Spear, 1982; Stone et al., 1979). The largest subdivision of the LGN consists of two laminae (A and A1), which receive inputs only from X and Y cells and project only to cortical areas 17 and 18. There are four smaller laminae, called the C-laminae, which receive inputs from all three classes of ganglion cells and project to cortical areas 17, 18, and 19. Another subdivision of the LGN, the medial interlaminar nucleus, receives Y cell, W cell, and possibly X cell inputs and also projects to all three cortical areas. Finally, a subdivision called the geniculate wing receives W cell and possibly X cell inputs and projects only to area 19. For simplicity, Figure 1(a) shows these geniculocortical projections as a single pathway that carries X, Y, and W cell information for both eyes to the visual cortex.

Among the many areas of the cortex, only the posteromedial lateral suprasylvian (PMLS) visual area has been studied after neonatal damage to areas 17, 18, and 19. The PMLS cortex is a relatively large region that extends along the posterior two thirds of the medial bank of the middle suprasylvian sulcus (Palmer *et al.*, 1978). Single-cell recording studies in normal cats (Camarda & Rizzolatti, 1976; Hubel & Wiesel, 1969; Spear & Baumann, 1975; Turlejski, 1975; Wright, 1969) indicate that most PMLS neurons have well-defined visual receptive fields, though they are much larger than the receptive fields of neurons in areas 17, 18, or 19. As shown in Figure 2(a) (right), about 70% of PMLS cells respond to stimulation of both eyes and about 30% respond only to the contralateral eye. Studies of receptive-field properties indicate that PMLS cells can be divided into four relatively distinct classes (Figure 2[a], left). The vast majority (about 80%) of the cells are direction selective. They respond better to moving than to stationary flashing stimuli, and the response is strongly dependent on the direction of stimulus movement. The remaining 20% of PMLS cortex cells are about evenly divided among the other three receptive field classes. Cells in the movement-sensitive class respond best to moving stimuli but are not sensitive to the direction of stimulus movement. Cells in the stationary class respond as well or better to stationary flashing stimuli as to moving stimuli. Cells in the indefinite class have diffuse, ill-defined receptive fields or give indefinite responses to light. In contrast to cells in cortical areas 17, 18, and 19, few or no cells in the PMLS cortex of normal cats respond selectively to the orientation of a moving or flashing stimulus (Camarda & Rizzolatti, 1976; Palmer *et al.*, 1978; Smith & Spear, 1979; Spear & Baumann, 1975).

As shown in Figure 1(a), the PMLS cortex receives inputs from the visual cortex, including areas 17, 18, and 19. These inputs come directly through corticocortical projections as well as through various corticothalamocortical loops (Sherman & Spear, 1982; Spear, in press). Lesion studies (to be described in more detail later) indicate

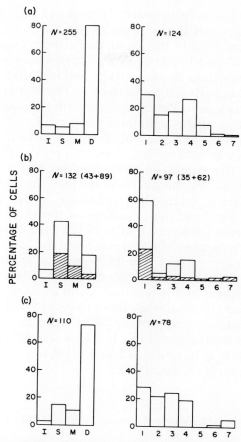

Figure 2. Summary of effects of visual cortex damage on response properties of posteromedial lateral suprasylvian cortex cells. (Left) the percentage of responsive cells (N, number of responsive cells in the sample) in each of four receptive-field classes. (I) indefinite; (S) stationary; (M) movement sensitive; (D) direction selective. (Right) the percentage of cells in each of seven ocular-dominance groups: (1) driven exclusively by the contralateral eye; (2) strongly dominated by the contralateral eye; (3) slightly dominated by the contralateral eye; (4) driven about equally by either eye or driven only by binocular stimulation; (5) slightly dominated by the ipsilateral eye; (6) strongly dominated by the ipsilateral eye; (7) driven exclusively by the ipsilateral eye. In the ocular-dominance analysis, only those cells that had their entire receptive field within the binocular-overlap field are considered. (a) normal adult cats. (b) cats with damage to areas 17, 18, and 19 received as adults. Crosshatched portions of each bar are results from cats with long-term lesions (6.5–8-month survival, $N = 43$), and open portions are results from cats with shorter survival times (0.5–1-month, $N = 89$). The height of each bar represents the sum of the crosshatched and open portions. (c) cats with damage to areas 17, 18, and 19 received on the day of birth (6–8.5-month survival). Both neonatal and adult lesions were unilateral, and recordings were made in the ipsilateral hemisphere. (From Spear, Kalil, & Tong, 1980.)

that removal of inputs from ipsilateral areas 17 and 18 produce several immediate changes in the responses of PMLS cortex cells (additional removal of area 19 has no further effect). These changes indicate that areas 17 and 18 provide PMLS cortex neurons with information for producing direction selectivity and inhibition of responses to stationary flashing stimuli for both eyes. The inputs from the visual cortex also provide most PMLS neurons with the ability to respond to visual stimulation of the ipsilateral eye.

Thalamic pathways to the PMLS cortex arise from a variety of nuclei (Sherman & Spear, 1982; Spear, in press). The major projections are from the lateral posterior nucleus, the posterior nucleus, and to a lesser extent the pulvinar nucleus. In addition, there are weaker projections from the geniculate wing, the medial interlaminar nucleus, and the C-laminae of the LGN. There normally are no inputs from laminae A and A1 of the LGN to the PMLS cortex. There have been no physiological studies of the extent to which X, Y, and W cell pathways from the LGN project to the PMLS cortex. However, anatomical studies suggest that the PMLS cortex receives W and Y cell inputs, and little or no X cell input. Lesion studies (see following section) indicate that these thalamic pathways, in the absence of the visual cortex, provide PMLS neurons with the ability to respond to the contralateral eye but lack information necessary to produce direction selectivity and inhibition of responses to stationary flashing stimuli (Figure 1[a]).

Effects of Visual Cortex Damage in Adult Cats

Many of the neural consequences of visual cortex damage in adult cats are shown schematically in Figure 1(e). Damage to areas 17, 18, and 19 produces marked retrograde degeneration in the LGN (Chow & Dewson, 1966; Garey & Powell, 1967; Niimi & Sprague, 1970). In addition, there is some transneuronal retrograde degeneration of ganglion cells in the retina. The retinal degeneration is confined to neurons of the X cell functional class and results in a loss of about 22% of those cells (Tong, Spear, Kalil, & Callahan, 1982). Because this is a relatively small loss, the X, Y, and W cell pathways from the retina have been depicted as essentially normal in Figure 1(e).

In addition to the retrograde changes that occur following visual cortex damage in adult cats, the damage of course results in a loss of efferent projections to various areas of the brain. One such pathway that is lost is that to the PMLS cortex (Figure 1[e]). Physiological studies indicate that three changes in the response properties of PMLS neurons occur following visual cortex damage in adult cats (Spear & Baumann, 1979a). These are summarized in Figure 2(b). First, there is a marked reduction in the percentage of direction-selective cells, from about 80% in normal adult cats to about 20% in cats with adult visual cortex lesions. Second, there is a marked increase in the percentage of cells that respond best to stationary flashing stimuli (cells in the stationary receptive-field class). Third, there is a decrease in the proportion of cells that respond to the ipsilateral eye, from about 70% in normal adult cats to about 40% in cats with adult visual cortex damage. Correspondingly, the percentage of cells that respond exclusively to the contralateral eye increases. These changes occur immediately after the visual cortex damage (Spear & Baumann, 1979a) and remain unaltered over long survival times, even if visual discrimination training is given (Spear & Baumann, 1979b; Spear, Kalil, & Tong, 1980). Thus there is no evidence that functional compensation for the loss of visual cortex inputs can occur in the PMLS cortex of adult cats.

The response properties that remain in the PMLS cortex after visual cortex has been removed reflect the functional properties that are formed on the basis of remaining thalamic–PMLS cortex inputs. As shown in Figure 1(e), these inputs provide information primarily for the contralateral eye and lack information for the formation of direction selectivity and for inhibition of responses to stationary flashing stimuli.

Anatomical studies using retrograde tracing methods confirm the presence of thalamic–PMLS cortex projections after visual cortex damage in adult cats (Kalil, Tong, & Spear 1980). They show that even after long survival times, relatively normal projections remain from the pulvinar, lateral posterior, and posterior nuclei, and from the geniculate wing, medial interlaminar nucleus, and C-laminae of the LGN. These results, plus those of anterograde tracing studies (Tong, Kalil, & Spear, 1984), suggest that the remaining thalamocortical projections to the PMLS cortex do not increase or otherwise compensate for the damage to visual cortex in adult cats.

EFFECTS OF VISUAL CORTEX DAMAGE
ON THE DAY OF BIRTH

The consequences of damage to areas 17, 18, and 19 in newborn kittens are very different from those of damage in adult cats (Figure 1[b]). One of the most striking effects of neonatal visual cortex damage is a marked transneuronal retrograde degeneration of retinal ganglion cells. This was first noted by Ganser (1882), who carried out anatomical studies of the ganglion cell fiber layer of cats that had received large cortical lesion at birth. More recent anatomical studies have confirmed this finding and have shown that the ganglion cell loss is restricted to the medium-size ganglion cells (Kalil, 1980; Pearson, Labar, Payne, Cornwell, & Aggarwall, 1981). Physiological studies have shown that the loss is restricted to ganglion cells of the X cell functional class and that about 78% of these cells are lost following neonatal damage to areas 17, 18, and 19 (or just areas 17 and 18). Y and W cells in the retina are unaffected (Tong *et al.*, 1982).

Degeneration of retinal ganglion cells also has been reported to occur following visual cortex damage in dogs, squirrel monkeys, owl monkeys, rhesus monkeys, and humans (Cowey, 1974; Dineen & Hendrickson, 1981; Van Buren, 1963a,b; von Monakow, 1889; Weller & Kaas, 1982; Weller, Kaas, & Wetzel, 1979), so it appears to be a relatively general occurrence. The reason that X cells are affected selectively by visual cortex damage may be related to differences in axon branching patterns among the three classes of retinal ganglion cells (Tong *et al.*, 1982; Weller *et al.*, 1979). However, it is not clear why the loss of retinal X cells is so much more severe after neonatal lesions than after adult lesions (Tong *et al.*, 1982).

The retinal ganglion cells that remain after neonatal visual cortex damage provide at least two anomalous projections to the thalamus. First, the projections to the geniculate wing are larger and denser than normal (Labar, Berman, & Murphy, 1981). Detailed developmental studies indicate that this is due to an active invasion of excess retinal terminals during development and possibly also to some failure of initially exuberant projections to retract (Labar *et al.*, 1981). It is known that the geniculate wing projects to the PMLS cortex in cats with neonatal visual cortex damage; however, it is not known if this projection differs from normal (Kalil, Tong, & Spear, 1979). It also is not known if the physiological properties of neurons in the geniculate wing differ from normal in cats with neonatal visual cortex damage.

The second anomalous retinal projection is to the laminated portion of the LGN (laminae A and A1 and the C-laminae). Before describing this projection, it is necessary to describe the state of the LGN itself. Following visual cortex damage in newborn kittens, there is a marked retrograde degeneration of neurons in the LGN that is in many respects more severe than that following damage in adults (Cornwell *et al.*, 1978; Doty, 1961; Mize & Murphy, 1976; Spear *et al.*, 1980). Despite this, many large, dark-staining cells remain within otherwise degenerated portions of the C-laminae and laminae A and A1. These large, surviving cells are not related to localized sparing within areas 17, 18, or 19 (Cornwell *et al.*, 1978; Mize & Murphy, 1976; Spear *et al.*, 1980; Tucker *et al.*, 1968).

Anatomical studies indicate that both retinae send projections to the degenerated LGN, and that their terminals tend to cluster around the large surviving cells (Kalil, 1978; in press). This projection is anomalous in that the inputs are not as well organized as normal (Kalil, 1978). In addition, electron microscopic analysis indicates that the retinogeniculate synaptic connectivity differs from that in both normal cats and cats with adult visual cortex damage (Kalil & Behan, 1982). Physiological recordings indicate that these retinogeniculate connections are functional, inasmuch as the surviving LGN cells respond to visual stimulation (Murphy & Kalil, 1979). Many of the response properties of these cells are like those of normal LGN. For example, all of the cells are monocularly driven, with about equal numbers driven by the contralateral and ipsilateral eyes. In addition, the basic center-surround receptive-field organization is normal for most of the cells. However, the centers of the receptive fields appear to be 3–4 times larger than normal and, although a gross visuotopic organization is present, the finegrain topographic organization is abnormal. These physiological abnormalities are in general accord with the anatomical anomalies in retinogeniculate termination patterns.

Anatomical studies indicate that these large surviving cells in the LGN form part of an enhanced pathway to the PMLS area of the cortex. Kalil (in press) first demonstrated the existence of an enhanced projection from retina to thalamus to PMLS cortex using transneuronal autoradiographic techniques. Additional experiments using retrograde tracing methods confirmed this finding (Kalil *et al.*, 1979). They showed that the large, surviving neurons in the C-laminae and in laminae A and A1 of the LGN send a projection to the PMLS cortex, and that this projection is much heavier than normal. In the C-laminae, there is a tenfold increase in the number of cells that project to the PMLS cortex in cats with neonatal visual cortex damage compared to normal cats. In laminae A and A1, many cells project to the PMLS cortex in cats with neonatal visual cortex damage, whereas these laminae appear to have no projection to the PMLS cortex in normal adult cats. Developmental studies suggest that this enhanced geniculo–PMLS cortex projection is due to an active invasion of terminals into the PMLS cortex (Tong, Kalil, and Spear, 1983).

A question of some interest is whether these enhanced projections

from the thalamus to the PMLS cortex are of physiological significance. Single-cell recording experiments suggest that they are. Spear
et al. (1980) found that PMLS cortex cells have normal receptive-field
properties and binocularity in cats that had areas 17, 18, and 19
removed on the day of birth. This result is summarized in Figure 2(c).
Note that the percentage of direction-selective cells and the percentages of cells in the other receptive-field classes are similar to those in
normal cats (Figure 2[a]), but very different from those in cats with
visual cortex damage received as adults (Figure 2[b]). Likewise, a
normal percentage of cells respond to the ipsilateral eye in cats with
neonatal visual cortex damage, whereas such cells are reduced in
frequency following adult visual cortex damage (Figure 2, right). No
evidence was found for a massive appearance of anomalous properties that might substitute for those of the damaged visual cortex. For
example, the receptive fields are as large as normal and few cells
(about 5%) are orientation selective.

Detailed histological analysis indicates that these results occur in
animals with complete neonatal removal of areas 17, 18, and 19; the
appearance of normal response properties is not due to remaining
inputs from spared remnants of the visual cortex (Spear *et al.*, 1980). In
addition, the results are not due to inputs from the other hemisphere
via the corpus callosum (Tong, Spear, & Kalil, 1983). Therefore, following neonatal visual cortex damage, the ipsilateral thalamic–
PMLS cortex pathways provide PMLS neurons with responsiveness to
the ipsilateral as well as to the contralateral eye. In addition, they
provide information that enables PMLS cortex cells to develop direction selectivity and inhibition of responses to stationary flashing stimuli (Figure 1[b]). This is information normally provided by inputs
from the visual cortex (Figure 1[a]).

The results discussed thus far have several general implications
that deserve emphasis. First, it is clear that visual cortex damage in
both adult and neonatal cats has neural consequences that go well
beyond a simple loss of the cortical tissue that was damaged. Some of
these consequences are orthograde, due to a loss of important visual
cortical inputs to other structures. In addition, some of the consequences are retrograde, and these can affect the visual system as far
peripherally as the retina. Second, despite these direct orthograde
and retrograde consequences, the visual system is very plastic neonatally. Pathways between structures can be enhanced and, in at
least two cases, this enhancement is due to an active invasion of
excessive inputs. Furthermore, these anomalous inputs can form synaptic connections that are of physiological significance. In the case of

the PMLS cortex, this leads to a physiological compensation for the lost visual cortex inputs.

There are instances, however, in which physiological compensation does not occur following neonatal visual cortex damage. An example is the superior colliculus. In normal cats, superior colliculus neurons have receptive-field properties and binocularity that are very similar to those of PMLS cortex neurons (Berman & Cynader, 1972; Rosenquist & Palmer, 1971; Stein & Arigbede, 1972; Sterling & Wickelgren, 1969). In addition, adult visual cortex damage produces very similar effects on superior colliculus and PMLS neurons. There is a loss of response to the ipsilateral eye, a loss of direction selectivity, and an increased response to stationary flashing stimuli (Berman & Cynader, 1972, 1975, 1976; Mize & Murphy, 1976; Rosenquist & Palmer, 1971; Stein, 1978; Wickelgren & Sterling, 1969). However, unlike the PMLS cortex, the superior colliculus shows no compensation for the loss of visual cortex inputs in newborn kittens; similar changes are seen following visual cortex lesions in adult and neonatal cats (Berman & Cynader, 1976; Flandrin & Jeannerod, 1977; Mize & Murphy, 1976; Stein & Magalhaes-Castro, 1975). The reason that some pathways and recipient structures are capable of neural plasticity following neonatal brain damage while others are not is an important question that remains to be answered.

Finally, results for the PMLS cortex indicate that when neural plasticity occurs, it is very orderly, and this can provide important information about some of the rules of visual system development. For example, comparison of Figures 1(a) and 1(b) shows that the inputs to the PMLS cortex are very different in normal adult cats and cats with visual cortex lesions made at birth. The most obvious difference is that inputs from cortical areas 17, 18, and 19 are present in one case and absent in the other. Nevertheless, the receptive-field properties of PMLS neurons are the same in the two conditions. This suggests that the receptive-field properties of neurons are not determined simply by the nature of their afferents. Rather, information contained within the recipient neurons in some way influences what their receptive-field properties will be.

Critical Periods

The preceding section showed that many of the neural consequences of visual cortex damage differ for newborn and adult cats. It is of

interest to determine the range of ages, or critical period of development, during which visual cortex damage produces effects that are
characteristic of those in the newborn organism. A determination of
the length of the critical period for these effects can provide very
useful information toward an understanding of their neural mechanisms. Several studies have investigated the critical periods for effects of neonatal visual cortex damage, with somewhat surprising
results. These findings are discussed in the following and are summarized schematically in Figure 1(b–e).

Physiological studies of the retina indicate that the period of life
during which visual cortex damage produces a marked loss of ganglion cells is quite limited (Callahan, Tong, & Spear, 1982). There is a
much smaller loss of X cells following lesions made at 2 weeks of age
(a 38% loss) than at birth (78% loss), and following lesions made at 4
weeks of age the loss is minimal (20%), just as in adults. Thus, Figure
1(c–e) shows that following visual cortex damage made at 2 weeks of
age or later, nearly normal percentages of X, Y, and W cells are
present in the retina.

Unfortunately, it is not known when the critical period is over for
the enhanced retinal projections to the geniculate wing or for the
anomalous retinal synaptic connections in the laminated portion of
the LGN. However, some information is available concerning the
enhanced pathway to the PMLS cortex. Transneuronal autoradiographic studies indicate that the increased projection from retina to
thalamus to PMLS cortex is present in animals that received visual
cortex lesions at 18 weeks of age, but little or no increase is seen
following damage at 26 weeks of age (Tong et al., 1984). Thus, the
critical period for development of this pathway following visual cortex damage ends between 18 and 26 weeks of age. This indicates that
the anomalous projection to the PMLS cortex is not related to the
retinal X cell loss.

The physiological compensation that occurs in the PMLS cortex
also is present following visual cortex damage incurred relatively
late in life (Tong et al., 1984). However, the critical period differs for
different response properties. Normal binocularity develops following lesions made at 18 weeks of age (Figure 1[d]), whereas following
lesions at 26 weeks of age there is a reduction in response to the
ipsilateral eye similar to that seen after lesions made in adult cats
(Figure 1[e]). Thus the critical period for development of binocularity
corresponds well with that for the development of enhanced projections to the PMLS cortex. In contrast, the critical period for development of normal direction selectivity and inhibition of responses to

stationary flashing stimuli is shorter. Normal percentages of PMLS cells develop these properties following lesions made at 12 weeks of age (Figure 1[c]), but not at 18 weeks of age (Figure 1[d]). Together these results suggest that the enhanced projections to the PMLS cortex are more related to binocular inputs than to the development of specific receptive-field properties. The specific receptive-field properties, on the other hand, may be a reflection of internal cortical connections. Consistent with this suggestion is the observation that the LGN cells, which contribute to the enhanced projection to the PMLS cortex, are not direction selective in cats with early visual cortex damage (Murphy & Kalil, 1979).

A particularly surprising result concerns the appearance of orientation selectivity among PMLS neurons following visual cortex damage at some ages. Recall that in normal adult cats, few or no PMLS cells respond selectively to the orientation of a moving or flashing stimulus. Similarly, few orientation-selective cells (5% or less) are found in the PMLS cortex of cats that received visual cortex damage on the day of birth or as adults (Spear & Baumann, 1979a,b; Spear et al., 1980). In contrast, about 30% of the PMLS cells display orientation selectivity in cats that received lesions at 2, 4, or 8 weeks of age, and about 11% display this property following lesions made at 12 weeks of age (Tong et al., 1984). Lesions made at 18 and 26 weeks of age yield results that are similar to those following lesions in adult cats. Thus, visual cortex damage at some ages results in the appearance of orientation selectivity for many PMLS neurons. The critical period for the appearance of this property begins later than that for other properties of PMLS neurons and ends at about the same time as (or slightly earlier than) that for direction selectivity and inhibition of responses to stationary flashing stimuli (Figure 1[c]).

These results have a number of important implications and raise a number of questions. Because few or no orientation-selective cells are found in the PMLS cortex of normal cats, it appears that an anomalous property can develop for many PMLS neurons after early visual cortex damage. Why and how does this occur? Presumably, the loss of numerous orientation-selective neurons when areas 17, 18, and 19 are damaged in some way triggers neurons within the PMLS cortex to develop orientation selectivity. However, the mechanisms by which neurons are induced to develop anomalous functional properties are a mystery.

Given that anomalous orientation selectivity does develop in the PMLS cortex following early visual cortex damage, why does it develop only in animals given lesions at 2 weeks of age or older and not in animals given lesions at birth? The answer to this question may be related to the state of the retina and the X cell pathways. It is possible that X cell pathways to the thalamus and the PMLS cortex are necessary for the development of orientation selectivity. That is, the mechanisms for development of anomalous orientation selectivity may be active following visual cortex lesions made as early as the day of birth, but few cells develop the property in these animals because there has been a massive degeneration of the retinal X cells and their inputs to the thalamus. Following lesions made at 2 weeks of age or later, however, many X cells and their central projections remain, making it possible for orientation selectivity to develop.

A third question is why the brain is able to alter its projections and physiological response properties afer damage incurred early in life but not later. That is, what are the mechanisms that allow or produce neuronal plasticity and what are the events that bring plasticity to an end, resulting in a critical period? This is, of course, a question of general importance to the understanding of mechanisms of neural development. Work on the effects of visual deprivation on the developing visual pathways suggests that neuronal plasticity is controlled, at least in part, by the widespread catechlamine-containing system of the brain (Daw, Rader, Robertson, & Ariel, 1983; Kasamatsu & Pettigrew, 1979; Kasamatsu, Pettigrew, & Ary, 1979, 1981). However, it is not clear how or why this system might have different effects at different ages. Moreover, it is not known if this system plays any role in the neuronal plasticity observed after early visual cortex damage. Whatever the mechanisms of the onset and offset of neuronal plasticity, it is clear from results of studies of the PMLS cortex that they are more complex than a general pharmacological switch that turns plasticity on and off. At least within the PMLS cortex, plasticity remains possible later in life for some properties (binocularity) than for others (specific receptive-field characteristics).

Relationships between Brain and Behavior

It was shown earlier that cats with neonatal lesions of areas 17, 18, and 19 are superior to cats with adult lesions in performance of a variety of visual behaviors. Indeed, in some cases cats with neonatal lesions can perform visual tasks normally whereas cats with adult lesions are severely deficient. It is of considerable interest to know if the functional compensation that occurs in the PMLS cortex of cats with neonatal visual cortex lesions is involved in this behavioral sparing. Unfortunately, there is no direct evidence on this question. However, several findings suggest that it may be.

First, there is direct evidence that cortex in the medial bank of the middle suprasylvian sulcus, including the PMLS area, is involved in behavioral recovery from damage to cortical areas 17, 18, and 19 in adult cats. Thus, removal of the PMLS and adjacent cortex in otherwise intact adult cats has no effect on retention or new learning of brightness, form, or pattern discriminations (Spear, Miller, & Ohman, 1983; Sprague, Levy, DiBerardino, & Berlucchi, 1977). However, if adult cats receive damage to areas 17, 18, and 19 and then are trained on form and pattern discriminations to establish behavioral recovery, subsequent lesions of the PMLS and adjacent cortex produce profound deficits in the recovered performance (Baumann & Spear, 1977). These results indicate that the PMLS area plays little essential role in form- and pattern-discrimination ability in normal cats but is part of a region that is involved in recovery of this ability after areas 17, 18, and 19 have been damaged. This by itself is an interesting finding. Because there is no functional compensation in either the PMLS or the adjacent cortex following visual cortex damage in adult cats (Spear & Baumann, 1979b), this finding indicates that the behavioral recovery in adult cats is based on residual abnormal function in this region. In addition, the demonstration that the PMLS cortex is part of the region involved in recovery from visual cortex damage in adults adds support to the suggestion that it is involved in recovery from neonatal visual cortex damage as well.

Certain behavioral results in cats with neonatal visual cortex damage also are consistent with this suggestion. Both Doty (1961) and Cornwell et al. (1978) reported that cats with neonatal damage to areas 17, 18, and 19 plus the suprasylvian gyri are much more impaired on form- and pattern-discrimination performance than cats with neonatal damage confined to areas 17, 18, and 19. Furthermore, Cornwell et al. (1978) found that the presence or absence of reliable visual-evoked potentials recorded over the suprasylvian cortex is significantly related to the ability of cats with neonatal visual cortex lesions to learn a form-discrimination task. Several aspects of the evoked potentials suggested that they arise from the middle suprasylvian sulcus rather than from polysensory cortical areas on the crown of the suprasylvian gyrus. Thus, these results suggest that some region in the middle suprasylvian sulcus is involved in the performance of visual discrimination tasks when areas 17, 18, and 19 have been damaged neonatally.

Clearly, what is needed is a study directly aimed at determining whether the presence of the PMLS cortex is important for the superior visual performance of cats with neonatal visual cortex damage. Only then will it be possible to reach firm conclusions about whether the enhanced thalamocortical projections and functional compensation in the PMLS cortex are part of the neural mechanisms of behavioral compensation from neonatal damage to areas 17, 18, and 19.

If the PMLS cortex is involved in the visual abilities of cats with neonatal visual cortex damage, then results discussed in this chapter provide an understanding of the neural mechanisms for the superior behavioral performance of these animals compared to animals with visual cortex damage received as adults. As pointed out earlier, cats with adult visual cortex damage use residual abnormal function in the PMLS and adjacent cortex as the neural basis for whatever sparing or recovery is possible (Spear, 1979). In contrast, animals with neonatal visual cortex damage appear to use the enhanced projections to the PMLS cortex and the more normal visual response properties of neurons there. Thus, the neural mechanisms of recovery appear to be very different following visual cortex damage incurred early life and in adulthood.

Even following visual cortex damage incurred early in life, however, the neural mechanisms of behavioral recovery and sparing may be very different following damage incurred at different ages. This is because, as emphasized earlier, different neural consequences of the early damage have different critical periods. Therefore, very different behavioral results might be expected from cats that received early visual cortex damage at different ages. For example, if the X cell pathways are involved in high spatial frequency resolution and visual acuity, as is commonly supposed (Sherman, 1979; Sherman & Spear, 1982; Stone et al., 1979), their loss following visual cortex lesions at birth might preclude the development of normal visual acuity. In contrast, animals that incurred damage at 2 weeks of age or later have only a small loss of retinal X cells and might be able to develop better visual acuity. In fact, psychophysical studies that have reported normal visual acuity in cats with early visual cortex damage used cats that received lesions between 2 and 4 weeks of age (Kaye & Mitchell, 1983). It would be of value to test visual acuity in animals that received visual cortex damage at birth.

Another example of behavioral differences that might be expected following early visual cortex damage at different ages is the extent of sparing of orientation-discrimination thresholds. These thresholds are known to be markedly increased following visual cortex lesions in adult cats (Berkley & Sprague, 1979), presumably because of the loss of orientation-selective neurons in the damaged cortex. If the PMLS cortex is involved in the psychophysical abilities of cats with early visual cortex damage, then one might expect orientation-discrimination thresholds to be lower in cats with lesions made at 2 to 8 weeks of age (in which many PMLS neurons are orientation selective) than in cats with lesions made at birth or at 18 weeks of age (in which few PMLS cells are orientation selective). On the other hand, tests of binocular function might reveal behavioral sparing following lesions made as late as 18 weeks of age, because these animals have normal binocularity in the PMLS cortex. Findings such as these would provide important information about the neural mechanisms of behavioral compensation from early visual cortex damage. In addition, they would have general implications for the understanding of the neural bases of orientation discrimination and binocular visual function.

Whatever the age at which the visual cortex damage occurs, however, it seems unlikely that completely normal visual function can be expected to develop. At their best (following lesions made between 2 and 8 weeks of age), the specificity of PMLS cortex neurons is not equivalent to that of neurons normally present in areas 17, 18, and 19. For example, a smaller proportion of PMLS cells is orientation selective and the sizes of the receptive fields are much larger than those of normal visual cortex cells. Therefore, orientation-discrimination thresholds might not reach normal levels, and other aspects of spatial vision that normally depend upon areas 17, 18, and 19 (such as vernier acuity, see Berkley & Sprague, 1979) might be impaired in animals with early visual cortex damage. Thus, unless some other region of the brain is capable of even greater physiological compensation than occurs in the PMLS cortex, neural substrates for complete behavioral compensation probably are not present following early visual cortex damage.

References

Baumann, T. P., & Spear, P. D. (1977). Role of the lateral suprasylvian visual area in behavioral recovery from effects of visual cortex damage in cats. *Brain Research, 138*, 445–468.

Berkley, M. A., & Sprague, J. M. (1979). Striate cortex and visual acuity functions in the cat. *Journal of Comparative Neurology, 187*, 699–702.

Berman, N., & Cynader, M. (1972). Comparisons of receptive-field organization of the superior colliculus in Siamese and normal cats. *Journal of Physiology, London, 224*, 363–389.

Berman, N., & Cynader, M. (1975). Receptive fields in cat superior colliculus after visual cortex lesions. *Journal of Physiology London, 245*, 261–270.

Berman, N., & Cynader, M. (1976). Early versus late visual cortex lesions: Effects on receptive fields in cat superior colliculus. *Experimental Brain Research, 25*, 131–138.

Callahan, E. C., Tong, L., & Spear, P. D. (1982). The critical period for effects of visual cortex lesions on retinal X-cells in cats. *Investigative Ophthalmology and Visual Science Supplement, 22*, 236.

Camarda, R., & Rizzolatti, G. (1976). Visual receptive fields in the lateral suprasylvian area (Clare-Bishop area) of the cat. *Brain Research, 401*, 425–443.

Chow, K. L., & Dewson, J. H. (1966). Numerical estimates of neurons and glia in lateral geniculate body during retrograde degeneration. *Journal of Comparative Neurology, 128*, 63–73.

Cornwell, P., & Overman, W. (1981). Behavioral effects of early rearing conditions and neonatal lesions of the visual cortex in kittens. *Journal of Comparative and Physiological Psychology, 95*, 848–862.

Cornwell, P., Overman, W., & Ross, C. (1978). Extent of recovery from neonatal damage to the cortical visual system in cats. *Journal of Comparative and Physiological Psychology, 92*, 255–270.

Cowey, A. (1974). Atrophy of retinal ganglion cells after removal of striate cortex in a rhesus monkey. *Perception, 3*, 257–360.

Daw, N. W., Rader, R. K., Robertson, T. W., & Ariel, M. (1983). Effects of 6-hydroxydopamine on visual deprivation in the kitten striate cortex. *Journal of Neuroscience, 3*, 907–914.

Dineen, J. T., & Hendrickson, A. E. (1981). Age-correlated differences in the amount of retinal degeneration after striate cortex lesions in monkeys. *Investigative Ophthalmology and Visual Science, 21*, 749–752.

Dineen, J., Vermeire, B., & Boothe, R. (1982). Contrast sensitivity changes in an infant monkey with extensive transsynaptic ganglion cell loss following striate cortex lesions. *Society for Neuroscience Abstracts, 8*, 295.

Doty, R. W. (1961). Functional significance of the topographical aspects of the retinocortical projection. In R. Jung & H. Kornhuber (Eds.), *The visual system: Neurophysiology and psychophysics* (pp. 228–247). Berlin: Springer.

Flandrin, J. M., & Jeannerod, M. (1977). Lack of recovery in collicular neurons from the effects of early deprivation or neonatal cortical lesions in the kitten. *Brain Research, 120*, 362–366.

Ganser, S. (1882). Über die periphere und zentrale Anordnung der Sehnervenfasern und uber das Corpus Bigeminum anterius. *Archives für Psychiatrie, 13*, 341–381.

Garey, L. J., & Powell, T. P. S. (1967). The projection of the lateral geniculate nucleus upon the cortex in the cat. *Proceedings of the Royal Society of London, Series B, 169*, 107–126.

Graybiel, A. M., & Berson, D. M. (1981). On the relation between transthalamic and transcortical pathways in the visual system. In F. O. Schmitt, F. G. Worden, G. Adelman, & F. Dennis (Eds.), *The organization of the cerebral cortex* (pp. 285–324). Cambridge: M.I.T. Press.

Heath, C. J., & Jones, E. G. (1971). The anatomical organization of the suprasylvian gyrus of the cat. *Ergebrisse der Anatomie, 45*, 1–64.

Hubel, D. H., & Wiesel, T. N. (1969). Visual area of the lateral suprasylvian gyrus (Clare-Bishop area) of the cat. *Journal of Physiology, London, 202*, 251–260.

Kaas, J. H. (1980). A comparative survey of visual cortex organization in mammals. In S. O. E. Ebbesson (Ed.), *Comparative neurology of the telencephalon* (pp. 483–502). New York: Plenum.

Kalia, M., & Whitteridge, D. (1973). The visual areas in the splenial sulcus of the cat. *Journal of Physiology, 232*, 275–283.

Kalil, R. E. (1978). Projection of the retina to the lateral geniculate nucleus in the cat following neonatal ablation of visual cortex. *Society for Neuroscience Abstracts, 4*, 633.

Kalil, R. E. (1980). Retrograde degeneration of retinal ganglion cells following removal of visual cortex in the newborn kitten. *Society for Neuroscience Abstracts, 6*, 790.

Kalil, R. E. (in press). Removal of visual cortex in the cat: Effects on the morphological development of the retino-geniculo-cortical pathway. In J. Stone, B. Dreher, & D. H. Rapaport (Eds.), *Development of Visual Pathways in Mammals* New York: A. R. Liss.

Kalil, R. E., & Behan, M. (1982). Synaptic organization of the lateral geniculate nucleus of the cat after removal of visual cortex. *Investigative Ophthalmology and Visual Science Supplement, 22*, 45.

Kalil, R. E., Tong, L., & Spear, P. D. (1979). Reorganization of the geniculocortical pathway in the cat following neonatal damage to visual cortex. *Investigative Opthalmology and Visual Science Supplement, 18*, 157.

Kalil, R. E., Tong, L., & Spear, P. D. (1980). [Observations on projections from the thalamus to lateral suprasylvian visual cortex in cats with adult removal of areas 17, 18, and 19]. Unpublished raw data.

Kasamatsu, T., & Pettigrew, J. D. (1979). Preservation of binocularity after monocular deprivation in the striate cortex of kittens treated with 6-hydroxydopamine. *Journal of Comparative Neurology, 185*, 139–162.

Kasamatsu, T., Pettigrew, J. D., & Ary, M. (1979). Restoration of visual cortical plasticity by local microperfusion of norepinephrine. *Journal of Comparative Neurology, 185*, 163–182.

Kasamatsu, T., Pettigrew, J. D., & Ary, M. (1981). Cortical recovery from effects of monocular deprivation: Acceleration with norepinephrine and suppression with 6-hydroxydopamine. *Journal of Neurophysiology, 45*, 254–266.

Kaye, M., & Mitchell, D. E. (1983). [Observations on the visual acuity of cats with damage of areas 17, 18, and 19 incurred early in life or as adults]. Unpublished raw data.

Kaye, M., Mitchell, D. E., & Cynader, M. (1981). Selective loss of binocular depth perception after ablation of cat visual cortex. *Nature, 293*, 60–62.

Kaye, M., Mitchell, D. E., & Cynader, M. (1982). Consequences for binocular depth perception of neonatal and adult lesions of cat visual cortex. *Investigative Ophthalmology and Visual Science Supplement, 22*, 175.

Labar, D. R., Berman, N. E., & Murphy, E. H. (1981). Short- and long-term effects of neonatal and adult visual cortex lesions on the retinal projection to the pulvinar in cats. *Journal of Comparative Neurology, 197*, 639–659.

Lehmkuhle, S., Kratz, K. E., & Sherman, S. M. (1982). Spatial and temporal sensitivity of normal and amblyopic cats. *Journal of Neurophysiology, 48*, 372–387.

Lennie, P. (1980). Parallel visual pathways: A review. *Vision Research, 20*, 561–594.

Mize, R. R., & Murphy, E. H. (1976). Alterations in receptive field properties of superior colliculus cells produced by visual cortex ablation in infant and adult cats. *Journal of Comparative Neurology, 168,* 393–424.

Murphy, E. H., & Kalil, R. E. (1979). Functional organization of lateral geniculate cells following removal of visual cortex in the newborn kitten. *Science, 206,* 713–716.

Murphy, E. H., Mize, R. R., & Schechter, P. B. (1975). Visual discrimination following infant and adult ablation of cortical areas 17, 18, and 19 in the cat. *Experimental Neurology, 49,* 386–405.

Niimi, K., & Sprague, J. M. (1970). Thalamocortical organization of the visual system in the cat. *Journal of Comparative Neurology, 138,* 219–250.

Olson, C. R., & Graybiel, A. M. (1981). A visual area in the anterior ectosylvian sulcus of the cat. *Society for Neuroscience Abstracts, 7,* 831.

Palmer, L. A., Rosenquist, A. C., & Tusa, R. J. (1978). The retinotopic organization of lateral suprasylvian visual areas in the cat. *Journal of Comparative Neurology, 177,* 237–256.

Pearson, H. E., Labar, D. R., Payne, B. R., Cornwell, P., & Aggarwal, N. (1981). Transneuronal retrograde degeneration in the cat retina following neonatal ablation of visual cortex. *Brain Research, 212,* 470–475.

Rodieck, R. W. (1979). Visual pathways. *Annual Reviews of Neuroscience, 2,* 193–226.

Rosenquist, A. C., & Palmer, L. A. (1971). Visual receptive field properties of cells of the superior colliculus after cortical lesions in the cat. *Experimental Neurology, 33,* 629–652.

Schneider, G. E. (1970). Mechanisms of functional recovery following lesions of visual cortex or superior colliculus in neonate and adult hamsters. *Brain, Behavior, and Evolution, 3,* 295–323.

Sherman, S. M. (1979). The functional significance of X- and Y-cells in visually deprived cats. *Trends in Neuroscience, 2,* 192–195.

Sherman, S. M., & Spear, P. D. (1982). Organization of visual pathways in normal and visually deprived cats. *Physiological Reviews, 62,* 738–855.

Smith, D. C., & Spear, P. D. (1979). Effects of superior colliculus removal on receptive field properties of neurons in lateral suprasylvian visual area of the cat. *Journal of Neurophysiology, 42,* 57–75.

Spear, P. D. (1979). Behavioral and neurophysiological consequences of visual cortex damage: Mechanisms of recovery. In J. M. Sprague & A. N. Epstein (Eds.), *Progress in psychobiology and physiological psychology* (Vol. 8, pp. 45–90). New York: Academic Press.

Spear, P. D. (in press). Neural mechanisms of compensation following neonatal visual cortex damage. In C. W. Cotman (Ed.), *Synaptic plasticity and remodeling.* New York: Guilford Press.

Spear, P. D., & Baumann, T. P. (1975). Receptive-field characteristics of single neurons in lateral suprasylvian visual area of the cat. *Journal of Neurophysiology, 38,* 1403–1420.

Spear, P. D., & Baumann, T. P. (1979a). Effects of visual cortex removal on receptive-field properties of neurons in lateral suprasylvian visual area of the cat. *Journal of Neurophysiology, 42,* 31–56.

Spear, P. D., & Baumann, T. P. (1979b). Neurophysiological mechanisms of recovery from visual cortex damage in cats: Properties of lateral suprasylvian visual area neurons following behavioral recovery. *Experimental Brain Research, 35,* 161–176.

Spear, P. D., Kalil, R. E., & Tong, L. (1980). Functional compensation in lateral suprasylvian visual area following neonatal visual cortex removal in cats. *Journal of Neurophysiology, 43,* 851–869.

Spear, P. D., Miller, S., & Ohman, L. (1983). Effects of lateral suprasylvian visual cortex lesions on visual localization, discrimination, and attention in cats. *Behavioural Brain Research, 10,* 339–359.

Sprague, J. M., Hughes, H. C., & Berlucchi, G. (1981). Cortical mechanisms in pattern and form perception. In O. Pompeiano & C. A. Marsan (Eds.), *Brain mechanisms of perceptual awareness and purposeful behavior* (pp. 107–132). New York: Raven Press.

Sprague, J. M., Levy, J., DiBerardino, H., & Belucchi, G. (1977). Visual cortical areas mediating form discrimination in the cat. *Journal of Comparative Neurology, 172,* 441–488.

Stein, B. E. (1978). Nonequivalent visual, auditory, and somatic corticotectal influences in cat. *Journal of Neurophysiology, 41,* 55–64.

Stein, B. E., & Arigbede, M. O. (1972). A parametric study of movement detection properties of neurons in the cat's superior colliculus. *Brain Research, 45,* 437–454.

Stein, B. E., & Magalhaes-Castro, B. (1975). Effects of neonatal cortical lesions upon the cat superior colliculus. *Brain Research, 83,* 480–485.

Sterling, P., & Wickelgren, B. G. (1969). Visual receptive fields in the superior colliculus of the cat. *Journal of Neurophysiology, 32,* 1–15.

Stewart, D. L., & Riesen, A. H. (1972). Adult versus infant brain damage: Behavioral and electrophysiological effects of striatectomy in adult and neonatal rabbits. *Advances in Psychobiology, 1,* 171–211.

Stone, J., Dreher, B., & Leventhal, A. (1979). Hierarchical and parallel mechanisms in the organization of visual cortex. *Brain Research Reviews, 1,* 345–394.

Symonds, L. L., Rosenquist, A. C., Edwards, S. B., & Palmer, L. A. (1981). Projections of the pulvinar-lateral posterior complex to visual cortical areas in the cat. *Neuroscience, 6,* 1995–2020.

Teuber, H.-L. (1961). Recent observation on the visual radiations and visual cortex. In R. Jung (Ed.), *The visual system: Neurophysiology and psychophysics* (pp. 256–274). Berlin: Springer-Verlag.

Tong, L., Kalil, R. E., & Spear, P. D. (1983). [Observations on the development of thalamic inputs to the cat's lateral suprasylvian visual cortex]. Unpublished raw data.

Tong, L., Kalil, R. E., & Spear, P. D. (in press). Critical periods for functional and anatomical compensation in the lateral suprasylvian visual area following removal of visual cortex in cats. *Journal of Neurophysiology.*

Tong, L., Spear, P. D., & Kalil, R. E. (1983). Role of the corpus collosum in functional compensation in the lateral suprasylvian visual area after early visual cortex damage in cats. *Investigative Ophthalmology and Visual Science Supplement, 24,* 228.

Tong, L., Spear, P. D., Kalil, R. E., & Callahan, E. C. (1982). Loss of retinal X-cells in cats with neonatal or adult visual cortex damage. *Science, 217,* 72–75.

Tucker, T. V., Kling, A., & Scharlock, D. P. (1968). Sparing of photic frequency and brightness discriminations after striatectomy in neonatal cats. *Journal of Neurophysiology, 31,* 818–932.

Turlejski, K. (1975). Visual responses of neurons in the Clare-Bishop area of the cat. *Acta Neurobiologica Experimentalis, 35,* 189–208.

Tusa, R. J., & Palmer, L. A. (1980). Retinotopic organization of areas 20 and 21 in the cat. *Journal of Comparative Neurology, 193,* 147–164.

Tusa, R. J., Palmer, L. A., & Rosenquist, A. C. (1978). The retinotopic organization of area 17 (striate cortex) in the cat. *Journal of Comparative Neurology, 177,* 213–236.

Tusa, R. J., Rosenquist, A. C., & Palmer, L. A. (1979). Retinotropic organization of areas 18 and 19 in the cat. *Journal of Comparative Neurology, 185,* 657–678.

Updyke, B. V. (1982). An additional retinotopically organized visual area (PS) within the cat's posterior suprasylvian sulcus and gyrus. *Society for Neuroscience Abstracts, 8,* 810.

Van Buren, J. M. (1963a). Trans-synaptic retrograde degeneration in the visual system of primates. *Journal of Neurology, Neurosurgery, and Psychiatry, 26,* 402–407.

Van Buren, J. M. (1963b). *The retinal ganglion cell layer.* Springfield, IL: Thomas.

Van Essen, D. C. (1979). Visual areas of the mammalian cerebral cortex. *Annual Reviews of Neuroscience, 2,* 227–263.

von Monakow, C. (1889). Experimentelle und pathologisch-anatomische Untersuchingen über die optischen Centren und Bahnen. *Archives für Psychiatrie und Nervenkrankheiten, 20,* 714–789.

Weller, R., & Kaas, J. H. (1982). Retinal degeneration and loss of retinogeniculate projections in infant and adult monkeys surviving variable times after lesions of striate cortex. *Investigative Ophthalmology and Visual Science Supplement, 22,* 46.

Weller, R. E., Kaas, J. H., & Wetzel, A. B. (1979). Evidence for the loss of X-cells of the retina after long-term ablation of visual cortex in monkeys. *Brain Research, 160,* 134–138.

Wetzel, A. B., Thompson, V. E., Horel, J. A., & Meyer, P. M. (1965). Some consequences of perinatal lesions of the visual cortex in the cat. *Psychonomic Science, 3,* 381–382.

Wickelgren, B. G., & Sterling, P. (1969). Influences of visual cortex on receptive fields in the superior colliculus of the cat. *Journal of Neurophysiology, 32,* 16–23.

Wright, M. J. (1969). Visual receptive fields of cells in a cortical area remote from the striate cortex in the cat. *Nature, 223,* 973–975.

13

Olfactory Bulb Control
of Sexual Function

Robert L. Meisel,
Benjamin D. Sachs,
and Augustus R. Lumia

Introduction

For many years olfaction has been viewed as an important sensory modality for the initiation of copulation, especially in rodents (Murphy, 1976). Numerous studies have demonstrated a role for the olfactory bulbs in the control of both male and female mating patterns. For example, with respect to male copulatory behavior, olfactory bulbectomy eliminates copulatory responding in hamsters (Devor, 1973; Doty, Carter, & Clemens, 1971; Lisk, Zeiss, & Ciaccio, 1972; Murphy, 1980; Murphy & Schneider, 1970; Winans & Powers, 1974) and mice (Rowe & Edwards, 1972; Rowe & Smith, 1973), and severely disrupts copulation in rats (see following section) and guinea pigs (Beauchamp, Magnus, Shmunes, & Durham, 1977).

The olfactory system of these species possesses a substantial regenerative capacity that lasts throughout the animal's life. In adult rats and mice, for example, olfactory receptors have a relatively short life span, with new receptors continually being formed to replace lost cells (Graziadei & Monti Graziadei, 1978). Consequently, in the olfactory bulb there is an ongoing turnover of synapses as contacts from the degenerating receptors are reinnervated by terminals from the newly maturing cells (Graziadei & Monti Graziadei, 1978). In addition, at least one olfactory bulb cell type, the granule cell, proliferates (apparently without any cell loss) in the adult rat (Kaplan & Hinds, 1977).

The regenerative ability of the peripheral receptors and the olfactory nerve is not diminished by removal of their target organ, the olfactory bulbs. Following olfactory bulbectomy in either neonatal or adult mice, the olfactory nerve regenerates and innervates the frontal cortex, with a pattern of synaptic connections resembling that seen in the normal olfactory bulb (Graziadei, Levine, & Monti Graziadei, 1978; Wright & Harding, 1982). In the adult mouse, the recovery of olfactory capability coincides with the timing of the innervation of the frontal cortex by the regenerating olfactory nerve (Wright & Harding, 1982).

Our interests in the neural control of copulatory function led us initially to examine the effects of olfactory bulbectomy on the copulatory behavior of male and female rats, and subsequently led to questions concerning the recoverability of copulatory function following bulbectomy incurred at different ages. Our approach to studying these problems is reflected in the organization of this chapter. We first review what is known about the effects of olfactory bulbectomy on sexual behavior in adult rats, information necessary for understanding the effects of the early lesions, which are considered next. Table 1 summarizes the available literature on olfactory bulbectomy at different ages. And finally, we offer some speculations on possible neural events associated with the development of reproductive function in animals bulbectomized at these earlier ages. Our decision to focus this chapter on data obtained from studies using rats is based on the paucity of data from neonatally bulbectomized animals of other species.[1]

Olfactory Bulbectomy and Masculine Copulatory Behavior

EFFECTS ON MALE RATS

Following bilateral removal of the olfactory bulbs of adult male rats, there commonly is a marked reduction in the percentage of these males that copulate to ejaculation (Larsson, 1969, 1975; Meisel,

---

[1] For a review of his excellent studies on morphological and behavioral plasticity following damage to the olfactory tract of hamsters, the reader should refer to Devor (1977).

TABLE 1

Copulatory Behavior of Adult Rats after Olfactory Bulbectomy

Age at bulbectomy	Masculine behavior	Feminine behavior
Day 2		
Male	Reduced proportion copulating	Not tested
Female	Reduced proportion copulating	Normal
Days 5 or 10		
Male	Normal	Not tested
Female	Not tested	Not tested
Juvenile (Days 30–42)		
Male	Reduced proportion copulating; increased ejaculation latency	Not tested
Female	Not tested	Normal
Adult (> Day 80)		
Male	Reduced proportion copulating; increased intromission and ejaculation latencies	Enhanced lordotic responsivity
Female	Reduced proportion copulating?	Enhanced precopulatory and lordotic responsivity

Lumia, & Sachs, 1980, 1982; Wang & Hull, 1980). In most cases, this ejaculatory deficit is due to an inability of these males to initiate copulation (Larsson, 1969, 1975; Meisel *et al.*, 1980; Wang & Hull, 1980). Among those studies in which a high proportion of bulbectomized males retain the ability to copulate to ejaculation (Bermant & Taylor, 1969; Cain & Paxinos, 1974; Heimer & Larsson, 1967), considerable test–retest variability in copulatory performance may exist (Cain & Paxinos, 1974; Heimer & Larsson, 1967). For example, in one study, all bulbectomized males ejaculated at least once postoperatively (Heimer & Larsson, 1967), yet on any given test only 50–75% of the bulbectomized males copulated to ejaculation.

Even when bulbectomized male rats copulate to ejaculation, evidence of copulatory impairment is still discernible. Bulbectomized males generally take longer to initiate copulation (increased intromission latency), and subsequently to ejaculate (increased ejaculation latency) (Bermant & Taylor, 1969; Cain & Paxinos, 1974; Heimer & Larsson, 1967; Larsson, 1969). In addition, at least one study has reported an increase in the time from ejaculation to the resumption of copulation (increased postejaculatory interval) (Heimer & Larsson, 1967). In contrast to the observed changes in temporal measures, other parameters of copulation, such as number of mounts and intromission patterns preceding ejaculation, appear to be unaffected by olfactory bulbectomy.

Several attempts have been made to reverse the debilitating effects of olfactory bulbectomy in adult male rats. Unlike the behavioral consequences of some lesions (e.g., septal lesion-induced hyperemotionality; Yutzey, Meyer, & Meyer, 1964), the effects of olfactory bulb removal on copulation do not dissipate over time. For example, Larsson (1969) found no recovery of copulatory behavior as long as 130 days postoperatively. Furthermore, exogenous administration of testosterone does not counteract the effects of bulbectomy (Larsson, 1969, 1975; Meisel et al., 1980), suggesting that the copulatory dysfunction suffered by bulbectomized males is not a secondary consequence of reduced testosterone levels.

At least one type of manipulation, however, can transiently activate sexual behavior in previously noncopulating bulbectomized male rats. Based on the assumption that the copulatory deficits in bulbectomized male rats result from a reduction in intrinsic sexual arousal (Cain & Paxinos, 1974), it seemed likely that procedures that enhance an animal's level of arousal should promote copulation (Barfield & Sachs, 1968; Caggiula, Shaw, & Antelman, 1976). Indeed, two such procedures, tail pinch (Wang & Hull, 1980) and flank shock (Meisel et al., 1980), will stimulate copulation in bulbectomized males. Working with sexually experienced male rats, we found that the percentage of male rats copulating to ejaculation was reduced by bulbectomy from 100% preoperatively to between 0 and 22% postoperatively. When mild electric shock was delivered to the flanks of the noncopulating bulbectomized males, 5 of 6 of these males subsequently copulated to ejaculation. It is notable that even though the bulbectomized males were shocked every 30 sec following the introduction of the female, they took significantly longer to initiate copulation than similarly shocked sham-lesioned males. Furthermore, the bulbectomized males copulated to a second ejaculation without additional flank shock. However, when retested 1 week later without shock, none of the bulbectomized males copulated. Thus, the effectiveness of flank shock or tail pinch to stimulate copulation can continue following cessation of the treatment, but these procedures cannot effect a long-term change in the copulatory responsiveness of bulbectomized males (Meisel et al., 1980; Wang & Hull, 1980).

The effectiveness of exogenous stimuli to (temporarily) ameliorate the effects of olfactory bulbectomy on copulation is consistent with the idea that these males are sexually underaroused. However, other activities of these animals suggest that reduced sexual arousal may be an inappropriate characterization of bulbectomized male rats. That is, upon introduction of the stimulus female rat, the precopulatory activities of bulbectomized and control males are often indistinguishable. Bulbectomized males actively pursue and investigate the anogenital region of receptive female rats (e.g., Meisel *et al.*, 1980), but then most males seem to lose interest in the female after a short period of time, although as noted previously a number of males will ultimately initiate copulation. Thus, it is unclear whether bulbectomized males are underaroused, or whether they are unable to make the transition from precopulatory arousal to the initiation of copulation. In a similar context, Sachs and Barfield concluded, "Such a deficit may be viewed as inadequate net sexual arousal, but it may also indicate an inability to gate adequate arousal into appropriate copulatory behavior" (1976, p. 102).

EFFECTS ON FEMALE RATS

As would be expected, far fewer studies have been done on the effects of olfactory bulb removal on mounting by female rats. We found that bulbectomized female rats that were ovariectomized and treated with testosterone were less likely (1/11) than sham-lesioned females (5/8) to mount receptive female rats (Lumia, Meisel, & Sachs, 1981), a finding that parallels the results of our experiments with males (e.g., Meisel *et al.*, 1980). However, Coniglio and Clemens (1972) were unable to detect any copulatory deficits in bulbectomized females maintained on testosterone. Given the interexperiment variability in the rate of mounting in normal female rats (Coniglio & Clemens, 1972; Södersten, 1972), it may prove difficult to obtain reliable effects of olfactory bulbectomy on mounting in female rats.

Olfactory Bulbectomy and Feminine Copulatory Behavior

EFFECTS ON FEMALE RATS

Whereas olfactory bulb removal in adult male (and possibly female) rats interferes with the ability of these animals to display masculine copulatory behavior (see previous section), olfactory bulbectomy in adult female rats enhances their sexual responsiveness. Moss (1971) found that following priming with estrogen and progesterone, bulbectomized female rats assumed the receptive posture, lordosis, to a copulating male rat more readily than did control-lesioned females. Subsequent studies also found an enhanced lordotic potential in estrogen–progesterone-treated females (Edwards & Warner, 1972; Lumia et al., 1981), as well as in estrogen-primed (Edwards & Warner, 1972; McGinnis, Nance, & Gorski, 1978; Tyler & Gorski, 1980) and even intact, cycling bulbectomized female rats (Al Salti & Aron, 1977). These studies indicate that lordotic responsivity to estrogen (and possibly progesterone) is elevated by olfactory bulb removal.

We pursued the question of how the olfactory bulbs are involved in the regulation of female sexual responsiveness and expanded our analyses (Lumia et al., 1981) to include the precopulatory (darting, ear wiggling) components of the female sexual mating pattern (Dewsbury, 1979; Madlafousek & Hliňák, 1977). In our first experiment, bilaterally bulbectomized and control-lesioned female rats were tested for sexual responsivity to increased doses of estrogen, each followed by a fixed dose of progesterone. The frequency of lordosis for both groups of females increased as a function of estrogen dose, yet at all doses, estrogen-treated bulbectomized females had higher levels of lordosis than did control females. Darting and ear wiggling were also enhanced in bulbectomized females at all doses of estrogen, although there was no change in these measures as a function of estrogen dose. Whereas lordosis is generally considered to be an estrogen-sensitive response, darting and ear wiggling are dependent on the presence of both estrogen and progesterone (Tennent, Smith, & Davidson, 1980; Whalen, 1974). Thus the facilitation of darting and ear wiggling by olfactory bulbectomy suggested an enhanced responsivity to progesterone as well. To test this possibility, we treated bulbectomized and control female rats with a fixed dose of estrogen and varying doses of progesterone. Once again we found elevated lordosis in bulbectomized females, but there was no change in lordosis across progesterone doses. These bulbectomized females had high levels of darting and ear wiggling, with a dose-dependent relationship between progesterone and amount of darting.

From the evidence reviewed so far, we would agree with Edwards and Warner (1972) that the olfactory bulbs normally inhibit neural systems involved in the display of lordosis, and we would extend their hypothesis to include a tonic inhibition of the female rat's precopulatory behavior as well. It should be noted, however, that the generalization of these effects to other hormone-sensitive response patterns, or even to copulatory responsiveness outside the context of the vigorously mounting male rat, may be limited. For example, we placed our bulbectomized and control female rats in an open-field apparatus that contained a caged, gonadally intact male rat in its center (Lumia *et al.*, 1981). Estrogen and progesterone treatment increased the number of squares entered and the number of contacts the female made with the cage containing the male. However, there were no differences between bulbectomized and control females on these hormone-sensitive measures. Furthermore, at the highest dose of estrogen (with progesterone), females were observed to dart in this testing situation, with no group differences in darting frequency. Finally, the enhanced lordotic responsivity of bulbectomized females can occur under conditions of hormone priming that do not promote the induction of hypothalamic progestin receptors (McGinnis, Lumia, & McEwen, 1981). The potentiation of hormone-sensitive responses by olfactory bulbectomy, therefore, may be restricted to mating responses only, and moreover to mating responses in specific contexts.

EFFECTS ON MALE RATS

There has been only one report on the effects of olfactory bulb removal on female mating behavior in male rats (Edwards & Warner, 1972). These authors reported that olfactory bulbectomy enhanced both the lordosis quotient and lordosis intensity of male rats treated with estrogen and progesterone. Although higher than that of control males, the lordotic responsiveness of the bulbectomized males did not approach the levels seen in control female rats.

Effects of Olfactory Bulbectomy in Juveniles and Neonates

MASCULINE COPULATORY BEHAVIOR

Like the effects of olfactory bulb removal in adult male rats (see previous sections), bulbectomy in juvenile males (30 days old) also disrupts copulation when these males are tested in adulthood (Wilhelmsson & Larsson, 1973). In this study only 50% of the group-

reared bulbectomized males copulated to ejaculation as adults, compared to 90% of the sham-lesioned males. Again reminiscent of adult
bulbectomized males, those juvenile bulbectomized males that copulated to ejaculation had longer ejaculation latencies than the sham-
lesioned controls; other copulatory parameters appeared to be normal.

The first evidence that copulatory function could be spared in male
rats receiving bilateral olfactory bulb removal came from a study by
Pollak and Sachs (1975). In this instance, there was no difference
between male rats bulbectomized at 6 days of age and sham-lesioned
males in the proportions copulating to ejaculation, and quantitative
measures of their copulatory behavior were similar.

We attempted to further delineate the critical ages at which sparing of copulatory function following olfactory bulbectomy could be
obtained and found some interesting results (Meisel *et al.*, 1982). Copulatory behavior in male rats bulbectomized at 10 days of age was
quite normal, with 94% of these males copulating to ejaculation (versus 86% for the control males). In contrast, males bulbectomized at 2
days of age showed a reduced copulatory potential, as 50% (compared to 92% of the control males) copulated to ejaculation. On their
five tests, from 31% (Test 2) to 44% (Test 1) of the Day 2 bulbectomized males ejaculated, owing to the variable responsiveness of
these males. Copulatory latencies of the ejaculating Day 2 bulbectomized males were normal, a characteristic distinguishing these
males from those bulbectomized as juveniles or adults.

Interestingly, Day 2 bulbectomy also reduces the masculine copulatory potential of female rats (Lumia *et al.*, 1981). As noted earlier,
mounting can be elicited from androgen-treated female rats, and
bulbectomy in adulthood may reduce this mounting potential. Only
23% (6/26) of our Day 2 bulbectomized females mounted receptive
female rats, a proportion significantly smaller than the 63% (5/8) of
our control females that mounted. Masculine copulatory behavior
has not been tested in females bulbectomized at other neonatal or
juvenile periods, limiting comparisons with males. However, the
available data suggest that bulbectomy in female rats produces effects on mounting in a manner similar to that seen in male rats
bulbectomized at equivalent ages.

FEMININE COPULATORY BEHAVIOR

Removal of the olfactory bulbs in 42-day-old female rats, about the
time of sexual maturity (in this strain), resulted in normal sexual

responsiveness when these animals were tested at about 100 days of age (Al Salti & Aron, 1977). Similar results were obtained by Larsson (1977), who bulbectomized female rats at an unspecified age between 21 and 30 days. In this experiment bulbectomy produced an initial reduction in lordosis responsivity, after which time normal levels of lordosis were attained.

The effects of neonatal olfactory bulbectomy on female sexual behavior have been studied in female rats bulbectomized at only one age. Female rats bulbectomized at 2 days of age did not exhibit the enhanced behavioral responsivity to estrogen and progesterone characteristic of female rats bulbectomized in adulthood (Lumia et al., 1981). Levels of lordosis, as well as darting and ear wiggling, in neonatally bulbectomized females are comparable to control-lesioned females. We can rule out differences in the amount of time between bulbectomy and testing as a factor in the recovery of the neonatally bulbectomized females, because lordosis in female rats bulbectomized as adults remains enhanced 120 days after bulbectomy (Tyler & Gorski, 1980). Thus, it appears that female reproductive behavior is unaffected by olfactory bulbectomy if the operation is performed at any time up to sexual maturity. However, investigations of the effects of olfactory bulbectomy at various preweaning ages are necessary to validate this conclusion. In addition, since male rats bulbectomized in adulthood display elevated levels of lordosis, it would be interesting to discover whether male rats bulbectomized prior to sexual maturity recover normal levels of lordosis. The effects of olfactory bulbectomy on the copulatory behavior of male and female rats are summarized in Table 1 (see p. 255).

Conclusions

FUNCTIONAL SPECIFICITY

After reviewing the literature on the effects of olfactory bulb removal on a wide range of functional systems, Cain (1974) concluded that the olfactory bulbs are part of a forebrain arousal system and that olfactory bulbectomy eliminates both olfactory information and an important source of excitatory neural inputs to the limbic system. Although Cain's hypothesis is consistent with much of the literature on bulbectomy-induced behavioral changes, we have argued (Meisel et al., 1980) that alterations in arousal mechanisms alone cannot account for the varied effects of olfactory bulbectomy on reproductive behavior. The limitations of arousal as an explanatory construct is best illustrated by the behavior of bulbectomized female rats. In this case, olfactory bulbectomy increased both the precopulatory (proceptivity) and receptivity components of the female mating pattern. In contrast, neurochemical alterations that reduce the arousability of female rats eliminate precopulatory responsivity without affecting the receptivity of these females (Caggiula, Herndon, Scanlon, Greenstone, Bradshaw, & Sharp, 1979). We have already discussed the difficulty of interpreting the copulatory deficit of bulbectomized males in the context of reduced sexual arousal. Although a model of male rat sexual behavior could include several arousal mechanisms (e.g., investigation of the female rat, initiation of copulation, reinitiation of copulation after ejaculation), such a system becomes conceptually unwieldy.

Rather than a single mechanism for the effects of bulbectomy on reproductive behavior, there seems to be a functional specificity related to bulbectomy (Lumia et al., 1981; Tyler & Gorski, 1980). Some hormone-sensitive response patterns (e.g., mounting) may be disrupted by olfactory bulbectomy, whereas others (e.g., lordosis and darting) may be enhanced, or unaffected (e.g., open-field activity) by bulbectomy. Further complicating matters is the observation that the effects of bulbectomy may be context dependent (e.g., bulbectomy-enhanced darting in the presence of an accessible male rat, but not a caged male). The notion that olfactory bulb efferents to different functional systems may be qualitatively distinct is supported by the patterns of behavioral recovery of our neonatally bulbectomized animals. In both males and females, bulbectomy at 2 days of age disrupted mounting behavior, whereas the receptivity and precopulatory behavior of the neonatally bulbectomized females (the only sex tested) was normal. Also, male rats bulbectomized at either 2 or 10 days of age showed evidence of an olfactory deficit neonatally, but not in adulthood (Meisel et al., 1982). Yet adult copulatory behavior was impaired only in males bulbectomized at 2 days of age. This dissociation between the patterns of recovery of copulatory behavior and of olfactory capability points to a nonsensory effect of olfactory bulbectomy on copulation. However, we should point out that the relative contributions of olfactory and nonsensory functions of the olfactory bulbs on copulatory behavior in rats remains unknown. Filling the gaps in Table 1, particularly with respect to feminine copulatory behavior, is necessary for establishment of the between-sex consistency in the recovery of copulatory function following bulbectomy in rats.

POSSIBLE NEURAL LOCI AND MECHANISMS MEDIATING BEHAVIORAL RECOVERY

The results of lesion studies have established that neural pathways between the olfactory bulbs and the hypothalamus have a functional role in the control of copulation in both males and females. For male copulatory behavior, lesions of the corticomedial amygdala, stria terminalis, or bed nucleus of the stria terminalis share the ability to lengthen the intromission latency, often to the point of creating noncopulators (Sachs, 1978). Inasmuch as these structures together with the olfactory bulbs form an afferent pathway to the medial preoptic region (Berk & Finkelstein, 1981; Scalia & Winans, 1976), it seems likely that these connections form a functional system for the activation of masculine copulatory behavior (Sachs, 1978). In the female rat, lesions of either the olfactory bulbs or the caudal part of the lateral amygdala (Mascó & Carrer, 1980) facilitate lordotic responding, leading to the conclusion that these structures normally inhibit female copulatory behavior. These structures probably exert their effects on the ventromedial hypothalamus, a nucleus critical for the activation of female copulatory behavior (Pfaff, 1980; Rubin & Barfield, 1980). The failure of lesions of the stria terminalis to affect lordosis in female rats (Brown-Grant & Raisman, 1972) indicates that the ventral amygdalofugal pathway transmits this inhibition to the ventromedial hypothalamus (Mascó & Carrer, 1980).

Clearly, any hypothesis concerning the neural basis for copulatory recovery following early olfactory bulbectomy must take into account the potential reorganization of the projection areas of the olfactory bulbs (and other distal regions), as well as the regenerative capacity of the olfactory tissues. We can conceive of at least three nonexclusive mechanisms by which neural reorganization can contribute to the patterns of copulatory recovery outlined in this chapter. In the first and simplest case, the olfactory bulbs may regenerate. This is an unlikely possibility inasmuch as there are no reports of regeneration following neonatal olfactory bulbectomy. Second, there is some support in the literature (Graziadei et al., 1978; Wright & Harding, 1982) for a related mechanism in which another brain region may assume the role of the olfactory bulbs, possibly reestablishing the anatomical connections of the ablated tissue. Last, because the olfactory bulbs share first-order reciprocal connections with a number of structures, the elimination of afferent and efferent projections of these regions may promote a subsequent sprouting of fibers influencing the animal's potential for copulation (e.g., Devor, 1975). Similar changes in second- or third-order connections might also occur.

We first consider the recovery of feminine copulatory behavior. A common observation concerning the brains of neonatally bulbectomized rodents, when analyzed in adulthood, is the presence of neural tissue in the olfactory bulb capsule (Graziadei et al., 1978; Leonard, 1978; Lumia et al., 1981; Meisel et al., 1982). This tissue, which is an extension of the frontal cortex, becomes innervated by the olfactory nerve, forming glomeruli, though these glomeruli do not assume the laminar arrangement of the normal olfactory bulb (Graziadei et al., 1978; Leonard, 1978). Although we might be tempted to correlate the growth and innervation of the frontal cortex with the recovery of female copulatory responsiveness, we should keep in mind that female rats bulbectomized as juveniles show patterns of behavioral recovery analogous to neonatally bulbectomized females (Table 1), but without the cortical growth and innervation. A reasonable mechanism, therefore, for the recovery of female rats bulbectomized as neonates or juveniles might include a compensation by other brain regions also inhibitory to lordosis, such as the amygdala (Mascó & Carrer, 1980), the medial preoptic area (Powers & Valenstein, 1972), the septum (McGinnis et al., 1978), or the neocortex (Clemens, Wallen, & Gorski, 1967). In this instance, one would predict that "rebulbectomy" of neonatally bulbectomized female rats in adulthood should not alter their lordotic responsiveness.

For masculine copulatory behavior, such neurologizing is complicated by the different patterns of recovery between the males bulbectomized at 2 days of age and those bulbectomized at 10 days. The olfactory bulbs are quite mature soon after birth (Roselli-Austin & Altman, 1979), and intrinsic spontaneous activity can be recorded on the day of birth (Math & Davrainville, 1980). In contrast, the functional activity of the primary olfactory bulb projections (as measured by 2-deoxyglucose uptake) does not develop until rather late in the neonatal period. For example, activity in the amygdala does not develop until Day 9 postnatally (Astic & Saucier, 1982). We would propose that recovery in this system is unrelated to the maturation of the olfactory bulbs and may be possible only after the initial connections have been established. These functional connections could, for example, form a channel facilitating the reformation of connections from the newly reorganized "olfactory bulbs" (i.e., frontal cortex). Olfactory bulbectomy prior to the establishment of the primary olfactory projections (e.g., Day 2) may result in regenerating fibers making contacts detrimental to or irrelevant to the recovery of copulatory potential. As with the females, rebulbectomy of the neonatally bulbectomized males would reveal any contribution of the regrowth of the frontal cortex to the recovery of copulatory function. Alternatively, rebulbectomy might be without effect, suggesting that the copulatory recovery is related to changes in regions downstream from the olfactory bulbs.

Acknowledgments

Our research was supported by USPHS research Grant HD-08933 (to B. D. Sachs), and a grant from the University of Connecticut Research Foundation (to B. D. Sachs and A. R. Lumia). Preparation of this chapter was supported by a USPHS postdoctoral fellowship HD-06240 (to R. L. Meisel).

References

Al Salti, M., & Aron, C. (1977). Influence of olfactory bulb removal on sexual receptivity in the rat. *Psychoneuroendocrinology, 2,* 399–407.
Astic, L., & Saucier, D. (1982). Metabolic mapping of functional activity in the olfactory projections of the rat: Ontogenetic study. *Developmental Brain Research, 2,* 141–156.
Barfield, R. J., & Sachs, B. D. (1968). Sexual behavior: Stimulation by painful electric shock to skin in male rats. *Science, 161,* 392–395.
Beauchamp, G. K., Magnus, J. G., Shmunes, N. T., & Durham, T. (1977). Effects of olfactory bulbectomy on social behavior of male guinea pigs (*Cavia porcellus*). *Journal of Comparative and Physiological Psychology, 91,* 336–346.
Berk, M. L., & Finkelstein, J. A. (1981). Afferent projections to the preoptic area and hypothalamic regions in the rat brain. *Neuroscience, 6,* 1601–1624.
Bermant, G., & Taylor, L. (1969). Interactive effects of experience and olfactory bulb lesions in male rat copulation. *Physiology and Behavior, 4,* 13–17.
Brown-Grant, K., & Raisman, G. (1972). Reproductive function in the rat following selective destruction of afferent fibers to the hypothalamus from the limbic system. *Brain Research, 46,* 23–42.
Caggiula, A. R., Herndon, J. G., Jr., Scanlon, R., Greenstone, D., Bradshaw, W., & Sharp, D. (1979). Dissociation of active from immobility components of sexual behavior in female rats by central 6-hydroxydopamine: Implications for CA involvement in sexual behavior and sensorimotor responsiveness. *Brain Research, 172,* 505–520.
Caggiula, A. R., Shaw, D. H., & Antelman, S. M. (1976). Interactive effects of brain catecholamines and variations in sexual and non-sexual arousal on copulatory behavior of male rats. *Brain Research, 111,* 321–336.
Cain, D. P. (1974). The role of the olfactory bulb in limbic mechanisms. *Psychological Bulletin, 81,* 654–671.

Cain, D. P., & Paxinos, G. (1974). Olfactory bulbectomy and mucosa damage: Effects on copulation, irritability, and interspecific aggression in male rats. *Journal of Comparative and Physiological Psychology, 86,* 202–212.

Clemens, L. G., Wallen, K., & Gorski, R. A. (1967). Mating behavior: Facilitation in the female rat after cortical application of potassium chloride. *Science, 157,* 1208–1209.

Coniglio, L., & Clemens, L. G. (1972). Stimulus and experiential factors controlling mounting behavior in the female rat. *Physiology and Behavior, 9,* 263–267.

Devor, M. (1973). Components of mating dissociated by lateral olfactory tract transection in male hamsters. *Brain Research, 64,* 437–441.

Devor, M. (1975). Neuroplasticity in the rearrangement of olfactory tract fibers after early olfactory tract lesions. *Science, 190,* 998–1000.

Devor, M. (1977). Central processing of odor signals: Lessons from adult and neonatal olfactory tract lesions. In D. Müller-Schwarze & M. M. Mozell (Eds.), *Chemical signals in vertebrates* (pp. 529–545). New York: Plenum.

Dewsbury, D. A. (1979). Description of sexual behavior in research on hormone–behavior interactions. In C. Beyer (Ed.), *Endocrine control of sexual behavior* (pp. 3–32). New York: Raven.

Doty, R. L., Carter, C. S., & Clemens, L. G. (1971). Olfactory control of sexual behavior in the male and early androgenized female hamster. *Hormones and Behavior, 2,* 325–335.

Edwards, D. A., & Warner, P. (1972). Olfactory bulb removal facilitates the hormonal induction of sexual receptivity in the female rat. *Hormones and Behavior, 3,* 321–332.

Graziadei, P. P. C., Levine, R. R., & Monti Graziadei, G. A. (1978). Regeneration of olfactory axons and synapse formation in the forebrain after bulbectomy in neonatal mice. *Proceedings of the National Academy of Science USA, 75,* 5230–5234.

Graziadei, P. P. C., & Monti Graziadei, G. A. (1978). The olfactory system: A model for the study of neurogenesis and axon regeneration in mammals. In C. W. Cotman (Ed.), *Neuronal plasticity* (pp. 131–153). New York: Raven.

Heimer, L., & Larsson, K. (1967). Mating behavior of male rats after olfactory bulb lesions. *Physiology and Behavior, 2,* 207–209.

Kaplan, M. S., & Hinds, J. W. (1977). Neurogenesis in the adult rat: Electron microscopic analysis of light radioautographs. *Science, 197,* 1092–1094.

Larsson, K. (1969). Failure of gonadal and gonadotrophic hormones to compensate for an impaired sexual function in anosmic male rats. *Physiology and Behavior, 4,* 733–737.

Larsson, K. (1975). Sexual behavior of inexperienced male rats following pre- and postpubertal olfactory bulbectomy. *Physiology and Behavior, 14,* 195–199.

Larsson, K. (1977). Transient changes in the female rat estrous cycle after olfactory bulbectomy or removal of the olfactory epithelium. *Physiology and Behavior, 18,* 261–265.

Leonard, C. M. (1978). Maturational loss of thermotaxis prevented by olfactory lesions in golden hamster pups (*Mesocricetus auratus*). *Journal of Comparative and Physiological Psychology, 92,* 1084–1094.

Lisk, R. D., Zeiss, J., & Ciaccio, L. A. (1972). The influence of olfaction on sexual behavior in the male golden hamster (*Mesocricetus auratus*). *Journal of Experimental Zoology, 181,* 69–78.

Lumia, A. R., Meisel, R. L., & Sachs, B. D. (1981). Induction of female and male mating patterns in female rats by gonadal steroids: Effects of neonatal or adult olfactory bulbectomy. *Journal of Comparative and Physiological Psychology, 95,* 497–511.

McGinnis, M. Y., Lumia, A. R., & McEwen, B. S. (1981). Effects of a minimal estradiol stimulus on sexual receptivity and progestin receptor induction following olfactory bulb removal. *Society for Neuroscience Abstracts, 7*, 721.

McGinnis, M. Y., Nance, D. M., & Gorski, R. A. (1978). Olfactory, septal and amygdala lesions alone or in combination: Effects on lordosis behavior and emotionality. *Physiology and Behavior, 20*, 435–440.

Madlafousek, J., & Hliňák, Z. (1977). Sexual behaviour of the female laboratory rat: Inventory, patterning, and measurement. *Behaviour, 63*, 129–174.

Mascó, D. H., & Carrer, H. F. (1980). Sexual receptivity in female rats after lesion or stimulation in different amygdaloid nuclei. *Physiology and Behavior, 24*, 1073–1080.

Math, F., & Davrainville, J. L. (1980). Electrophysiological study on the postnatal development of mitral cell activity in the rat olfactory bulb. *Brain Research, 190*, 243–247.

Meisel, R. L., Lumia, A. R., & Sachs, B. D. (1980). Effects of olfactory bulb removal and flank shock on copulation in male rats. *Physiology and Behavior, 25*, 383–387.

Meisel, R. L., Lumia, A. R., & Sachs, B. D. (1982). Disruption of copulatory behavior of male rats by olfactory bulbectomy at two, but not ten, days of age. *Experimental Neurology, 77*, 612–624.

Moss, R. L. (1971). Modification of copulatory behavior in the female rat following olfactory bulb removal. *Journal of Comparative and Physiological Psychology, 74*, 374–382.

Murphy, M. R. (1976). Olfactory impairment, olfactory bulb removal, and mammalian reproduction. In R. L. Doty (Ed.), *Mammalian olfaction, reproduction processes, and behavior* (pp. 95–117). New York: Academic Press.

Murphy, M. R. (1980). Sexual preferences of male hamsters: Importance of preweaning and adult experience, vaginal secretion, and olfactory or vomeronasal sensation. *Behavioral and Neural Biology, 30*, 323–340.

Murphy, M. R., & Schneider, G. E. (1970). Olfactory bulb removal eliminates mating behavior in the male golden hamster. *Science, 167*, 302–304.

Pfaff, D. W. (1980). *Estrogens and brain function.* New York: Springer Verlag.

Pollak, E. I., & Sachs, B. D. (1975). Male copulatory behavior and female maternal behavior in neonatally bulbectomized rats. *Physiology and Behavior, 14*, 337–343.

Powers, J. B., & Valenstein, E. S. (1972). Sexual receptivity: Facilitation by medial preoptic lesions in female rats. *Science, 175*, 1003–1005.

Roselli-Austin, L., & Altman, J. (1979). The postnatal development of the main olfactory bulb of the rat. *Journal of Developmental Physiology, 1*, 295–313.

Rowe, F. A., & Edwards, D. A. (1972). Olfactory bulb removal: Influences on the mating behavior of male mice. *Physiology and Behavior, 8*, 37–41.

Rowe, F. A., & Smith, W. E. (1973). Simultaneous and successive olfactory bulb removal: Influences on the mating behavior of male mice. *Physiology and Behavior, 10*, 443–449.

Rubin, B. S., & Barfield, R. J. (1980). Priming of estrous responsiveness by implants of 17β-estradiol in the ventromedial hypothalamic nucleus of female rats. *Endocrinology, 106*, 504–509.

Sachs, B. D. (1978). Conceptual and neural mechanisms of masculine copulatory behavior. In T. E. McGill, D. A. Dewsbury, & B. D. Sachs, (Eds.), *Sex and behavior* (pp. 267–295). New York: Plenum.

Sachs, B. D., & Barfield, R. J. (1976). Functional analysis of masculine copulatory behavior in the rat. In J. S. Rosenblatt, R. A. Hinde, E. Shaw, & C. G. Beer (Eds.), *Advances in the study of behavior* Vol. 7, (pp. 91–154). New York: Academic Press.

Scalia, F., & Winans, S. S. (1976). New perspectives on the morphology of the olfactory system: Olfactory and vomeronasal pathways in mammals. In R. L. Doty (Ed.), *Mammalian olfaction, reproductive process, and behavior* (pp. 7–28). New York: Academic Press.

Södersten, P. (1972). Mounting behavior in the female rat during the estrous cycle, after ovariectomy, and after estrogen or testosterone administration. *Hormones and Behavior, 3,* 307–320.

Tennent, B. J., Smith, E. R., & Davidson, J. M. (1980). The effects of estrogen and progesterone on female rat proceptive behavior. *Hormones and Behavior, 14,* 65–75.

Tyler, J. L., & Gorski, R. A. (1980). Bulbectomy and sensitivity to estrogen: Anatomical and functional specificity. *Physiology and Behavior, 24,* 593–600.

Wang, L., & Hull, E. M. (1980). Tail pinch induces sexual behavior in olfactory bulbectomized male rats. *Physiology and Behavior, 24,* 211–215.

Whalen, R. E. (1974). Estrogen–progesterone induction of mating in female rats. *Hormones and Behavior, 5,* 157–162.

Wilhelmsson, M., & Larsson, K. (1973). The development of sexual behavior in anosmic male rats reared under various social conditions. *Physiology and Behavior, 11,* 227–232.

Winans, S. S., & Powers, J. B. (1974). Neonatal and two-stage olfactory bulbectomy: Effects on male hamster sexual behavior. *Behavioral Biology, 10,* 461–471.

Wright, J. W., & Harding, J. W. (1982). Recovery of olfactory function after bilateral bulbectomy. *Science, 216,* 322–324.

Yutzey, D. A., Meyer, P. M., & Meyer, D. R. (1964). Emotionality changes following septal and neocortical ablations in rats. *Journal of Comparative and Physiological Psychology, 58,* 463–465.

14

Organismic Set-Point System in Dorsomedial Hypothalamic Nuclei

Lee L. Bernardis
and Larry L. Bellinger

Introduction

Injury to almost any part of the brain in both infant and mature animals and man is followed by temporary or long-term functional deficits. Experimental destruction of specific loci in the brain of infant animals severely affects growth and development by interfering with the functional and structural integrity of neuroendocrine and neuroautonomic control systems that are crucial for orderly growth. Such systems include energy and body water homeostasis. They are connected with two hypothalamic areas: the ventromedial (VMN) and the dorsomedial (DMN) hypothalamic nuclei.

THE DMNL SYNDROME

Whereas experimental destruction of several hypothalamic areas in the weanling and mature rat, such as the lateral (LHA), the paraventricular, and the zona incerta, bring about gross regulatory deficits in digestive behavior, body-weight control, and neuroendocrine function, experimental destruction of the DMN in both weanling and mature rats results in a functionally normal animal that is, however, greatly reduced in body weight and size. Evidently the DMN is part of a circuitry that plays an important integrative role in growth and development, at least in the model studied, the infant rat.

269

The DMN exerts a complex but poorly understood influence on feeding, drinking, growth, and body composition. It was first observed in the early 1960s and subsequently confirmed (Bernardis, 1970) that destruction of the DMN in both weanling and mature rats of both sexes resulted in reduced food and water intake and ponderal and linear growth. However, the most puzzling observation was the coexistence of these changes with normal body composition. This finding clearly distinguished the DMN-lesioned (DMNL) rat from the rat with LHA lesions. This condition also results in reduced food intake and body weight, but the decrease of the latter is due to the loss of body fat (Bellinger & Bernardis, 1979). Figure 1 shows a microphotograph of a typical DMNL in a weanling rat in which damage does not extend into the LHA. A distinction between body-weight and body-fat control is discussed later.

The notion of a participation of the DMN and its circuitry in food-intake control has its beginnings in the older literature; these have been discussed in a previous review article (Bernardis, 1975).

In addition to the just-mentioned changes, the weanling rat DMNL syndrome is characterized by normal plasma concentrations of both growth hormone (GH) and insulin. These data make it quite evident that the DMNL rat is not simply a hypophagic-hypodipsic-debilitated animal, and they suggest a broader and more complex role for the DMN area in body-weight regulation. Specifically, these findings suggest that the DMNLs simultaneously both reduce ingestive behavior and via some undefined mechanism(s) reduce body size: Body compartments of protein and fat are reduced to the same degree and with a general and commensurate reduction in the size of all organs.

THE RESETTING HYPOTHESIS

These findings and the fact that the weanling DMNL rat adapts more efficiently to its lower caloric (substrate) influx than control rats fed the same (low) amounts of food made us suggest that the lesions bring about a resetting of the somatic–metabolic machinery of the DMNL rat (Bernardis & Goldman, 1972).

It is generally accepted that stimulation of a neuroendocrine or autonomic system has the opposite effects as its destruction. Whether or not stimulation of the DMN in growing rats—perhaps by implanted electrodes or by chemicals—could produce an animal with

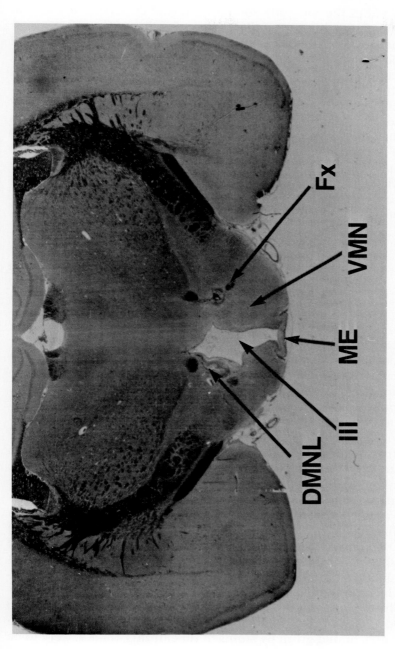

Figure 1. Microphotograph showing dorsomedial hypothalamic lesions. (DMNL) dorsomedial hypothalamic nucleus lesions; (III) third ventricle; (ME) median eminence; (VMN) ventromedial hypothalamic nucleus; (FX) fornix. (cresyl violet and Luxol fast blue, 13.5×).

larger size but normal body composition is of considerable interest. Such a result would support the concept that the DMN is a regulator of ultimate body size in the developing animal. Inasmuch as classical hormones do not seem to play a role in the DMN body-size control, other unknown physiological mechanisms must influence body size. In addition to these academic considerations, the implications of the prospect of creating faster growing and larger animals of normal body composition for agricultural and commercial applications would be staggering.

Since the first description of the syndrome in weanling rats, we and others have studied the DMNL syndrome in more detail. Most of the work was performed in the areas of ingestive behavior and body-weight control, but here we also present neuroendocrine, metabolic, and neuroanatomical findings.

Food Intake

SHORT-TERM FOOD-INTAKE CONTROLS:

In attempts to elucidate the DMNL syndrome we first directed our attention to the possibility that DMNL rats suffer from a deficit in short-term food-intake control. Compensatory reduction of ad libitum food intake following stomach intubation of extra calories in intact rats had been reported earlier. This demonstrated that normal rats can regulate caloric intake. Weanling DMNL rats and sham-lesioned controls were given additional calories by stomach tube (Bernardis & Border, 1975). Both groups reduced their ad libitum food intake to the same degree. In a second study, weanling DMNL rats were preloaded with either glucose, corn oil, egg white, or saline following a 24-hour fast. Their subsequent caloric intake was recorded at various time intervals over the next 24 hours. After data normalization to take into account the inherently lower food intake of the DMNL rats, there was no difference between them and control rats in the ability of the nutrients to suppress feeding. The only exception was during the 1st hour of refeeding following the glucose preload, when the DMNL rats showed greater suppression than the controls. This suggests that DMNL rats may be initially more sensitive to the food intake-suppressing effect of glucose when it is offered as a single nutrient and given by stomach tube. If this, in fact, were to be true, one might predict that DMNL rats reduce their meal size. This question is under study.

In a subsequent study, food intake in weanling DMNL rats was stimulated by acute insulin injection (Bellinger & Bernardis, 1979). Following a period of initial hyperphagia, DMNL rats reduced their food intake such that their 24-hour food intake was comparable to that of the controls.

The general tenor of these studies is that DMNL rats, despite their inherent hypophagia, show no deficits in their ability to regulate 24-hour caloric intake, although they do so at a reduced caloric level compared to the controls. This is an important finding, more so because these are very young, growing animals.

Because stomach preloading with glucose did suppress food intake in weanling DMNL rats, we undertook a series of studies to examine this phenomenon further. One of these experiments investigated the feeding response of DMNL rats to manipulation of circulating glucose and glucose availability by employing insulin, 2-deoxy-D-glucose (2DG), and glucose injections.

Quite strikingly, weanling DMNL rats with electrolytic lesions did not increase their food intake following the injection of 150 to 500 mg/kg of 2DG, whereas controls showed increased feeding by the 1st hour of measurement.

KAINIC ACID LESIONS

These results were subsequently confirmed in mature DMNL rats with electrolytic lesions (Dalton, Carpenter, & Grossman, 1981) and, also in mature rats, following kanic acid lesions of the DMN area (Bellinger & Williams, 1983). Because kainic acid is thought to destroy cell bodies and not fibers of passage, the latter study suggests that it is the destruction of cell bodies in the DMN that is responsible for the loss of 2DG-induced feeding. This notion is supported by other findings that in food-deprived mature rats DMN implants of 2DG enhanced feeding, whereas it did not increase feeding in rats fed ad libitum. Evidently, some glucose-sensitive elements are called upon in some nutritional states and not in others.

Quite remarkably, intraperitoneally injected glucose after an overnight fast failed to decrease food intake in weanling DMNL rats during the 1st hour of refeeding, but it did decrease it in controls. Whereas this finding is complementary to the results of the 2DG study, it contrasts the food intake-depressing effect observed in DMNL rats given glucose intragastrically. This inconsistency may be reconciled by invoking the possibility that preabsorbed glucose, as in the case of gastric intubation, initiated satiety through activation of gastric or intestinal receptors or through the release of satiety hormones such as cholecystokinin. Intraperitoneally injected glucose or 2DG, on the other hand, would bypass these receptors and act centrally. In a preliminary study, we tested the ability of cholecystokinin to affect feeding in weanling DMNL rats. Notably, the injections (3–6 µg/kg) suppressed eating in controls by 50% but was ineffective in DMNL rats. If preabsorptive satiety is enhanced in DMNL rats, it must be the result of preabsorptive food-intake control mechanism(s) other than cholecystokinin.

It is noteworthy that destruction in mature rats of two other anatomically close areas, the zona incerta and the LHA, also results in a loss of 2DG-induced glucoprivic feeding. Thus, the possibility exists that the three areas may be functionally joined, such that loss of any one area eliminates 2DG-induced glucoprivic feeding (Bellinger & Williams, 1983). In this connection it should be recalled that LHA-lesioned rats do not increase food intake after insulin administration but rather die in hypoglycemic shock. On the other hand, zona incerta-lesioned rats respond normally to insulin challenge.

In view of these findings, we explored the short-term feeding response of weanling DMNL rats to insulin. After normalization of the data to take into account the lower baseline food intake of the DMNL rats, it was evident that after insulin injection the lesioned rats increased their food intake similar to the controls. The ability of insulin to enhance feeding in DMNL rats that were unresponsive to 2DG was subsequently confirmed in mature DMNL rats by Dalton et al., (1981). Nevertheless, weanling DMNL rats responded differently than did controls, inasmuch as significantly more controls than DMNL rats began eating during the 1st hour after insulin injection (Bellinger & Bernardis, 1979). The controls also ate more during the 1st hour of testing than did the DMNL rats. The slower feeding response of the lesioned rats was reflected in a more pronounced hypoglycemia after insulin injection than was observed in the controls. A subsequent study demonstrated that, following long-term insulin injections. weanling DMNL rats increased food intake, body weight, and Lee index. However, in absolute terms, insulin-injected DMNL rats remained consistently hypophagic and weighed less than insulin-injected controls. After discontinuation of insulin administration, both groups comparably reduced their food intake, body weight, and body fat.

The question arises as to why DMNL and zona incerta-lesioned rats eat in response to insulin and not following 2DG, although both compounds produce neuronal intracellular glucopenia. It has been suggested that insulin and 2DG may act through two anatomically distinct glucoreceptors. Furthermore, because feeding in DMNL rats is unresponsive to intraperitonelly injected glucose, insulin may affect feeding by direct interaction with neuronal tissue. Lastly, insulin may enhance feeding by altering some metabolite other than glucose. The possibility that insulin affects feeding behavior through one of several mechanisms may explain the initially reduced eating of the DMNL rats following insulin injection as well as their normal response over several hours of measurement.

We do not feel that DMNL-induced hypophagia is due to destruction of glucoreceptive tissue. (Bellinger, Bernardis, & Brooks, 1978). Rather, as previously suggested for the LHA-lesioned and for the medial forebrain bundle-lesioned rat, glucoprivic control is probably unnecessary for normal feeding but rather plays a role in emergency situations. This view is supported by the observation that weanling DMNL rats adequately meter and regulate calories: A loss of glucoprivic feeding cannot explain their hypophagia.

DIETARY SELECTION

The hypophagia in DMNL rats could conceivably be due to an aversion to chewing dry, hard food or to some particular diet preference. However, weanling DMNL rats do not prefer powdered lab chow (which is easier to chew) over chow pellets, powdered cookies over cookies, or the presumably tastier cookies over chow pellets. They also compensate adequately for the different caloric content of food items by ingesting more or less of other foods, and they select a nutrionally complete but bland diet (chow) over nutritionally empty but tastier items (marshmallows) (Bernardis, Bellinger, Spinner, & Brooks, 1978).

In an additional investigation into a possible chewing aversion, DMNL rats and controls were fed a liquid diet, and other groups the same diet in powder form. If our aforementioned resetting hypothesis is correct, DMNL rats should respond like controls, only at a lower absolute level of caloric intake. This was indeed the case. Although the liquid diet-fed DMNL rats remained hypophagic compared with controls fed the liquid diet, both DMNL rats and controls fed the liquid diet ingested more calories and became heavier than their counterparts fed the diet in powder form (i.e., DMNL did not affect the body-fat set point or its manipulation, see following). In a similar experiment, we noted that both weanling DMNL rats and controls ate more of a mash (moistened lab chow) diet than powdered lab chow. Nevertheless, the DMNL rats were again hypophagic relative to their respective controls and also gained less weight. The data demonstrate that the DMNL rat is capable of responding to the "catalytic" effect of the hydration water, albeit at a lower level, apparently appropriate for its reduced body size. The data also indicate that the DMNL rat responds appropriately to diets of various hardness.

Destruction of hypothalamic areas has been shown to interfere with the appropriate choice of nutrients (Andik, Bank, & Donhoffer, 1957; Bernardis, Luboshitsky, Bellinger, & McEwen, 1982). We performed two experiments to assess whether weanling DMNL rats were hypophagic because they had an aversion to a particular macronutrient in their diet.

In one experiment, the rats were given a choice between three equicaloric diets—a high-carbohydrate (75.7%), a high-fat (18.4%), and a high-protein (43.2%) diet—and their intake from each was compared to that of controls.

Again, because of the inherent hypophagia, the data of the DMNL rats had to be normalized. In percentage of total food intake, lesioned and control animals ate similar percentages of the high-fat and high-carbohydrate diet, but both groups found the high-protein diet aversive, this being more evident in the DMNL rats. Calculation of macronutrient intake as percentage of total caloric intake revealed, however, no difference between lesioned and control rats. The DMNL rats were subsequently forced to eat only the high-protein diet. Quite remarkably, they consumed as many calories of the latter as they had during the choice from all three diets. Evidently, DMNL rats show no gross abnormalities in their ability to select or utilize various diets of different nutrient composition and have the capacity to handle a high-protein diet when forced to consume it. Our data also support the notion that dietary selection deficits—none of which are evident in the weanling DMNL rat—are attributable to metabolic alterations (Kanarek & Beck, 1980. We have not revealed metabolic alterations in the DMNL rat. Again, the above findings gain more significance when one considers that the animals in question are very young at the time of the hypothalamic injury.

The above studies indicate that the weanling DMNL rat responds normally to diets of various consistencies and to diet manipulations while growing at a reduced rate that is apparently normal for its reduced size. This notion is supported by the DMNL rat's chemically determined normal body composition. The above data also suggest that the metabolism of the DMNL rat should be relatively normal and appropriate for a smaller animal. We have performed several experiments to test this aspect of the DMNL syndrome.

Intermediary Metabolism

Both hepatic and adipose tissue metabolism (Shimazu, 1981) are under the control of the hypothalamic-autonomic outflow: Animals with lesions in the ventromedial, anterior, or paraventricular nuclei have shown dramatic changes in the activities of certain enzymes. Thus, there was reason to suspect that DMN destruction might also result in metabolic alterations. Therefore, we have performed a series of studies to examine certain aspects of intermediary metabolism and enzyme patterns in rats with DMNL.

The incorporation of [^{14}C]glucose into DMNL diaphragm lipid, CO_2, and glycogen is normal or slightly greater than that of controls. Glucose incorporation into liver lipid and glycogen is similar in DMNL and control rats. Finally, glucose incorporation into epididymal fat-pad lipid, CO_2, and fatty acids of weanling DMNL rats is slightly less than normal.

Because destruction of the immediately adjacent VMN produces dramatic increases in gluconeogenesis, we investigated this aspect of protein metabolism in the weanling DMNL rat (Bernardis, Goldman & Bellinger, 1976). We found normal incorporation of [^{14}C]alanine into total lipid, fatty acids, glycogen, and tissue protein of both liver and diaphragm as well as plasma glucose and protein. These findings add to the puzzling coexistence in DMNL rats of growth retardation and hypophagia with normal GH, insulin levels and body composition.

CIRCULATING SUBSTRATES

Plasma substrate concentrations of various metabolites generally correlate well with the lack of gross changes in tissue metabolism. In the weanling DMNL rat, plasma glucose, glycerol, free fatty acids, and total protein are in the normal range (Bernardis & Bellinger, 1982).

ADIPOSE TISSUE AND LIVER ENZYMES

An analysis of the activities of several key enzymes in liver, adipose tissue, and diaphragm in weanling DMNL rats 2 weeks after lesion revealed a depression of liver glucose-6-phosphate dehydrogenase, citrate cleavage enzyme, glycerol phosphate dehydrogenase, and malic enzyme. However, 6-phosphogluconate dehydrogenase, fatty acid synthetase, alanine aminotransferase, fructose disphosphatase, pyruvate kinase, and protein (Lowry) were normal.

The changes in citrate cleavage enzyme, malic enzyme, and glycerol phosphate deydrogenase suggest a depression of hepatic lipogenesis, yet the activity of fatty acid synthetase is unaltered in DMNL rats. The elevated activity of alanine aminotransferase in the diaphragm suggests enhanced protein metabolism, which is, however, at variance with normal body composition, liver protein, and plasma protein. The normal activities in epididymal fat pads of glucose-6-phosphate dehydrogenase, phosphogluconate dehydrogenease, citrate cleavage enzyme, glycerol phosphate dehydrogenase, malic enzyme, and pyruvic kinase involved in the conversion of dietary carbohydrate into fatty acids, are in excellent agreement with previous findings of generally normal glucose incorporation into fatty acids in weanling DMNL rats. This suggests that, whatever the specific neural disruption that is brought about by DMN lesions, it does not grossly affect lipid storage and de novo fatty acid synthesis in adipose tissue cells (Martin & Bernardis, 1980).

BASAL AND EPINEPHRINE-STIMULATED LIPOLYSIS

In view of the findings of normal plasma free fatty acid levels in short-term experiments and decreased free fatty acid levels in a long-term study, we examined basal and epinephrine-stimulated lipolysis in both epididymal and brown adipose tissue (BAT) of weanling DMNL rats. Epididymal fat-pad basal lipolysis was increased and epinephrine-stimulated lipolysis was greatly decreased in DMNL rats, whereas BAT basal lipolysis and epinephrine-stimulated lipolysis were normal in weanling DMNL rats, as was BAT weight in percentage of body weight, lipid, and protein. With a view of the involvement of BAT in dietary-induced and non-shivering thermogenesis, we concluded that BAT function is normal in DMNL rats. This appears in accord with the earlier-discussed normal body composition, plasma glycerol, and free fatty acid levels that were also noted in this study. The enhanced basal lipolysis and the normal plasma fatty acid levels, although inconsistent at first sight, are conceivably due to enhanced uptake of fatty acids by other depots.

In agreement with the generally normal intermediary metabolism in the weanling DMNL rat is the normal efficiency of food utilization (weight gained per food eaten). These data lend support to previous findings that DMN destruction produces a rat that, except for its reduced size, is metabolically normal. This is the more significant in view of the very young age of the experimental animals.

Extra- and Intracellular Thirst Mechanisms

The pronounced hypodipsia in the weanling DMNL rat was conceivably a reflection of a disrupted water regulatory system. However, water–food intake ratios were comparable to that of the controls, which argues against this notion. Similarly, plasma osmolality was normal in the weanling DMNL rat.

Extensive studies (Bellinger & Bernardis, 1982) have investigated water intake in weanling DMNL rats and noted that they will eat in the absence of water and drink in the absence of food, indicating that they are not prandial drinkers. In contrast, rats with LHA and zona incerta lesions are prandial drinkers. Tests for intra- and extracellular thirst and a combination of the two in DMNL rats elicited normal responses. In contrast, animals with LHA lesions responded to intracellular thirst challenges only when tested during the dark phase of the diurnal cycle, and zona incerta-lesioned rats did not respond at all. Furthermore, injection of angiotensin II brought about similar water intake in both DMNL rats and controls. These data indicate that DMN lesions, although causing hypodipsia, do not disrupt—or bring about a deficit in—classic thirst-regulatory mechanism(s), a finding that is of great significance in growing animals; the importance of proper hydration in human infants is well established.

Hormones

CIRCULATING HORMONE LEVELS

One of the most puzzling findings in the weanling DMNL rat is the normal plasma GH and insulin levels in the face of reduced ponderal and linear growth. It will be recalled that lesions in the adjacent VMN result in reduced pituitary and plasma GH levels that are still noticable 198 days after lesion production, whereas normal (or slightly elevated!) GH levels are found in the DMNL rat. The immediate proximity of the VMN and DMN and the profound difference in GH levels following their destruction cannot be enough emphasized. We are investigating somatomedin and somatomedin inhibitory activity in DMNL rats to see if the growth defect lies beyond GH.

THE DMN AS PART OF THE INCERTO–HYPOTHALAMIC DOPAMINERGIC SYSTEM

In contrast to normal GH and insulin levels, DMN lesions are followed by hyperprolactinemia. This could be attributable to the elimination of an inhibiting effect by catecholamines on prolactin release. High levels of norepinephrine and dopamine have indeed been found in the DMN, with the latter being part of the extrainfundibular incerto–hypothalamic dopaminergic system (Bjorklund, Lindvall, & Nobin, 1975). Dopamine has been suggested as the prolactin-inhibiting factor; thus removal of dopamine by DMN lesions could increase prolactin secretion. Indications of high prolactin levels following arcuate nucleus, VMN, and DMN lesions, that is, prolonged diestrus and active corpora lutea, have been previously reported and are thus in accord with our findings.

PITUITARY HORMONE DYNAMICS

Previous quantitative electron microscopy studies have suggested different roles for the DMN and VMN in GH dynamics. Stachura, Bernardis, Kent, Farmer, and Tyler (1983), using an in vitro perifusion-immunoprecipitation system, have confirmed such a differential role and in addition have provided strong evidence for a similar role in prolactin dynamics. In weanling rats, VMNLs inhibited and DMNLs stimulate early (20–30 minutes) and late-phase (40–60 minutes and later) GH release. Prolactin release was also inhibited from pituitaries of VMNL rats, whereas in pituitaries of DMNL rats early release was slightly suppressed and late release was moderately stimulated. Intracellular transit time of both newly synthesized hormones was decreased after both types of hypothalamic lesion. The authors emphasize that in addition to simple increases or decreases of total hormone-release rates, the hypothalamic tone from both VMN and DMN differentially influences cellular events such as synthesis and release via direct or indirect action.

The DMN could also be involved in adenhypophysial control via an indirect route, that is, the VMN, the latter being an intergal part of the hypophysiotrophic area. Direct connections between the VMN and DMN have been discussed in a previous review article (Bernardis, 1975) and have received persuasive support from the findings by Luiten and Room, (1980).

Circadian Feeding and Hormone Rhythms

Prolactin injections have been reported to increase feeding of female but not male rats, and circadian rhythms of prolactin and corticosterone have been shown to influence body-fat stores in birds and mammals. We have noted that the plasma corticosterone rhythm is altered in wealing DMNL rats. To what extent these hormonal changes may or may not influence feeding, development, and weight gain in these animals is uncertain.

Lesions in the suprachiasmatic area disrupt circadian rhythms of feeding and drinking, locomotor activity, and plasma corticosterone levels. These and other findings suggested that the suprachiasmatic area may be the critical part of a system that drives all other circadian rhythms. It could bring to bear its influence on the medial hypothalamic nuclei by pathways identified between these areas. Indeed, it was shown some time ago that lesions in either DMN or VMN in weanling rats disrupt diurnal feeding and weight-gain cycles. We (Bellinger, Bernardis, & Mendel, 1976) noted that DMNL weanlings failed to exhibit the AM–PM differences in plasma corticosterone that characterize the intact rat, and we have also observed higher AM and PM levels than in controls in both DMNL and VMNL rats. DMNLs may have interrupted suprachiasmatic area connections that influence corticosterone secretion.

Organismic Resetting Hypothesis

THE DMN AND BODY-WEIGHT
AND BODY-FAT SET POINTS

Because both as weanlings and mature the DMNL rats eat sufficient calories for their reduced size, appear competent to meter and
regulate calories, show normal body composition, have a generally
normal intermediary metabolism, evince normal thirst and body-
water regulation, and exhibit normal GH and insulin levels, the suggestion was made that the lesions produce a resetting of a central
autonomic control system that makes it possible for DMNL rat to
adapt more efficiently to a reduced inflow of substrate (Bernardis &
Goldman, 1972). Later this resetting hypothesis was expanded into
the concept that DMNLs bring about a body-*weight* set-point reduction and not merely the *fat* set-point reduction that is observed in the
LHA-lesioned rat. With a body-weight set-point reduction the DMNL
rat experiences an organismic resetting in body fat, protein, intermediary metabolism, food and water intake, and growth.

The normal body composition, anabolic hormone levels (GH and
insulin), intermediary metabolism, caloric regulation, and water regulation in an animal that is so much smaller than a control rat is
most perplexing, because it is generally thought that body growth
and size under adequate access to nutrients are controlled by an
animal's genetic makeup. How a central nervous system lesion can
change food and water intake and body growth without commen-
surately affecting—or being reflected in—these parameters is also
puzzling.

There is a notable and quite important difference between body-
weight and body-fat set points. Whereas the LHA-lesioned rat loses
body weight primarily because of body-fat reduction that subsequently lowers the body-fat set point around which the animal will
regulate (Bellinger, Bernardis, & Brooks, 1979), the DMNL rat, also
showing reduced body weight, exhibits normal body composition.

From a developmental point of view it is worthy of note that 6
months after lesion production at weaning, DMNL rats still show
greatly reduced growth parameters (body weight 74%, length 88%)
but normal body composition as shown by both indirect (Lee index)
and chemical determination. Furthermore, mean food intake in this
study was 60% of that of the control rats. Some of these data are
shown in Figure 2.

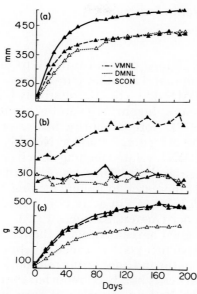

Figure 2. Time course of (a) body length, (b) Lee index (obesity), and (c) body weight in rats with dorsomedial, ventromedial and sham lesions produced shortly after weaning and maintained for 6 months. (From Bernardis *et al.*, *J. Neuroscience Research* 1:95–108, 1975, with permission from Alan Liss, Inc., 150 Fifth Avenue, New York, NY 10011.)

The body-fat set point of the DMNL rat is apparently intact, but it may lack sensitivity: When weanling DMNL rats were ovariectomized, they, like their sham-lesioned ovariectomized counterparts, increased body fat, that is, they responded by elevating the body-fat set point. DMNL weanlings also increased their body fat to a greater degree than even control rats when offered a palatable cafeteria diet or a palatable liquid diet.

These findings have led us to hypothesize that the DMN belong to a medial hypothalamic zone that is critical for the initiation of excessive caloric intake under appropriately palatable and high-caloric diet conditions. The existence of hypothalamic zones, irrespective of the nuclei situated in these zones, has been advanced and used by Ban (1975) in his analysis of the role of the septo–preoptico–hypothalamic system in neuroendocrine and neuroautonomic homeostasis.

THE DMN AND CATECHOLAMINERIGIC CONTROL OF FEEDING

Just what type of change occurs centrally to bring about such a resetting of body weight and all other parameters measured is uncertain. However, the DMN does contain relatively high concentrations of norepinephrine and epinephrine (Van der Gugten, deKloet, Versteeg, & Slangen, 1977). Norepinephrine has several times been implicated in the control of feeding behavior. Notably, a norepinephrine involvement in the DMNL-related feeding deficits has been suggested by the work of these authors. They reported that norepinephrine turnover in the DMN increased following feeding and suggested that these changes reflect increases of activity of a feeding, rather than a satiety system (Van der Gugten, Slangen, 1975).

These data are in good agreement with the findings by Grossman (1960) in which consistently good or excellent effects on feeding were noted after noraderenalin and adrenaline microinjection into or adjacent to the DMN. Earlier it had been reported that the feeding effect of 2DG could be inhibited by injection of an α-adrenergic blocker. This is of particular interest because subsequent work had failed to observe increased feeding after 2DG administration in DMNL rats. Thus, impairment of a norepinephrine system may possibly be implicated in producing the DMNL-induced feeding deficit. It is most important to consider that the DMNL syndrome cannot be the manifestation of the loss of only a feeding system, because this would merely produce a semistarved animal (with reduced body-fat stores), not a smaller animal with normal body composition. Thus, although the possibility exists that the loss of norephinephrine feeding system is involved in producing the DMNL syndrome, it is probably one of several factors that produces it.

ENDORPHINERGIC FEEDING SYSTEM IN THE DMN

It has been proposed that opiates influence both feeding and drinking behavior with the opiate antagonist naloxone suppressing both these parameters. Because the DMN contains opiate cells and fiber tracts, we have explored the effects of naloxone in DMNL rats (Bellinger and Bernardis, submitted). The ability of naloxone to suppress feeding in DMNL rats was either eliminated or attenuated. The effect on water intake in DMNL rats was more variable but was also attenuated. These data suggest that the DMN may be part of an opiate feeding system, the loss of which may be—at least to some extent— responsible for the hypophagia.

Several other lines of evidence suggest a role of opiates in DMN function. Naloxone in continuous doses elevates corticosterone, and we had noted previously that plasma corticosterone is elevated in morning samples of DMNL rats. Loss of 2DG but not of insulin-induced feeding has been attributed to a disruption of opiate systems. Again, it will be recalled that a loss of 2DG but not insulin-induced feeding occurs in weanling DMNL rats.

A link between opiate-induced feeding and norepinephrine release for the paraventricular nucleus has been proposed by Leibowitz and Hor (1982). A similar relationhip might conceivably exist in the DMN, according to which opiate released within this structure could affect—or act synergistically with—norepinephrine to influence feeding.

EXTENDED ORGANISMIC-RESETTING HYPOTHESIS

In summary, the above data demonstrate that the selective destruction of an area that has received little attention brings about a set of changes that appear inconsistent at first sight. However, all parameters studied have shown alterations that appear appropriate for an animal of smaller size, that are harmonious in relation to one another, and that are not specific for any particular homeostatic control compartment. We have therefore termed this phenomenon an organismic resetting of the animal's somatic–metabolic machinery (Bernardis & Bellinger, 1981). Thus, the development of an animal can be profoundly influenced by manipulation of the DMN through undefined mechanisms that do not appear to be the classic mechanisms that normally affect body size.

References

Andik, I., Bank, J., & Donhoffer, S. (1957). Über die Wirkung von Hypothalamusläsionen auf die Nahrungsaufnahme und Nahrungswahl der Ratte. *Archiv. für experimentelle Pathology und Pharmakologie, 231,* 55–62.

Ban, T. (1975). Fiber connections in the hypothalamus and some autonomic functions. *Pharmology, Biochemistry and Behavior (Suppl.), 3,* 3–13.

Bellinger, L. L., & Bernardis, L. L. (1979). Effect of insulin in rats with lesions of the dorsomedial hypothalamic nucleus. *Physiology and Behavior, 23* 1157–1161.

Bellinger, L. L., & Bernardis, L. L. (1982). Water regulation in weanling hypo dipsic dorsomedial hypothalamic-lesioned rats. *American Journal of Physiology, 242,* R285–R295.

Bellinger, L. L., Bernardis, L. L., & Brooks, S. (1978). Feeding responses of rats with dorsomedial hypothalamic lesions given ip 2DG or glucose. *American Journal of Physiology, 235,* R168–174.

Bellinger, L. L., Bernardis, L. L., & Brooks, S. (1979). The effect of dorsomedial hypo-thalamic nuclei lesions on body weight regulation. *Neuroscience, 4:* 659–665.

Bellinger, L. L., Bernardis, L. L., & Mendel, V. E. (1976). Effect of ventromedial and dorsomedial hypothalamic lesions on circadian corticosterone rhythms. *Neuroendocrinology, 22,* 216–225.

Bellinger, L. L., & Williams, F.E. (1983). Aphagia and adipsia after kainic acid lesion-ing of the dorsomedial hypothalamic area. *American Journal of Physiology, 244,* R389–R399.

Bernardis, L. L. (1970). Participation on the dorsomedial hypothalamic nucleus in the "feeding center" and water intake circuitry of the weanling rat. *Journal of Neurovisceral Relations, 31,* 387–398.

Bernardis, L. L. (1975). The dorsomedial hypothalamic nucleus in autonomic and neuroendocrine homeostasis. *Canadian Journal of Neurological Sciences, 2,* 45–60.

Bernardis, L. L., & Bellinger, L. L. (1981). Dorsomedial hypothalamic hypophagia: Self-selection of diets and macronutrients, efficiency of food utilization, "stress eating", response to high-protein diet and circulating substrate concentrations. *Appetite, 2,* 103–113.

Bernardis, L. L., & Bellinger, L. L. (1982). Effect of diet hydration on food and water intake, efficiency of food utilization and response to fast, and realimentation in rats with dorsomedial hypothalamic hypophagia and growth retardation. *Appetite, 3,* 35–52.

Bernardis, L. L., Bellinger, L. L., Spinner, L. I., & Brooks, S. P. (1978). Feeding studies in weanling rats with dorsomedial hypothalamic lesions: Effect of high fat and high carbohydrate diet and nutrient completeness on food choice and intake. *Journal of Nutrition, 108,* 753–758.

Bernardis, L. L., & Border, J. R. (1975). Feeding studies in weanling rats with dor-somedial hypothalamic lesions:Maintenance of competence to compensate for ad-ditional calories. *Physiology and Behavior, 15,* 37–40.

Bernardis, L. L., & Goldman, J. K. (1972). Growth and metabolic changes in weanling rats with lesions in the dorsomedial hypothalamic nuclei. *Experimental Brain Research, 15,* 424–429.

Bernardis, L. L., Goldman, J. K., & Bellinger, L. L. (1976). Failure to demonstrate alterations in gluconeogenesis in growth-retarded weanling rats with dorsomedial hypothalamic lesions. *Journal of Neuroscience Research, 2,* 395–399.

Bernardis, L. L., Goldman, J. K., Chlouverakis, C. & Frohman, L. A. (1975). Six-month follow-up in weanling rats with ventromedial and dorsomedial hypothalamic le-sions:somatic, endocrine, and metabolic changes. *Journal of Neuroscience Research, 1,* 95–108.

Bernardis, L. L., & Luboshitzky, R. (in press). White and brown adipose tissue lipolysis in weanling rats with dorsomedial hypothalamic lesions. *Neurological Research.*

Bernardis, L. L., Luboshitsky, R., Bellinger, L. L., & McEwen, G. (1982). Nutritional studies in the weanling rat with normophagic hypothalamic obesity. *Journal of Nutrition, 112*, 1441–1455.

Bjorklund, A., Lindvall, O., & Nobin, A. (1975). Evidence of an incerto–hypothalamic dopamine neurone system in the rat. *Brain Research 89*, 29–42.

Dalton, L. D., Carpenter, R. G., & Grossman, S. P. (1981). Ingestive behavior in adult rats with dorsomedial hypothalamic lesions. *Physiology and Behavior, 26*, 117–123.

Grossman, S. P. (1960). Eating and drinking elicited by direct adrenergic and cholinergic stimulation of the hypothalamus. *Science, 132*, 301–302.

Kanarek, R., & Beck, J. H. (1980). Role of gonadal hormones in diet selection and food utilization in female rats. *Physiology and Behavior, 24*, 381–396.

Leibowitz, S. F., & Hor, L. (1982). Endorphinergic and alpha-noradrenergic systems in the paraventricular nucleus: Effects on eating behavior. *Peptides, 3:* 421–428.

Luiten, P. G., & Room, P. (1980). Interrelations between lateral, dorsomedial and ventromedial hypothalamic nuclei in the rat. An HRP study. *Brain Research, 190*, 321–332.

Martin, R. J., & Bernardis, L. L. (1980). Characterization of tissue enzyme activities in rats with dorsomedial hypothalamic lesions and their sham-operated controls. *Physiology and Behavior, 24*, 855–858.

Nakayama, I., Bernardis, L. L., & Tseng, M. T. (1974). Ultrastructural studies of adenohypophyseal somatotrophs in weanling rats with ventromedial and dorsomedial hypothalamic lesions. *Laboratory Investigation, 30*, 119–128.

Shimazu, T. (1981). Central nervous system regulation of liver and adipose tissue metabolism. *Diabetolgia Supplement, 20*, 343–356.

Satchura, M. E., Bernardis, L. L., Kent, P. G., Farmer, P. K., & Tyler, J. M. (1983, January). Growth hormone (GH) and prolactin (PRL) synthesis and release by rat pituitaries in vitro predict in vivo hypothalamic lesions placement. *Southern Society for Clinical Investigation Meeting*, New Orleans.

Van der Gugten, J., deKloet, R., Versteeg, J. H., & Slangen, J. L. (1977). Regional hypothalamic catecholamine metabolism and food intake regulation in the rat. *Brain Research, 135*, 325–336.

Van der Gugten, J., & Slangen, J. L. (1975). Norepinephrine uptake by hypothalamic tissue from the rat related to feeding. *Pharmacology, Biochemistry and Behavior, 3*, 855–860.

III

Variables Interacting with Early Brain Damage

15

Roots to the Future: Gene–Environment Coaction and Individual Vulnerability to Neural Insult

Peter J. Donovick
and Richard G. Burright

General Overview

The balance between stability and vulnerability of the individual is the result of ongoing, dynamic gene–environment coactions that occur throughout life. The complexity of such interactions is illustrated in the following example. In humans, individuals with a 47,XXX karyotype are phenotypically female. Unlike several other sex-chromosome anomolies, 47,XXX individuals frequently do not exhibit readily apparent phenotypic disturbances. However, 47,XXX females are over represented in retarded, psychopathological, and criminal populations, even though such behavioral dysfunctions are seen in less than half of the individuals with this genotype. Of course, less than 100% penetrance (the proportion of individuals exhibiting a trait) and lack of uniform expressivity (variability in expression of a trait) are common in the translation of genotype to phenotype. Robinson and his co-workers (e.g., Pennington, Puck, & Robinson, 1980) have discussed developmental markers of 47,XXX females that may predict retardation. Not surprisingly, early delays in motor development and language acquisition are correlated with subsequent behavioral and learning disorders in the school-age population.

The focus of this chapter is on issues that influence vulnerability of the organism to neural insult and as such serve to determine the paths the individual follows through life. We review how genetic–environment interactions and correlations throughout the life span of the individual (cf. Donovick & Burright, 1982) are critical in developing predictors of behavior and a better understanding of those roots that influence the individual's future.

GENETIC CONSIDERATIONS

Knowledge concerning the role of genetic factors in the regulation of behavior is changing rapidly. In the first place, the premise that genetic transcription to phenotype is based on stable genetic material is being modified. Specifically, the concept that the transcription of DNA through RNA to amino acids is a highly stable, immutable process must be reconsidered. Although all cells share in their DNA complement, gene expression is altered through the differentiation process. In this context, the difference between potential and actualized genetic information must be recognized. Genetic expression is highly complex and influenced by a variety of external and internal environmental factors. Certainly, the hormonal milieu of the individual affects the process, but feedback on the basic genetic material is not limited to hormones, or for that matter to viruses that may effect the host. The receptor system(s) of individual cells are acutely sensitive and the enzymatic production of the cell, for example, is responsive to the microenvironment. Cellular reactivity determines what portion of the gene is expressed as reflected in protein production (cf. Campbell & Zimmerman, 1982). Thus, the production of proteins may be responsive to a variety of internal and external environmental factors including sensory stimulation. Commonality in genetic expressivity may be seen in response to similar environmental challenges. For instance, several forms of stress have been shown to lead to a common group of "stress" proteins (Hammond, Lai, & Markert, 1982). Genetic expression involves the interaction of DNA with many proteins, so that DNA itself, through feedback, may become a dynamic participant in the expression of its potential information. Advances in molecular biology have dramatically altered notions concerning the constancy of expression of genetic material. The task for those of us interested in behavior is to uncover the ways in which molecular processes translate to behavioral variation. Behavior provides feedback to the system, and the more behavioral options an organism has, the more varied is the feedback. These dynamic processes operate within complex boundary conditions to sustain life such that the potential genetic information that defines any given species serves to limit the process—a mouse is not a fish, nor even a small rat.

Gene–Environment Interactions and Correlations

The translation from genetic material to phenotype is a product of the continuous coaction of genome and environment. Such coactive processes may induce even "minor" genetic differences among individuals that will be magnified through time, producing life-span effects. In this sense, genotype is only an invitation to developmental processes that will be acted on by the environment. Although several aspects of gene–environment interactions and gene–environment correlations have been discussed in detail elsewhere, some points are worth review.

In the case of a gene–environment interaction, the behavior observed in response to an independent variable of choice is a joint product of the individual's genetic substrate and the stimulus conditions. For instance, lesions of the septal region of the forebrain may lead to increased saccharin consumption in C57 mice but may fail to do so in either HET or RF mice (Donovick, Burright, Fanelli, & Engellenner, 1981a). In the case of gene–environment correlations, the genotype of the individual leads it along a developmental life-span path that differs from that of an individual with a different genetic constitution. Although at least three variants of such correlations may be discussed, here we need only restate that such coactive processes may lead the individual through a unique life experience (genetically blind organisms experience a very different world than do normal or genetically deaf individuals). Thus, experience may act to further differentiate (and perhaps isolate) an individual from others who may have varied only subtly during the earliest stages of development. Because one may expect such factors to influence the individual throughout its life, it is easy to imagine the magnification that may occur in response to "minor" genetic or environmental differences.

ENVIRONMENTAL CHALLENGE–
ORGANISMIC RESPONSE

Obviously, the organism is faced with a variety of environmental challenges. All living systems are designed to respond to change. Physiological stability and reliability must be balanced against adaptability and variability of response pattern. Phylogenetically simple organisms often appear to respond to challenge by over-production of young—diversity of their response pattern(s) is obviously limited and the cost of species survival is the death of many individuals. Enhanced capacity for behavioral plasticity associated with more complex organisms allows for learning that may buffer environmental disturbances. Stability must be viewed across time. Such a longitudinal view may provide the best indication of the degree of buffering provided the individual and may best describe the results of the individual's interaction with the environment. Wilson (1978) noted, for instance, that as one examines the developmental spurts and lags of IQ scores of monozygotic twins relative to those of dizygotic twins, the agreement across time is remarkable and far more impressive than data from single points in time.

PERINATAL INFLUENCES

Some buffering against environmental perturbations, especially in altricial animals, may be provided by early postpartum behavior of the parents; the consequence of parental behavior may be to reduce subsequent phenotypic variance that might have been expressed had the individual not been protected. Relative to natural conditions, both the constancy of the laboratory and the frequent use of random-bred stocks of animals may provide additional buffering that could mask further potential phenotypic variance. Despite the limits imposed by the laboratory, variability between and within subjects is the hallmark of behavioral data. Indeed, even the selection of inbred strains of animals often does not reduce this variation. Under many conditions, behavior of inbred stocks of animals is as variable as that of outbred animals. Even though a variety of challenges may reduce coping strategies of the organism, they do not necessarily reduce the variability of behavior in all situations.

The choice of experimental animal may dramatically influence the outcome of our experiments, and a failure to recognize either genetic or environmental history may play havoc with interpretation of our data. For instance, in selecting animals, the history of the dam is frequently ignored even though parity can have dramatic influences on anatomy as well as behavior of the animal. Wahlsten (1982) for example, reported that BALB/c mice frequently show deficiencies of the corpus callosum. The frequency of this deficiency increases if the male is left in the cage with the female, a procedure that typically produces another pregnancy at the first postpartum estrus. Differential responsiveness to the environment by pups of primiparous and multiparous rats as a function of environmental stress has been shown as well. Such effects may be due in part to differential responsiveness of the mother to stress signals emitted by the young (Wright, Bell, Schreiber, Villescas, & Conely, 1977).

Even in the absence of profound anatomical changes such as those reported by Wahlsten, perinatal factors may have prolonged behavioral effects; when tested at 2 years of age, rats from the second mating were superior on a passive avoidance task to those derived from the primaparous mating (Elias, Nau, Villescas, & Bell, 1982). And at least some forms of early experience may have multigenerational effects. For instance, caloric (Chandra, 1975) deprivation may alter immune responsivity through at least three generations. Similarly, stressing female rats may alter the behavioral reactivity of their subsequent offspring even when those pups are tested as adults. In some cases it may be assumed that maternal behavior is critical in mediating such effects (Denenberg, Holloway, & Dollinger, 1967), but autoregulatory effects on the genes themselves could be "mechanistically" responsible. Obviously, when portions of the genome are turned on (or off), the impact may be profound and prolonged, lasting for many generations (Campbell & Zimmermann, 1982).

Clearly then, perinatal environmental experience dramatically alters subsequent brain organization and behavior. The relative plasticity of young organisms may be observed both in reports of greater response to a variety of early manipulations and in reports of greater recovery from such influences. Some aspects of these effects are mediated by the dam's own life experience as expressed in maternal behavior. For instance, Denenberg et al. (1967) cross-fostered pups at birth either to a female whose own pups were 10 days old, or to one who had just given birth; pups grew more poorly if cross-fostered to females with 10-day-old pups. Denenberg attributed these results to changes in maternal behavior across the postpartum period. Such results, of course, are not surprising—one expects nursing time to change as the pup develops. However, even within a litter, maternal behavior will not be identical for all pups. Furthermore, subtle aspects of maternal behavior and physiology may be incorporated into a variety of aspects of the pups own behavioral repertoire. An example of the potentially extraordinary power of altered maternal behavior is illustrated in a report in which young bonnet monkeys were subjected to a period of separation from their mothers (Laudenslager, Reite, & Harbeck, 1982). In addition to exhibiting behavioral separation anxiety, the young monkeys showed decreased immune activity. One might expect that even minor perturbations of maternal–young interactions might have profound and lasting consequences on the young. Such reactions also depend on the genotype of both the pup and the mother (Wainwright, 1981).

Enrichment–Deprivation

Reactions of the young to the environment are clearly influenced by maternal behavior and other aspects of the environment in which they were reared. The importance of early olfactory environment on subsequent behavior has been nicely illustrated in the work of Spear and his co-workers. They showed that young rats tested in the presence of odors from their home cages were facilitated in the acquisition of spatial discrimination (Smith & Spear, 1981) relative to age mates that were tested without such familiar cues. However, the presence of home-cage odors interfered with the acquisition of a taste-aversion task in similarly aged rats (Infurna, Steinert, & Spear, 1979), suggesting the complexity of interaction between background stimulation and performance of specific behavioral problems. There is evidence that at least some aspects of the home cage-odor effects may be mediated by the catecholamine systems, and that these odors may effectively reduce stress of the testing situation (Barrett, Caza, Spear, & Spear, 1982).

Work such as this has led to the suggestion that young organisms are most responsive to environmental manipulations, including environmental enrichment or restriction and brain damage. Such manipulations of experience must be considered in relation to the organism's genetic and rearing history. Sackett (1967) suggested that rats would explore more complex objects in their environment as a function of their prior experience with complex environmental stimuli. And although virtually all living organisms are capable of response to change, the elegant work of Fuller and Harlow suggests that animals may be poorly buffered against sudden exposure to complex environments.

In the past we have tended to work under the assumption that effects of environmental enrichment or deprivation lead to relatively permanent phenomena. It also has become obvious that even brief exposures to environmental enrichment may impact intact (Studelska & Kemble, 1979) and brain-damaged organisms (Will, Rosenzweig, Bennett, Herbert, & Morimoto, 1977). Furthermore, as the early work by Fuller (1967) suggested, some aspects of the response to enrichment may be transitory, and sudden changes in environmental conditions may be reflected immediately in the response pattern of brain-damaged animals (Goodlett, Engellenner, Burright, Donovick, 1982). Finally, environmental enrichment may not benefit the organism under all conditions. For instance, Parsons and Spear (1972) found that rats with a history of enrichment were impaired on the retention of an avoidance task.

Environmental enrichment has been shown to alter a wide variety of anatomical and biochemical aspects of the brain. These changes appear to necessitate active interaction with the environment (e.g., Ferchmin, Bennett, & Rosenzweig, 1975). Not surprisingly, a number of changes similar to those seen in environmental enrichment are associated with experimental testing (Greenough, Juraska, & Volkmar, 1979).

Of course, the other side of environmental enrichment is a deprivation of stimulation. However, even this concept is complex. Although visual input under some circumstances can be enriching, continuous exposure to light has detrimental effects on retinal receptors and, as might be expected, can cause deficiencies in visual discrimination tasks (Bennett, Dyer, & Dunn, 1973). These findings are paralleled by those that have shown sensory deficits as a function of visual deprivation. Results such as those discussed in this section indicate both the difficulty and the importance of specifying environmental characteristics that influence experience.

Vulnerability to Brain Insult

Evidence of sensitive periods abounds. Although windows of vulnerability may be limited in time, the impact of the environment may not always be observable immediately. For instance, there are suggestions that prenatal lead administration may have profound effects on cortical cell development (McCauley *et al.*, 1982), but the translation of such cortical impact into behavioral consequences is not simple. We have reported the results from a series of experiments that compared the impact of lead administration during several stages of pre- and perinatal development (Dolinsky, Burright, & Donovick, 1983). We administered lead to dams (1) prenatally only, (2) beginning on the day of birth and through the end of testing, (3) both pre- and postnatally, or (4) not at all. Mice that were administered lead only postnatally showed hyperactivity as measured by the number of squares crossed in an open field relative to the other three groups; mice that were presented lead both pre- and postnatally were least active. In contrast, measures of aggression showed decreased latencies to fight regardless of when lead was administered. Unfortunately, description of the interactive effects of environmental enrichment and lesions or toxins are frequently limited to one point in time. Such procedures may fail to detect differences if the impact of the insult is delayed. Limited ontogenetic descriptions may be misleading, because effects of the manipulation may change over time or age. For instance, lead administration to young and older adult mice has dramatically different effects on male agonistic behavior (Burright, Engellenner, Donovick, 1983).

The detection and apparent nature of environmental manipulation may depend on the age at which both the procedure is initiated and the tests are conducted. Oppenheim (1981) suggests that not only are there limited periods of sensitivity for specific environmental factors, but that both structures and behaviors may play a critical organizational role for limited periods of time. If a tissue-specific environmental event occurs after that structure has played its main organizing role, one might expect the results to be minimized. Similarly then, mechanisms of gene–environment correlations involving manipulations early in development may have cascading effects that profoundly alter ontogeny. That is, the organizational development of the central nervous system (CNS) may be constrained by the genotype and environment for certain limited periods of time. Environmental impact on a given behavior may alter the future coping options available to the organism. Of course, in the same vein, one can speculate that early environmental events that precede a period of vulnerability may also be relatively ineffective.

GENE–ENVIRONMENT INFLUENCES
ON RECOVERY FUNCTIONS

Clearly, genotype of an individual may alter responsiveness to a variety of environmental insults, including X-ray radiation (Nash, 1973), lead toxicity (Burright, Donovick, Michaels, Fanelli, Dolinsky, 1982) and specific brain lesions (Donovick *et al.*, 1981a)—but the mechanisms producing differential sensitivity are not well understood. Similarly, environmental stimulation has been shown to impact several forms of neurological insult, ranging from thyroid deficiency (Davenport, Gonzalez, Carey, Bishop, & Hagquist, 1976) and X-ray radiation (Shibagaki, Seo, Asano, & Kiyono, 1981) to specific brain lesions (Greenough, Fass, & DeVoogd, 1976). Again, the relationship between environmental manipulation and responsivity to neurological insult is clearly complex. A genetically dominant response to environmental enrichment appears to be increased brain size (e.g., Rosenzweig, 1979). A variety of molecular and cellular structures are changed by environment as well (e.g., Globus, Rosenzweig, Bennett, & Diamond, 1973). Although active contact with an enriched environment may be necessary, stimulus specification of enrichment remains elusive. For instance, some of the anatomical changes associated with general enrichment (e.g., increased dendritic branching) may occur in response to specific behavioral testing as well (Greenough *et al.*, 1979). Furthermore, to uniquely characterize such changes as beneficial may be difficult: Unlike increased brain size following environmental enrichment, brain hypertrophy associated with adrenalectomy (e.g., Devenport & Devenport, 1983) is unlikely to be interpreted in favorable terms.

A further example of the complexity of the relationship between apparent neurological change and performance was presented by Kolb, Sutherland, and Whishaw (1983a). These investigators examined the differential impact of hemidecortication and bilateral removal of the frontal cortex in both perinatal and adult rats. When tested as adults, the impact of perinatal lesions was less than that of adult lesions. Furthermore, the extent of behavioral deficits seen was similar in the two perinatal lesions; however, whereas frontal lesions reduced the thickness of the remaining neocortex, hemidecortication increased the thickness of the remaining contralateral cortex. Thus, although the specific behaviors measured were quite similar, the neurological response was not.

To further complicate interpretation of the finding that environmental enrichment enhances recovery from neurological insult, events that clearly are not beneficial to the organism may at times minimize the obtained behavioral response to neurological insult. We investigated the impact of the neurotrophic parasite *Toxocara canis*. This nematode is the common roundworm parasite of domestic dogs and may infect between one third and two thirds of all such animals. Other mammals, including humans and mice, may be infected by the eggs of this parasite, which then develop into second-stage larvae and migrate through somatic tissues, including the brain. The potential health problem of toxocariasis may be indicated in data that suggest that between 2 and 5% of all humans tested in the United Kingdom gave positive reactions to an immunodiagnostic test (Jacobs, 1979). Although ocular and motor disturbances have been associated with infection in humans, the difficulty in diagnosis has limited our understanding of the impact of this parasite on human behavior. In mice, severe and profound changes in behavior following infection with *T. canis* have been observed (Dolinsky *et al.*, 1981; Donovick *et al.*, 1981b); they include changes in a variety of motor exploratory tasks as well as in consummatory behavior. Extensive neurological damage, particularly in major fiber pathways, results from such infection (Summers, Cypess, Dolinsky, Burright, & Donovick, 1983). Interestingly, infection and simultaneous ingestion of lead, which in its own right may disturb both CNS and behavior when administered to perinatal (e.g., Dolinsky *et al.*, 1983) or adult animals (e.g., Burright *et al.*, 1983), was found to reduce the behavioral impact of *T. canis* in many cases; however, lead did not alter the gross morphological brain destruction associated with the parasite itself (Summers *et al.*, 1983).

This protective impact of simultaneous administration of two neurotoxic substances is not unique, as is illustrated by the impact of alcohol on dentate gyrus sprouting (West *et al.*, 1982). As a further example, we examined the impact of a sodium-depleted diet on brain-damaged rats. In this case, rats were exposed to a sodium-depleted diet for 4 weeks and then a standard laboratory chow diet for 2 weeks. This was followed by surgical manipulations in which half the animals received septal lesions and the remainder underwent control surgery. After 16 weeks of a replete diet, the animals were tested on a passive avoidance task. Those lesioned animals with a history of sodium depletion failed to show the typical passive avoidance deficits associated with septal lesions (Bengelloun, Burright &

Donovick, 1976). Clearly, the relationship between the sodium-depleted diet and the observed behavior of the rats with brain damage is less than obvious. In the same experiment we manipulated the temporal aspects of testing, and we also found that limiting the animal to one shock per day selectively improved performance of lesioned animals. It may be easier to discuss temporal aspects of information processing in the brain-damaged and intact animal and to concentrate on this aspect of the data. But such temptation does not necessarily lead to better insight regarding the mechanisms involved in the relationship between experience and performance. Obviously there are a multitude of examples in which combined assaults on the organism are additive or worse than either lone assault (e.g., Mangold, Bell, Gruenthal, & Finger, 1981). Unfortunately we lack explanation for either the paradoxical lessening or enhancing effects of such manipulations.

SPECIFYING ENVIRONMENTS

Most experiments that have manipulated environment have not attempted to compare general with specific features. In the literature that concerns exposure to environments not identical to the test situation but nonetheless containing specific sets of stimuli that one might expect to be related to the test environment, experiential effects are sometimes seen. For instance, hoarding behavior in rats is enhanced by perinatal food deprivation (Marx, 1952). Exposure to a variety of experimentally presented odors when the animal is young has been shown to increase acceptance of novel substances at later periods in the animal's life (Hennessy, Smotherman, & Levine, 1977). The complexity of the potential effects of early experience on later behavior is well illustrated in a study by Bainbridge (1973) in which he exposed female rats to unsolvable visual discrimination problems. After 20 days, when these animals were compared to controls, the experienced animals were shown to be deficient. Evidently response strategies adopted during the earlier phase of training interfered with subsequent performance.

A most obvious specific environmental manipulation involves the overlearning effect. In drug-induced state dependency an individual trained under one pharmacological state may not display the information under another state (e.g., Bliss, 1972). However, the degree of this phenomenon is dependent on the experience with the problem;

Bliss (1972) showed that if an animal was overtrained, state dependency was reduced. Similarly, when animals have been overtrained on a task preoperatively, their postoperative performance may be improved (Thatcher & Kimble, 1966).

Such transfer effects may be sensory-modality or task specific and thus not apparent in all conditions. For instance, Gabriel, Freer, and Finger (1979) trained rats on a tactile discrimination task prior to cortical lesions. This training did not reduce deficits on this task following frontal or somatic cortex lesions. Similarly, when rats were trained on a spatial discrimination task prior to lesions of the septum, the reversal deficit normally associated with this brain lesion was observed (Sikorszky, Donovick, Burright, & Chin, 1977). Furthermore, postoperative training on a brightness discrimination task did not reduce subsequent reversal deficits on a spatial discrimination pattern. However, it should be noted that in the latter study, the reversal deficit was most pronounced on early reversals, thus indicating that the specific experience and the training situation could reduce the lesion-induced deficit. LeVere and Morlock (1973) found that reversal of a brightness discrimination task following neodecortication was impaired relative to control animals, suggesting multiple representations of the original information.

In light of the extensive literature suggesting that early social behavior may be important in the development of normal heterosexual behavior, the impact of experience on response to brain lesions of structures related to such behavior is a natural area for research. Thus, Meisel (1982) reared male rats either (1) in isolation, (2) in isolation plus daily handling, or (3) in pairs with daily handling. The socially housed animals showed best recovery from medial preoptic–anterior hypothalamic lesions as reflected in copulatory behavior. However, other attempts to relate specific presurgical manipulations to altered responses to brain damage have not always been successful. Albert et al. (1981) found that preoperative gentling did not reduce hyperreactivity following septal lesions. Although generalized environmental enrichment may reduce this hyperreactivity, return to isolation may reinstate the hyperreactive response pattern (Goodlett et al., 1982). Similarly, although novel gustatory experiences prior to surgery may reduce taste reactivity normally associated with septal lesions in rats (Donovick, Burright, & Bentsen, 1974), so does exposure to a much more general environmental enrichment condition (Donovick, Burright, & Swidler, 1973). Not surprisingly, the general postoperative environment is critical in recovery from brain damage (e.g., Will, 1981) as well, and such manipulations also may effect normal animals. Many studies have manipulated specific experience and shown facilitated performance under a number of conditions (Hennessy, Smotherman, & Levine, 1977). However, few if any have directly attempted to compare general environmental enrichment effects to those of more specific exposure to relevant stimuli.

Serial-Lesion Effect

To understand the mechanism(s) through which environmental manipulations alter recovery from brain damage, it may be useful to examine several other experiential factors that effect the outcome of neurological insult. The differential response to brain lesions as a function of whether the destruction was produced in a single stage or in multiple steps has received considerable attention. Typically, one notes a greater impact of lesions produced in a single step. This serial-lesion effect is relatively robust and has been observed following destruction of a number of brain structures, including the visual cortex (Spear & Barbas, 1975), the medial frontal cortex (Corwin, Nonneman, Goodlett, 1981), and the hypothalamus (Gruenthal, 1981). However, not all studies have found protection from serial lesions relative to the effects produced by single-stage destruction. For instance, Fass, Wreg, Greenough, and Stein (1980) found essentially equivalent changes in open-field behavior and in the acquisition of an active avoidance task in rats with serial and simultaneous lesions of the septal region. Gruenthal (1981) suggested that the relative behavioral sparing of serial lesions depends on the response measure employed. When measured in a swim test at 37°C, rats with serial lesions of the posterior hypothalamus were quite comparable to controls, but animals with single-stage lesions were higly impaired. However, when tested in a dry open field, no serial-lesion advantage was observed originally, although one developed through the course of the experiment. Obviously, one issue raised has been whether the experience of the organism during the interoperative period provides some form of buffering analogous to pre- and postsurgical enrichment procedures. Support for the proposition that the serial effect may be related to the experiential history of the lesioned animal during the interoperative period was provided by Patrissi and Stein (1975). They observed that the differential reaction to surgery was minimized with a short interoperative interval (10 days), but that it was quite apparent with longer intervals (20 and 30 days) between surgical assault on the frontal lobes.

AGE EFFECTS

Parallel to the idea that the young brain is more plastic, a factor of concern has been the age at the time of insult and the relative vulnerability of the individual. The concept that the young brain is more susceptible to insult has been suggested for toxicological intrusions (e.g., Lagman, Webster, Rodier, 1975) as well as for specific lesions of the brain (e.g., Nonneman & Corwin, 1981). As might be expected, the response of the CNS to lesions varies as a function of age (Kolb et al., 1983b). Issues that complicate the interpretation of such age-related differences in sensitivity have been reviewed (Isaacson, 1975) and are not discussed here. However, several issues are clear. In the first place, the specific location of lesion and nature of the task often determine whether recovery of function is seen following early lesions. For instance, Kolb and Whishaw (1981) examined the impact of frontal cortical lesions in adult and perinatal rats on the subsequent performance of a variety of tasks. They found that some aspects of learned performance were spared, whereas other behaviors, such as burrowing and swimming, were not spared from the impact of early brain damage. These data may be suggestive of differential vulnerability to insult of various organizational systems. Even here, however, we must be cautious; a failure to detect differences between brain-damaged and intact animals may be a byproduct of the task employed, the time at which testing occurs (Goldman, 1974), or the genotype of the subject (Donovick et al., 1981a). Furthermore, even apparent recovery may be transitory in nature. Schallert (1983) reported that recovery from unilateral lesions in the posterior lateral hypothalamus, as measured in several orientation tasks, was not permanent; symptoms originally associated with the neural destruction reappeared with increasing age, particularly a year after surgery.

Obviously, consideration of stimulus conditions of testing of either brain-damaged or control animals is also critical. Spear and his coworkers examined the impact of the presence of odor stimuli from the home cage on a variety of behavioral tests. Training perinatal rats in environments that shared stimuli of the home nest facilitated performance on several learning tasks, as was discussed earlier. Interestingly, the spontaneous alternation deficit frequently observed following septal lesions in rats (Douglas & Raphelson, 1966) was eliminated when tests were conducted in the presence of home-cage shavings (Smith, Goodlett, Burright, Donovick, & Spear, 1983). Obviously, home-cage shavings are complex stimuli, and their presence during testing may reduce fear, perhaps minimizing the enhanced reactivity to novel or stressful situations associated with septal lesions (e.g., Brick, Burright, & Donovick, 1979).

General Overview Revisited

Considerations such as those presented in this chapter lead us to several conclusions. The elegant analysis by Pennington *et al.*, (1980) concerning the impact of the 47,XXX karyotype on behavior may be a prototype of the needed analysis of neurological trauma on behavior. We must better specify and predict changes in behavior across the life span of the organism and must follow the course of neurological insult over time. Research limited to a single genetic stock of animals, a particular age, or a specific task increases the probability of misleading descriptions. Even peripheral intervention may produce feedback to alter central substrates of behavior, including genotypic expression itself.

However, saying this is far easier than developing appropriate experimental designs to more fully appreciate roots to the future of either normal or brain-damaged individuals. We suggest that a starting place for the investigation of perinatal insult may be a choice of behaviors for which there has been genetic selection and temporal specification. For instance, in a series of studies, Henderson has plotted changes in activity of mouse pups at several stages during early postnatal development. At birth, mice are relatively inactive, perhaps ensuring that they remain in the nest (1978). By the time they are 11 days of age, there is strong genetic pressure for them to return to the nest after removal (1981a), but by the time they are 15 days of age, there is selection toward explosive escape behavior in the presence of startling stimuli (1981b). In each of his experiments, Henderson has shown genetic dominance for specific forms of activity; but, given our view of genotype as an invitation for response, one might expect that if neurological insult targeted such early behaviors, the impact would be profound, multifaceted, and life long.

The study of subtle aspects of complex, coactive processes (such as cognitive abilities comprise) may be powerfully benefited by the use of longitudinal designs (Wilson, 1978); and the specification of the impact of neurological insult on behavior necessitates consideration of the genotype of the subject (Donovick *et al.*, 1981a), of developmental factors (Goldman, 1974; Schallert, 1983), and of the subject's experience both prior to (Engellenner, Goodlett, Burright, & Donovick, 1982) and following (Will, 1981) trauma. From such considerations it seems reasonable to suggest that neurological insult, be it lesion or toxin, may increase vulnerability of the individual to subsequent environmental challenges by reducing available coping mechanisms. Indeed, if brain damage induces an individual to adopt what typically may be viewed as a nonoptimal strategy, demands for normal behavior may result in further deterioration of performance. The analyses of these complex interacting influences may require new approaches to our data, including the use of multivariate techniques (Fanelli, Burright, & Donovick, 1983) and general systems theory (Denenberg, 1980).

The exquisitely challenging problems regarding situational specificity and individual variation are to be expected in attempts to study the complex mechanisms of any living system. We must try to meet such idiographic challenges more directly, rather than simply casting them into the black hole of "experimental error," or attempting to reduce their influences by any means possible so that they may remain out of sight and out of mind. Instead, we must strive to understand the implications of vastly reduced or extreme variation in our data in the context of the very differential variables we would often rather ignore.

Acknowledgments

This chapter is dedicated to our friend, colleague, and teacher, John L. Fuller. We express our thanks to our students, who continually challenge us. The authors were supported in part by NSF (DAR 79 11233) while preparing this manuscript.

References

Albert, D. J., Chew, G. L., Tobani, A., Walsh, M. L., Lee, C. Y. S., & Ryan, J. (1981). Preoperative gentling does not attenuate septal lesion induced hyperreactivity. *Physiology and Behavior, 27,* 387–389.

Bainbridge, P. L. (1973). Learning in the rat: Effect of early experience with an unsolvable problem. *Journal of Comparative and Physiological Psychology, 82,* 301–307.

Barrett, B. A., Caza, P., Spear, N. E., & Spear, L. P. (1982). Wall climbing, odors from the home nest and catecholaminergic activity in rat pups. *Physiology and Behavior, 20,* 501–507.

Bengelloun, W. A., Burright, R. G., & Donovick, P. J. (1976). Nutritional experience and spacing of shock opportunities alter the effects of septal lesions on passive avoidance acquisition by male rats. *Physiology and Behavior, 16*, 583–587.

Bennett, M. H., Dyer, R. F., & Dunn, J. D. (1973). Visual dysfunction after long-term continuous light exposure. *Experimental Neurology, 40*, 652–660.

Bliss, D. K. (1972). Dissociated learning and state-dependent retention induced by pentobarbital in rhesus monkeys. *Journal of Comparative and Physiological Psychology, 84*(1), 149–161.

Brick, J., Burright, R. G., & Donovick, P. J. (1979). Stress responses of rats with septal lesions. *Pharmacology, Biochemistry and Behavior, 11*, 695–700.

Burright, R. G., Donovick, P. J., Michaels, K., Fanelli, M. J. & Dolinsky, Z. S. (1982). Effect of amphetamine and cocaine on seizure susceptibility in lead treated mice of different brain weights. *Pharmacology, Biochemistry and Behavior, 16*, 631–635.

Burright, R. G., Engellenner, W. J., & Donovick, P. J. (1983). Lead exposure and agonistic behavior of adult mice of two ages. *Physiology and Behavior, 30*, 285–288.

Campbell, J. H., & Zimmerman, E. G. (1982). Automodulation of genes: A proposed mechanism for persisting effects of drugs and hormones in mammals. *Neurobehavioral Toxicology and Teratology, 4*, 435–439.

Chandra, R. K. (1975). Antibody formation in first and second generation offspring of nutritionally deprived rats. *Science, 190*, 289–290.

Corwin, J., Nonneman, A., & Goodlett, C. (1981). Limited sparing of function on spatial delayed alternation after two-stage lesions of prefrontal cortex in the rat. *Physiology and Behavior, 26*, 763–771.

Davenport, J. W., Gonzalez, L. M., Carey, J. C., Bishop, S. B., & Hagquist, W. (1976). Environmental stimulation reduces learning deficits in experimental cretinism. *Science, 191*, 578–579.

Denenberg, V. H. (1980). General systems theory, brain organization and early experiences, invited opinion. *American Journal of Physiology, 238*, R3–R13.

Denenberg, V. H., Holloway, W. R., & Dollinger, M. J. (1967). Weight gain as a consequence of maternal behavior in the rat. *Behavioral Biology, 17*, 51–60.

Devenport, L. D., & Devenport, J. A. (1983). Brain growth: Interactions of maturation with adrenal steroids. *Physiology and Behavior, 30*, 313–315.

Dolinsky, Z. S., Burright, R. G., & Donovick, P. J. (1983). Behavioral changes in mice following lead administration during several stages of development. *Physiology and Behavior, 30*, 583–589.

Dolinsky, Z. S., Burright, R. G., Donovick, P. J., Glickman, L. T., Babish, J., Summers, B., & Cypess, R. H. (1981). Environmental neurotropic agents: Behavioral effects of lead and *Toxocara canis* in mice. *Science, 213*, 1142–1144.

Donovick, P. J., & Burright, R. G. (1982). Genetic influences on responses to brain lesions. In I. Lieblich (Ed.), *The genetics of the brain* (pp. 177–205). Amsterdam, The Netherlands. Elsevier.

Donovick, P. J., Burright, R. G., & Bentsen, E. O. (1974). Presurgical dietary history and the behavior of control and septal lesioned rats. *Developmental Psychobiology, 8*, 13–25.

Donovick, P. J., Burright, R. G., Fanelli, R. J., & Engellenner, W. J. (1981a). Septal lesions in avoidance behavior: Genetic, neurochemical and behavioral considerations. *Physiology and Behavior, 26*, 317–323.

Donovick, P. J., Burright, R. G., & Swidler, M. (1973). Influences of pre-surgical environment during rearing on exploration and consumption of both normal and septal lesioned rats. *Physiology and Behavior, 11*, 543–553.

Donovick, P. J., Dolinsky, Z. S., Perdue, V. P., Burright, R. G., Summers, B., & Cypess, R. H. (1981b). *Toxocara canis* and lead alter consummatory behavior in mice. *Brain Research Bulletin, 7,* 317–323.

Douglas, R. J., & Raphelson, A. C. (1966). Spontaneous alternation and septal lesions. *Journal of Comparative and Physiological Psychology, 62,* 320–322.

Elias, J. W., Nau, K. L., Villescas, R. X., & Bell, R. (1982). The effects of parity on passive avoidance conditioning on three age groups of Fischer 344 male rats. *Experimental Aging Research, 8*(4), 209–211.

Engellenner, W. J., Goodlett, C. R., Burright, R. G., & Donovick, P. J. (1982). Environmental enrichment and restriction: Effects on reactivity exploration, and maze learning in mice with septal lesions. *Physiology and Behavior, 29,* 885–893.

Fanelli, R. J., Burright, R. G., & Donovick, P. J. (1983). A multivariate approach to the analysis of genetic and septal lesion effects on maze performance in mice. *Behavioral Neuroscience, 97,* 354–369.

Fass, B., Wrege, K., Greenough, W. T., & Stein, D. G. (1980). Behavioral symptoms following serial or simultaneous septal-forebrain lesions: Similar syndromes. *Physiology and Behavior, 25,* 683–690.

Ferchmin, P. A., Bennett, E. L., & Rosenzweig, M. R. (1975). Direct contact with enriched environment is required to alter cerebral weights in rats. *Journal of Comparative and Physiological Psychology, 88*(1), 360–367.

Fuller, J. L. (1967). Experiential deprivation and later behavior. *Science, 158,* 1645–1652.

Gabriel, S., Freer, B., & Finger, S. (1979). Brain damage and the overlearning reversal effect. *Physiological Psychology, 7*(4), 327–332.

Globus, A., Rosenzweig, M. R., Bennett, E. L., & Diamond, M. C. (1973). Effects of differential experience on dendritic spine counts in rat cerebral cortex. *Journal of Comparative and Physiological Psychology, 82,* 175–181.

Goldman, P. S. (1974). An alternative to developmental plasticity: Heterology of CNS structures in infants and adults. In D. G. Stein, J. J. Rosen, & N. Butter (Eds.), *Plasticity and recovery of function in the central nervous system.* New York: Academic Press.

Goodlett, C. R., Engellenner, W. J., Burright, R. G., & Donovick, P. J. (1982). The influence of environmental rearing history and postsurgical environmental change on the septal rage syndrome in mice. *Physiology and Behavior, 28,* 1077–1081.

Greenough, W. T., Fass, B., & DeVoogd, T. J. (1976). The influence of experience on recovery following brain damage in rodents: Hypotheses based on development research. In R. N. Walsh and W. T. Greenough (Eds.), *Environments as therapy for brain dysfunction.* New York: Plenum.

Greenough, W. T., Juraska, J. M., & Volkmar, F. R.(1979). Maze training effects on dendritic branching in occipital cortex of adult rats. *Behavioral and Neural Biology, 26,* 287–297.

Gruenthal, M. (1981). Task dependent rate of recovery following serial posterior hypothalamic lesions. *Physiology and Behavior, 27,* 497–502.

Hammond, G. L., Lai, Y-K, & Markert, C. L. (1982). Diverse forms of stress lead to new patterns of gene expression through a common and essential metabolic pathway. *Proceedings of the National Academy of Sciences USA, Biochemistry, 79,* 3485–3488.

Henderson, N. D. (1978). Genetic dominance for low activity in infant mice. *Journal of Comparative and Physiological Psychology, 92,* 118–125.

Henderson, N. D. (1981a). Genetic influences on locomotor activity in 11-day-old housemice. *Behavior Genetics, 11,* 3, 209–225.

Henderson, N. D. (1981b). A fit mouse is a hoppy mouse: Jumping behavior in 14-day-old *Mus musculus. Developmental Psychobiology, 14,* 459–472.

Hennessy, M. B., Smotherman, W. P., & Levine, S. (1977). Early olfactory enrichment enhances later consumption of novel substances. *Physiology & Behavior, 19,* 481–483.

Infurna, R. N., Steinert, P. A., & Spear, N. E. (1979). Ontogenetic changes in the modulation of taste aversion learning by home environmental cues in rats. *Journal of Comparative and Physiological Psychology, 93,* 1097–1108.

Isaacson, R. L. (1975). The myth of recovery from early brain damage. In N. R. Ellis (Ed.), *Aberrant development in infancy: Human and animal studies* (pp. 1–26). Potomic, MD: L Erlbaum.

Jacobs, D. E. (1979). Man and his pets. In R. J. Donaldson (Ed.), *Parasites and western man* (pp. 171–200). Lancaster, England: MTP Press.

Kolb, B., Sutherland, R. J., & Whishaw, I. Q. (1983a). A comparison of the contributions of the frontal and parietal association cortex to spatial localization in rats. *Behavioral Neuroscience, 97,* 13–28.

Kolb, B., Sutherland, R. J., & Whishaw, I. Q. (1983b). Abnormalities in cortical and subcortical morphology after neonatal neocortical lesions in rats. *Experimental Neurology, 79,* 223–244.

Kolb, B., & Whishaw, I. Q. (1981). Neonatal frontal lesions in the rat: Sparing of learned but not species-typical behavior in the presence of reduced brain weight and cortical thickness. *Journal of Comparative and Physiological Psychology, 95,* 863–880.

Langman, J., Webster, W., & Rodier, P. (1975). Morphological and behavioural abnormalities caused by insults to the CNS in the perinatal period. In D. E. Poswillo (Ed.), *Teratology.* New York: Springer-Verlag.

Laudenslager, M. L., Reite, M., & Harbeck, R. J. (1982). Suppressed immune response in infant monkeys associated with maternal separation. *Behavioral Neural Biology, 36,* 40–48.

LeVere, T. E., & Morlock, G.W. (1973). Nature of visual recovery following posterior neodecortication in the hooded rat. *Journal of Comparative and Physiological Psychology, 83,* 62–67.

McCauley, P. T., Bull, R. J., Tonti, A. P., Lutkenhoff, S. D., Meister, M. V., Doerger, J. U., & Stober, J. A. (1982). The effects of prenatal and postnatal lead exposure on neonatal synaptogenesis in rat cerebral cortex. *Journal of Toxicology and Environmental Health, 10,* 639–651.

Mangold, R. F., Bell, J., Gruenthal, M., & Finger, S.(1981). Undernutrition and recovery from brain damage: A preliminary investigation. *Brain Research, 230,* 406–411.

Marx, M. H. (1952). Infantile deprivation and adult behavior in the rat: Retention of increased rate of eating. *Journal of Comparative and Physiological Psychology, 45,* 43–49.

Meisel, R. L. (1982). Effects of postweaning rearing condition on recovery of copulatory behavior from lesions of the medial preoptic area in rats. *Developmental Psychobiology 15,* 331–338.

Nash, D. J. (1973). Influence of genotype and neonatal irradiation upon open-field locomotion and elimination in mice. *Journal of Comparative and Physiological Psychology, 83,* 458–464.

Nonneman, A. J., & Corwin, J. V. (1981). Differential effects of prefrontal cortex ablation in neonatal juvenile and young rats. *Journal of Comparative and Physiological Psychology, 95,* 588–602.

Oppenheim, R. W. (1981). Ontogenetic adaptations and retrogressive processes in the development of the nervous system and behaviour: A neuroembryological perspective. In K. J. Connolly & H. F. R. Prechtl (Eds.), *Maturation and development: Biological and psychological perspectives* (pp. 73–109). Philadelphia: Lippincott.

Parsons, P. J., & Spear, N. E. (1972). Long-term retention of avoidance learning by immature and adult rats as a function of environmental enrichment. *Journal of Comparative and Physiological Psychology, 80,* 297–303.

Patrissi, G., & Stein, D. G. (1975). Temporal factors in recovery of function after brain damage. *Experimental Neurology, 47,* 470–480.

Pennington, B., Puck, M., & Robinson, A. (1980). Language and cognitive development in 47,XXX females followed since birth. *Behavior Genetics, 10,* 31–41.

Rosenzweig, M. R. (1979). Responsiveness of brain size to individual experience: Behavioral and evolutionary implications. In M. E. Hahn, C. Jensen, & B. C. Dudek (Eds.), *Development and evolution of brain size* (pp. 263–294). New York: Academic Press.

Sackett, G. P. (1967). Response to stimulus novelty and complexity as a function of rats' early rearing experiences. *Journal of Comparative and Physiological Psychology, 63,* 369–375.

Schallert, T. (1983). Sensorimotor impairment and recovery of function in brain damaged rats: Reappearance of symptoms during old age. *Behavioral Neuroscience, 97,* 159–164.

Shibagaki, M., Seo, M., Asano, T., & Kiyono, S. (1981). Environmental enrichment to alleviate maze performance deficits in rats with microencephaly induced by X-irradiation. *Physiology & Behavior, 27,* 797–802.

Sikorszky, R. D. Donovick, P. J., Burright, R. G., & Chin, T. (1977). Experimental effects on acquisition and reversal of discrimination tasks by albino rats with septal lesions. *Physiology & Behavior, 18,* 231–236.

Smith, G. J., Goodlett, C. R., Burright, R. G., Donovick, P. J., & Spear, N. E. (1983). The presence of home cage stimuli attenuate spontaneous alternation deficits in rats with septal lesions. *Physiological Psychology, 11,* 119–124.

Smith, G. J., & Spear, N. E.(1981). Home environment stimuli facilitate learning of shock escape spatial discrimination in rats 7–11 days of age. *Behavioral and Neural Biology, 31,* 360–365.

Spear, P. D., & Barbas, H. (1975). Recovery of pattern discrimination ability in rats receiving serial or one-stage visual cortex lesions. *Brain Research, 94,* 337–346.

Studelska, D. R., & Kemble, E. D.(1979). Effects of briefly experienced environmental complexity on open field behavior in rats. *Behavioral and Neural Biology, 26,* 492–496.

Summers, B., Cypess, R. H., Dolinsky, Z. S., Burright, R. G., & Donovick, P. J. (1983). Neuropathological studies of experimental toxocariasis in lead exposed mice. *Brain Research Bulletin, 10,* 547–550.

Thatcher, R. W., & Kimble, D. P. (1966). Behavior after cerebral lesions on retention of an avoidance response in overtrained and non-overtrained rats. *Psychonomic Science, 6,* 9–10.

Wahlsten, D. (1982). Genes with incomplete penetrance and the analysis of brain development. In I. Leiblich (Ed.), *Genetics of the brain* (pp. 367–391). New York: Elsevier.

Wainwright, P. (1981). Relative effects of maternal and pup heredity on postnatal mouse development. *Developmental Psychobiology, 13*, 493–498.

West, J. R., Lind, M. D., Demuth, R. M., Parker, E. S., Alkana, R. L., Cassell, M., & Black, A. C., Jr. (1982). Lesion-induced sprouting in the rat dentate gyrus is inhibited by repeated ethanol administration. *Science, 218*, 808–810.

Will, B. E. (1981). The influence of environment on recovery after brain damage in rodents. In S. Finger (Ed.), *Functional recovery from brain damage* (pp. 167–188). Amsterdam: Elsevier North-Holland.

Will, B. E., Rosenzweig, M. R., Bennett, E. L., Hebert, M., & Morimoto, H. (1977). Relatively brief environmental enrichment aids recovery of learning capacity and alters brain measures after postweaning brain lesions in rats. *Journal of Comparative and Physiological Psychology, 91*, 33–50.

Wilson, R. S. (1978). Synchronies in mental development: An epigenetic perspective. *Science, 202*, 939–948.

Wright, L. L., Bell, R. W., Schreiber, H. L., Villescas, R., & Conely, L. (1977). Stress on the maternal behavior of *Rattus norvegicus. Developmental Psychobiology, 10*, 331–337.

16

Sex-Steroid-Induced Alterations in the Behavioral Effects of Brain Damage[*]

Dwight M. Nance

Introduction

In the present study, a series of experiments on the psychoneuroendocrine effects of damage to the septum are reviewed. These experiments were initially motivated by an interest in the extrahypothalamic control of reproduction rather than by an interest in the more general problem of recovery of function or neural plasticity. However, it soon became apparent that the effects of septal destruction on sexual behavior were dependent on both the gender of the animal and the postlesion hormone environment. In order to appreciate the possible implications of these observations for recovery of function it is necessary to consider the effects of sex steroids on sexual differentiation of the brain, as well as the subsequent activational effects of these hormones on reproductive behavior.

EARLY ORGANIZATIONAL EFFECTS OF STEROIDS

As might be expected, the best documented examples of functional sex differences involve the control of reproduction (Gorski, 1980). In

[*]Supported by funds from USPHS, the Ford Foundation, and the Canadian Medical Research Council. The author gratefully acknowledges the comments and suggestions of David Hopkins and Michael Wilkinson during preparation of the present manuscript.

mammals, as typified by the rat, morphology of the reproductive system, neuroendocrine regulation, and brain are inherently female. Functionally this translates into a female phenotype, a cyclic pattern of gonadotropin release, and an ability to show high levels of female sexual behavior following hormone treatment. In contrast, males show an androgen-dependent shift in this inherently female system such that they develop a male phenotype, an acyclic pattern of gonadotropin release, an increased potential to show male copulatory behavior, and, importantly, a reduced capacity for ovarian hormones to induce female (lordotic) sexual behavior. These sexually dimorphic functions can be quantified by assessing an animal's ability to develop corpora lutea in intact ovaries (females) or subcutaneous ovarian grafts (males) and by measuring the levels of male and female sex behavior following appropriate hormone treatment.

NEONATAL CRITICAL PERIOD

In the rat, there is a perinatal critical period covering the first few days of life during which exposure to male sex hormones (regardless of the genetic sex of the animal) will masculinize (or defeminize) subsequent reproductive function. Consistent with the notion of a critical period, there is an interaction of age and dosage of androgens such that the ability of androgens to masculinize reproductive function is limited to a finite period in development. Even cavalier doses of testosterone will not modify the inherently female system if exposure to the hormone occurs after this critical period. By injecting various doses of androgens at different ages during the neonatal critical period (Gorski, 1980), it has been shown that androgenization is not a unitary phenomenon but rather involves the differentiation of several component processes. For example, the effects of early androgens on cyclicity can be dissociated from the effects on reproductive behavior by appropriate doses of testosterone at specific ages.

BRAIN FUNCTION AND MORPHOLOGY

There is evidence that functional sex differences in reproductive processes may actually reflect an underlying sex difference in brain morphology (see Gorski, Harlan, Jacobson, Shryne, & Southam, 1980). Reinforcing this conclusion are studies demonstrating that varying the amount of exposure to androgens during the neonatal critical period can produce morphological alterations in the same brain areas that are implicated in the control of reproduction of adult animals. Likewise, a number of sex differences in the levels of various brain neurotransmitters and receptors have been documented for a variety of specific brain areas, results that further indicate the potential extent of sex differences in the brain (Arimatsu, Seto, & Amano, 1981; Avissar, Egozi, & Sokolovsky, 1981; Egozi, Avissar and Sokolowsky, 1982; Orensanz, Guillamon, Ambrosio, Segovia, & Azuara, 1982).

PERMANENCE OF SEXUAL DIFFERENTIATION OF THE BRAIN

Although not usually explicitly stated, the long-term functional and anatomical consequences of androgenization are generally regarded as being permanent. No one has been able to reverse completely these early effects of androgenization, although, as will be shown, it appears possible to reverse partially the effects of androgenization on female sexual behavior.

Psychoneuroendocrine Functions of the Septum

It has been proposed that the septum, by serving as a major link between the rhinencephalon, diencephalon, and mesencephalon, functions as a nodal region for integrating endocrine control mechanisms with specific behavioral and motivational processes (Nance, 1983). In support of this hypothesis, septal damage alters gonadal feedback control mechanisms and at the same time dramatically alters the behavioral sensitivity to sex hormones. The presence of steroid-concentrating neurons (Pfaff & Keiner, 1973) as well as endocrine neuropeptide cell bodies in the septal region (Witkin, Paden, & Silverman, 1982) are consistent with this hypothesis. For the remaining discussion, the primary focus is on the effects of electrolytic septal lesions on female sexual behavior.

SEXUALLY DIMORPHIC RESPONSE TO SEPTAL LESIONS

The display of lordotic behavior is entirely hormone dependent when tested with sexually experienced male rats. Following appropriate priming with estrogen and progesterone, an unreceptive ova-riectomized female rat will display high levels of receptivity (proba-bility 90–100% that a lordotic response will occur each time the test animal is mounted by a stud male). An effective and typical hormone regimen consist of 2 μg of estradiol benzoate (EB) per day for 3 days followed by a single injection of 0.5 mg of progesterone (P) on Day 4 administered 4–6 hours prior to the behavior test. If, however, the animal is tested without the addition of P (i.e., 2 μg EB × 3 days, only), then lordotic behavior will be present, but at a greatly reduced level (probability of occurrence around 20%). Thus by using these two hormone regimens (EB alone and EB + P) it is possible to deter-mine whether specific brain lesions facilitate or inhibit the display of female sexual behavior.

BEHAVIORAL EFFECTS

Using the preceding general procedure it has been shown that bi-lateral electrolytic lesions in the lateral septum of adult female rats produce a dramatic increase in the display of female sexual behavior (EB only) (Nance, Shryne, & Gorski, 1974). The additional facilitory effects of P on lordotic behavior were less apparent in these lesioned rats than in control animals because their receptivity was already near maximal levels following treatment with EB alone. Additional studies demonstrated that this increased sensitivity to estrogen in female rats was not mediated by the adrenal glands (an endogeneous source of progesterone). Subsequently, dose-response data verified that septal lesions had a selective effect on behavioral sensitivity to estrogen in female rats (Nance, Shryne, & Gorski, 1975a).

In marked contrast to female rats, normal male rats typically show low levels of female sexual behavior when primed with EB + P (Nance et al., 1974). This sexually dimorphic response to ovarian hor-mones appears to reflect a selective decrease in the potentiating ef-fects of P on lordotic behavior in male rats, which show low levels of lordotic behavior following EB treatment alone as do female rats. However, unlike those in female rats, septal lesions in male rats were found to have no effect on the behavioral sensitivity to estrogen as indicated by lordotic behavior (Nance, Shryne, & Gorski, 1975b). Thus there appears to be a clear sexually dimorphic effect of septal lesions on female sexual behavior of rats. This behavioral sex dif-ference associated with septal lesions was also found to have several neurochemical correlates of septal damage.

NEUROCHEMICAL CORRELATES

An analysis of several neurotransmitter systems in septal-lesioned female rats revealed that relative to controls, changes in forebrain dopamine (DA) levels and turnover as well as in glutamic acid decarboxylase (GAD, the rate-limiting enzyme in γ-aminobutyric acid [GABA] synthesis) levels were systematically related to the facilitation of lordosis behavior (Gordon, Nance, Wallis, & Gorski, 1977). Interestingly, these neurochemical differences between septal-lesioned and control female rats were found to be estrogen dependent. Specifically, in the absence of EB priming, neurotransmitter function was similar between septal-lesioned and sham-lesioned rats. Moreover, in the absence of a septal lesion, EB injections had no detectable neurochemical effects on brain catecholamines in control female animals. However, the combination of a septal lesion and EB priming resulted in a relative decrease in DA levels and turnover in the striatum, nucleus accumbens septi, and amygdala relative to all other groups. Consistent with a GABA-activated feedback circuit onto DA cell bodies, GAD activity in the ventral tegmental area and substantia nigra was also significantly different between septal-lesioned and sham-operated rats. EB treatment reduced GAD levels in the ventral tegmental area and the substantia negra of sham-lesioned rats, whereas EB had no effect on GAD levels in animals with septal lesions. These latter results can be interpreted as follows: In normal animals, EB treatment reduces the postsynaptic efficiency of DA in areas containing DA terminals (Gordon, Borison, & Diamond, 1980). Thus the decrease in GAD levels in the region of DA cell bodies represents the feedback control of GABA neurons onto DA cells bodies in response to the estrogen-induced decrease in the postsynaptic efficiency of DA. Because septal lesions appear to eliminate this GABA-activated feedback onto DA cell bodies, these animals do not compensate for the estrogen-induced depression in DA function. It was also noted that DA levels in the striatum of septal-lesioned rats were inversely correlated with lordotic behavior, which supports the presumed inhibitory role of DA on lordotic behavior. Finally, brain levels of norepinephrine and serotonin were not consistently related to the effects of septal lesions.

The neurochemical effects of septal lesions in normal male rats can be briefly summarized. Septal damage, alone or in combination with EB treatment, had no major neurochemical effects in these animals, which is consistent with the lack of a significant effect of septal lesions on lordosis behavior of normal male rats. In the next section evidence is presented to demonstrate that these sexually dimorphic effects of septal lesions are due to the androgen-dependent process of sexual differentiation of the brain.

EARLY EXPOSURE TO ANDROGENS AND THE EFFECTS
OF SEPTAL LESIONS

As suggested in the introduction, androgenization appears to be a graded phenomenon, and this is verified by the effects of septal lesions on lordosis behavior of adult female rats treated neonatally with different doses of testosterone propionate (TP). For example, a single 90-μg injection of TP into 3-day-old female rats was capable of eliminating the facilitatory effects of P on lordosis behavior as well as producing an acyclic pattern of gonadotropin release (Nance et al., 1974). However, septal lesions in these rats exerted the same facilitory effect on behavioral sensitivity to estrogen as has been found in normal female rats. Thus 90 μg of TP on Day 3 of life was capable of androgenizing these female rats, but not to an extent sufficient to prevent the effects of septal lesions on lordosis behavior, as is the case with normal rats. Subsequently, these results were essentially replicated in androgenized adult female rats given a single 270-μg dose of TP on Day 3 of life (Nance, Shryne, Gordon, & Gorski, 1977b). However, in the same series of experiments, a dose of 1.0 mg of TP on Day 1 of life was found to block completely the effects of septal lesions on lordosis behavior of adult female rats. Thus these results (1) confirm that the sexually dimorphic response of rats to septal destruction is due to an androgen-dependent process of sexual differentiation of the brain and (2) suggest that in contrast to gonadotropin control and behavioral responsiveness to P, much higher doses of TP (or more chronic exposure, as is the case in normal male rats) are required to androgenize the behavioral response to septal lesions.

The effects of sex steroids on the behavioral consequences of septal lesions in both male and female rats is next considered. As can be seen, the long-term effects of septal damage can be permanently altered by chronic exposure to sex steroids during an apparent critical period following brain surgery.

Interaction of Estrogen and Septal Lesions
in Adult Male Rats

The discovery of the interaction of estrogen with septal lesions was based on the following observations: In our first investigation of the effects of septal lesions (Nance *et al.*, 1974), their possible effects on the sexually dimorphic pattern of gonadotropin release were also examined. This was indexed by recording vaginal cycles and the presence of recent corpora lutea in the normal and androgenized females. The septal-lesioned and sham-lesioned male rats (lacking ovaries) were given subcutaneous ovarian grafts for 1 month beginning 3 days after surgery. Septal lesions had no detectable effect on the sexually dimorphic pattern of gonadotropin release in that normal females continued to cycle and showed recent corpora lutea, whereas the androgenized female and male rats remained acyclic, showing no corpora lutea. In marked contrast to gonadotropin control, the suppressive effects of androgen-dependent sexual differentiation of the brain on female sexual behavior were functionally reversed by septal lesions. The high levels of female sexual behavior induced by EB in the male and androgenized female rats with septal lesions were indistinguishable from the behavior of normal female rats with septal lesions. However, in the next experiment, which consisted of establishing EB-dose response curves for female and male rats with septal lesions, we found that septal lesions had absolutely no effect on the lordosis behavior of male rats primed with EB. The dose-response data for the septal-lesioned females were reviewed earlier (Nance *et al.*, 1975a). These negative results with male rats led to a detailed examination of the differences between the two experiments.

CHRONIC EXPOSURE TO OVARIAN HORMONES

Major differences between the two experiments were the age of the animals at septal lesioning and castration and the presence of ovarian grafts in the earlier study (Nance *et al.*, 1974). Comparisons among combinations of pre- versus postpubertal ages at the time of castration, septal lesioning, and implantation of ovarian grafts provided the following results (Nance, Shryne, & Gorski, 1975b). The only group that showed a septal-lesion-induced facilitation of lordosis behavior was that of male rats that were given septal lesions, castrated, and then given subcutaneous ovarian grafts for 1 month beginning shortly after surgery. Animals exposed to ovarian grafts for 1 month prior to receiving a septal lesion (but not after) showed low levels of female sex behavior similar to control male rats. It is also of interest that the presence or absence of endogenous androgens (testes) for 1 month following a septal lesion had no detectable effect on the consequences of septal lesions. This specific requirement for exposure to ovarian hormones for an alteration in the behavioral effects of septal lesions in male rats was subsequently shown to be reproduced by daily injections of 2 μg of EB for 30 days. It was also observed that (1) the synergistic action of estrogen and septal lesions on female sexual behavior of male rats was actually more effective in older animals and (2) chronic exposure to EB for 30 days was ineffective if the treatment was initiated several months after septal destruction. These latter results, in particular, suggested the existence of a critical period that occurs following septal damage during which the behavioral consequences of the lesion are susceptible to estrogen treatment.

EVIDENCE FOR A POSTLESION CRITICAL PERIOD

In a further series of studies on the interaction of estrogen and septal lesions in male rats (Nance, Phelps, Shryne, & Gorski, 1977a), the effectiveness of (1) a single injection of 50 μg of EB given 48 hours postlesion, (2) 10 daily injections of 5 μg of EB given on postlesion Days 1–10, and (3) 10 daily injections of 5 μg of EB given on post lesion Days 11–20. Of these treatment regimens, chronic EB exposure on postlesion Days 1–10 had the greatest effect on the consequences of septal lesions, as was indexed by high levels of lordotic behavior displayed weeks later following acute EB priming. The single postlesion injection of 50 μg of EB was totally ineffective, whereas the rats exposed daily to EB (5 μg) on postlesion Days 11–20 showed a modest increase in subsequent responsiveness to EB. These latter results suggest that a period of susceptibility to estrogen intervention may extend for at least a few weeks after septal damage. The fact that the earlier regimen of 2 μg of EB per day for 30 days postlesion (Nance *et al.*, 1975b) was behaviorally more effective than the preceding hormone regimens reinforces this conclusion and reemphasizes the apparently essential requirement for postlesion EB exposure to be chronic in order to modify the effects of septal lesions. These results clearly indicate the presence of a finite critical period following a septal lesion during which the brain function of male rats can be permanently altered by chronic exposure to estrogen.

NEUROCHEMICAL CORRELATES OF ESTROGEN SENSITIZATION

As reviewed in the section "Neurochemical Correlates" septal lesions produce systematic changes in brain DA and GABA function in female rats, whereas they have no detectable neurochemical effect in male rats. Thus it is important to determine whether the feminizing effects of septal lesions combined with chronic EB treatment on lordosis behavior of male rats also result in a female pattern of neurotransmitter function. We found that adult male rats given septal lesions and exposed to EB for 30 days postlesion subsequently showed neurochemical changes in response to acute EB priming that were comparable to the pattern displayed by septal-lesioned female rats (Gordon, Nance, Wallis, & Gorski, 1979). That is, acute EB priming in estrogen-sensitized septal-lesioned males produced (1) high levels of lordotic behavior, (2) decreased tyrosine hydroxylase activity in the region of DA terminals, and (3) increased GAD activity in the region of DA cell bodies. This pattern is similar to that seen in female rats with septal lesions and is consistent with a lesion-induced change in GABA feedback control of DA function. These results support the hypothesis that septal lesions combined with chronic EB treatment actually reverse a major component of the androgen-dependent process of sexual differentiation of the brain. However, it was not known whether this EB–septal lesion interaction was specific to estrogen, or whether additional experimental interventions during the postlesion period would also modify the behavioral effects of septal lesions in male rats.

SPECIFICITY OF ESTROGEN ACTION

We hypothesized that estrogen treatment was interacting with a process initiated by a septal lesion in male rats that was associated with recovery of function following brain damage. To the extent that recovery recapitulates ontogeny, we speculated that experimental manipulations capable of modifying the developing brain would also influence the behavioral effects of septal lesions in male rats. Since hypothyroidism is known to have profound and deleterious effects on the developing nervous system, we examined the long-term consequences of hypothyroidism in male rats that had been made hypothyroid during the recovery phase following septal lesions either by feeding them a 0.15% diet of the goitergen propylthiouracil or else by surgical thyroidectomy (Nance *et al.*, 1977a). These studies verified that both chemical and surgical hypothyroidism during the postlesion recovery period following septal lesions in male rats produced alterations in the display of lordotic behavior that were essentially identical to the changes produced by chronic EB treatment. These results cast doubt on the possibility that estrogen is unique in its capacity to alter septal-lesion effects in male rats and indicate that both estrogen treatment and hypothyroidism act on a more generalized process associated with recovery from brain damage. In these same experiments we also verified that the relative insensitivity of male rats to the synergism between P and EB is unaltered by these manipulations.

Interaction of Testosterone and Septal Lesions in Adult Female Rats

As noted earlier, the effects of septal lesions on the lordosis behavior of adult female rats can be prevented by a single, androgenizing dose of TP (1.0 mg) on Day 1 of life. If, indeed, septal lesions initiate a critical period that shares common features with the earlier neonatal critical period, then it appeared possible that chronic exposure to TP following a septal lesion might attenuate the facilitatory effects of septal lesions on lordosis behavior of adult female rats. To test this possibility, adult female rats were given electrolytic septal lesions and received daily injections of 1.0 mg of TP or oil for 30 days following surgery (Nance *et al.*, 1977b). Subsequent tests for female sex behavior conducted 1–2 months following the termination of chronic TP treatment revealed that, similar to neonatal TP treatment, chronic exposure to TP following a septal lesion in adult female rats prevented the occurrence of high levels of lordotic behavior that is typically observed in septal-lesioned female rats.

This reversal in the behavioral effects of septal lesions in female rats by chronic TP treatment was specific to the behavior tests conducted following injections of EB alone, and the normal behavioral responsiveness of female rats to the synergism of P and EB remained normal in all groups. Thus, increased behavioral responsiveness to estrogen is not an inevitable consequence of septal lesions in female rats, but rather, the behavioral consequence of septal damage can be modified by the hormone environment during the postlesion recovery period in female rats. Also, unlike estrogen exposure, which may block or inhibit recovery from brain damage in septal-lesioned male rats, these results suggest that chronic exposure to androgen may facilitate recovery in septal-lesioned female rats.

Implications and Directions for Future Research

Although the mechanism underlying these lesion–hormone interactions remains to be explained, it is clear that hormones can have a powerful and possibly permanent effect on the behavioral consequences of septal damage in both male and female rats. In addition, these results provide considerable information regarding important dimensions along which recovery from brain damage may be directed. For example, recovery appears to share or rely on basic mechanisms that underlie normal brain development (recovery recapitulates ontogeny). Therefore variables capable of modifying brain development and maturation might be expected to alter the consequences of brain damage in older animals. Also, the demonstration of the existence of a critical period shortly following a brain lesion, a phenomenon so typical of earlier developmental stages, reinforces the analogy between developing animals and older brain-damaged rats. And finally, these results suggest that psychoneuroendocrine processes may provide a potentially powerful model system for studying recovery of function. There remain, however, a large number of critical and unanswered questions. For example, we do not know whether this interaction of hormones with a brain lesion is unique to the septal region. The effects of chronic sex steroids on other types of brain-lesion–behavior systems have not been tested. We have no information regarding the aspect of the recovery process on which sex steroids actually act, and we have only begun to establish some of the neurochemical manifestations of these hormone–lesion interactions. It would also be important to know and interesting to determine the morphological basis of these hormone-induced alterations in the effects of brain lesions. Work of Matsumoto and Arai (1979) testifies to the potential utility of more detailed neuroanatomical studies of this phenomenon. And finally, the potential implications of these results with reference to possible sex differences in the effects of central nervous system injury in humans or the contribution of endogeneous or exogeneous steroids to recovery from certain types of lesions has not been fully considered.

References

Arimatsu, Y., Seto, A., & Amano, T. (1981). Sexual dimorphism in α-bungarotoxin binding capacity in the mouse amygdala. *Brain Research, 213,* 432–437.

Avissar, S., Egozi, Y., & Sokolovsky, M. (1981). Studies on muscarinic receptors in mouse and rat hypothalamus: A comparison of sex and cyclic differences. *Neuroendocrinology, 32,* 295–302.

Egozi, Y., Avissar, S., & Sokolovsky, M. (1982). Muscarinic mechanisms and sex hormone secretion in rat adenohypophysis and preoptic area. *Neuroendocrinology, 35,* 93–97.

Gordon, J. H., Borison, R. L., & Diamond, B. I. (1980). Estrogen in experimental tardive dyskinesia. *Neurology, 30,* 551–554.

Gordon, J. H., Nance, D. M., Wallis, C. J., & Gorski, R.A. (1977). Effects of estrogen on dopamine turnover, glutamic acid decarboxylase activity and lordosis behavior in septal lesioned female rats. *Brain Research Bulletin, 2,* 341–346.

Gordon, J. H., Nance, D. M., Wallis, C. J., & Gorski, R. A. (1979). Effects of septal lesions and chronic estrogen treatment on dopamine, GABA and lordosis behavior in male rats. *Brain Research Bulletin, 4,* 85–89.

Gorski, R. A. (1980). Sexual differentiation of the brain. In D. T. Krieger & J. C. Hughes (Eds.), *Neuroendocrinology* (pp. 215–222). Sunderland, MA: Senauer Associates.

Gorski, R. A., Harlan, R.E., Jacobson, C.D., Shryne, J. E., & Southam, A. M. (1980). Evidence for the existence of a sexually dimorphic nucleus in the preoptic area of the rat. *Journal of Comparative Neurology, 193,* 529–539.

Matsumoto, A., & Arai, Y. (1979). Synaptogenic effect of estrogen on the hypothalamic arcuate nucleus of the adult female rat. *Cell Tissue Research, 198,* 427–433.

Nance, D. M. (1983). Psychoneuroendocrine effects of neurotoxic lesions in the septum and striatum of rats. *Pharmacology Biochemistry and Behavior. 18,* 605–609.

Nance, D. M., Phelps, C., Shryne, J. E., & Gorski, R. A. (1977a). Alterations by estrogen and hypothyroidism in the effects of septal lesions on lordosis behavior of male rats. *Brain Research Bulletin, 2,* 49–53.

Nance, D. M., Shryne, J. E., Gordon, J. H., & Gorski, R. A. (1977b). Examination of some factors that control the effects of septal lesions on lordosis behavior. *Pharmacology Biochemistry and Behavior, 6,* 227–234.

Nance, D. M., Shryne, J., & Gorski, R. A. (1974). Septal lesions: Effects on lordosis behavior and pattern of gonadotropin release. *Hormones and Behavior, 5,* 73–81.

Nance, D. M., Shryne, J., & Gorski, R. A. (1975a). Effects of septal lesions on behavioral sensitivity of female rats to gonadal hormones. *Hormones and Behavior, 6,* 59–64.

Nance, D. M., Shryne, J., & Gorski, R. A. (1975b). Facilitation of female sexual behavior in male rats by septal lesions: An interaction with estrogen. *Hormones and Behavior, 6,* 289–299.

Orensanz, L. M., Guillamon A., Ambrosio, E., Segovia, S., & Azuara, M. C. (1982). Sex differences in alpha-adrenergic receptors in the rat brain. *Neuroscience Letters, 30,* 275–278.

Pfaff, D., & Keiner, (1973). Atlas of estradiol-concentrating cells in the central nervous system of the female rat. *Journal of Comparative Neurology, 151,* 121–158.

Witkin, J. W. Paden, C. M., & Silverman, A. (1982). The luteinizing hormone-releasing hormone (LHRH) systems in the rat brain. *Neuroendocrinology, 35,* 429–438.

17

Some Factors Affecting Behavior After Brain Damage Early in Life

*Daniel Simons
and Stanley Finger*

The Kennard Principle

In 1936, Margaret Kennard published the first of a series of studies comparing the effects of cortical lesions in infant and adult monkeys (Kennard, 1936, 1938, 1940, 1942). She noted that when the cortical motor areas on one side of the brain were ablated early in life, the ability to use the contralateral limbs was far better than that seen in animals sustaining seemingly equivalent lesions after the period of infancy. The infant-lesioned monkeys were able to walk, climb, feed themselves, and perform movements of prehension. Kennard postulated that reorganization of function followed these early lesions. She believed that equivalent changes were less likely or unlikely to occur following brain damage after a certain level of development had been obtained.

Kennard's reports were not the first in which the effects of early brain damage were found to be less deleterious than those observed after later brain injuries. In fact she (Kennard, 1938) cited both Vulpian (1866) and Soltmann (1876), who described age-related differences in response to hemidecortication in much earlier experiments on laboratory animals. Kennard, however, was much more successful than any of her predecessors in drawing attention to these infant sparing effects. Her experiments inspired a wealth of new investigations on laboratory animals and stimulated more detailed observations on human case material to determine the extent to which these observations on the motor cortex would generalize to other brain lesions, behavioral tasks, and species.

At first, the papers that followed Kennard's initial reports seemed to provide strong support for her basic findings. In 1937, for example, Tsang reported the same sort of behavioral sparing in weanling rats subjected to hemidecortications before being tested for maze-learning abilities. A year later, Beach (1938) showed that nest building by brain-damaged female rats, an unlearned behavior, was also more disrupted by lesions in adult-lesioned as opposed to infant-lesioned animals. The contention that left hemispheric damage might be less disruptive of speech functions in children than in adults also received increased recognition at this time (Guttman, 1942; see also Lenneberg, 1967 and Hécaen, 1979). To account for the often remarkable recovery from aphasia that characterizes brain-damaged preschool-age children, it was suggested that the right hemisphere may compensate for the left hemisphere following brain damage early in life (see Milner, 1974).

The confirmations of Kennard's general findings seemed so broadly based that many scientists and practitioners began to look upon the greater behavioral sparing and compensation following brain damage in infancy as a rule or principle. In fact, on occasion this is referred to as the Kennard principle. Nevertheless, there now appear to be many exceptions to this "principle," and contemporary investigators have raised serious questions about the generality of the earlier findings (Isaacson, 1975).

Factors Affecting the Results of Infant-Lesion Studies

It is recognized that the dramatic sparing witnessed by Kennard has its limits and represents a situation considerably more complex than she and many investigators in the 1930s, 1940s, and 1950s had envisioned. That is, not only have infant-lesioned animals performed worse than sham-lesioned control subjects in some later experiments, but in a number of these reports the infant–lesioned subjects have been found to perform just as poorly as the adult-lesioned cases on certain behavioral tasks (see reviews by Finger & Stein, 1982; Johnson & Almli, 1978). For instance, no infant sparing effects were found with cats on a delayed-response task after hippocampal lesions

(Isaacson, Nonneman, & Schmaltz, 1968), on visual discriminations following posterior cortex lesions in rabbits (Murphy & Stewart, 1974), in social behavior after septal lesions in rats (Johnson, 1972), or in oddity-problem performance after dorsolateral prefrontal cortex lesions in infant monkeys (Thompson, Harlow, Blomquist, & Schiltz, 1971). Moreover, it is now clear that the young brain can be even more vulnerable than the adult brain to certain types of diffuse injury, such as may result from inadequate early nutrition. The behavioral consequences of poor prenatal and postnatal nutrition can be dramatic and have been well documented (Winick, 1976). If determintal nutritional conditions do not change before the period of rapid brain growth has ended, the chances of recovery from this type of insult (which can dramatically affect brain-cell number and physiology) may be very limited.

The response to early brain damage thus has not been consistent. In an attempt to account for this variability, some investigators have pointed out that many infant-lesion studies have lacked the necessary control groups and conditions needed to properly compare the effects of brain damage at different ages. As a case in point, only a small percentage of experiments have included adult comparison groups that are matched to the younger subjects for age at the time of testing as well as for recovery-period duration. Furthermore, as noted by Teuber and Rudel (1962), with human patients the lesions displayed by the children are often less known and more diffuse than those that characterize adult populations. Autopsied material may not even be available for study in many of these cases.

Still, many controlled laboratory studies are showing that even with appropriate control groups and rigorous testing conditions, the effects of early brain damage can differ from one set of conditions to the next. A number of factors that can account for this variability have now been studied in the laboratory and are becoming increasingly better understood.

AGE AT THE TIME OF TESTING
AND RECOVERY-PERIOD DURATION

Kennard herself noted that the behavioral sparing seen after motor cortex lesions in infant monkeys was in a sense limited in time. As the monkeys grew older they tended to develop more and more spasticity, although they still remained much less impaired than animals operated on later in life. The idea that deficits can appear or even worsen over time following early brain damage also has support in more recent, controlled laboratory studies dealing with other lesions and with tasks as varied as complex problem solving or reflexive movements of a limb in response to tactile stimulation (Almli, Golden, & McMullen, 1976; Goldman, 1974; Hicks & D'Amato, 1970, 1975).

One explanation for these later emerging deficits is that the aberrant behavior is appearing at a time when the part of the brain that has been damaged would normally begin to mediate or contribute to the function being assessed. For example, Hicks and D'Amato (1975) have hypothesized that subcortical areas can adequately mediate tactile placing responses prior to postnatal Day 17 in the rat. In their opinion, the deficit that consistently appears on Day 17 in neonatally lesioned rats reflects a major developmental change in the neural program for this behavior that normally occurs in the 3rd week after birth. Excitatory and inhibitory connections from the developing sensory–motor cortex play a major role in guiding tactile placing after Day 17, but not before then.

Just as there is increased recognition of the fact that posttraumatic performance can worsen with age, there is also greater appreciation of the possibility that for some types of lesion the ability to perform specific tasks may also improve significantly with age or the passage of time. This better recognized phenomenon has been described for monkeys that were given orbital prefrontal lesions in the first few weeks of life and were tested on a delayed-alternation task 1 and 2 years later (Miller, Goldman, & Rosvold, 1973). It has also been observed in brain-damaged children who are asked to sit in a tilted chair and to right themselves without visual or auditory cues (Teuber & Rudel, 1962). In these instances, the attenuation of symptoms could reflect many things, such as the acquisition of new behavioral strategies and compensations, the diminution of shock effects, or perhaps the achievement of other brain areas of the level of maturation needed to mediate the function in question (Finger & Stein 1982). Whatever the mechanisms may eventually prove to be, these studies show clearly that age at the time of testing and recovery-period duration can markedly affect the results obtained in infant-lesion studies.

AREA AND SYSTEM DAMAGED

There is no reason to believe that infant sparing effects must appear after a lesion in each and every system in the brain or at each level of a system. Even though such effects have been noted at both cortical and subcortical levels, with sensory systems in particular one may hypothesize that the closer one is to the sensory periphery, the less divergence one will find in the neural pathways and, concomitantly, the lower the probability that one will see control-level posttraumatic performance. In this context it is worth noting that the majority of infant sparing effects that have been reported after focal lesions have dealt with the cerebral cortex and perceptual learning paradigms, with much of the remaining work investigating components of the limbic system such as the amygdala. Very little research has been conducted on lesions early in life in midbrain, pontine, or medullary zones.

In addition, at each level of the nervous system there may be differences in the neural organization of the target area. Important considerations here might be whether the area is or is not topographically organized, how diffuse the input to the area is, and whether the target area is the only zone receiving projections from a specific lower region. The developmental status of the target area at the time of injury could also be an important determinant of behavior following brain damage, especially in cases where the area is not totally destroyed.

TASK AND DEMAND CHARACTERISTICS

A skeptic might be tempted to argue that insensitive tests could have been used in those experiments in which relatively normal behaviors were found following early brain lesions. Indeed, such a position must be given some consideration when infant-lesioned subjects are compared only to control cases without brain damage. Nevertheless, the notion of insensitive tests has little explanatory power in studies in which infant-lesioned subjects do better than adults that have sustained lesions in the same general regions. If the tests are sensitive enough to bring out deficits among the adult-lesioned subjects, the relatively good performance of the infant-lesioned group cannot be attributed to insensitive behavioral measurements.

This, of course, is not to say that the probability of detecting deficits in the infant-lesioned group does not increase as the task and demand characteristics of the behavioral tests become more challenging. Benjamin and Thompson (1959), for example, noted that adult cats performed poorly on a variety of rough–smooth and rough–rough tactile discriminations following extensive bilateral le-

sions of the cortical sensory–motor zones. Their matched infant-lesioned group performed significantly better on the easier problems in
the series (rough vs. smooth). Nevertheless, the infant-lesioned cats
performed just as poorly as the adults when attempting to dis-
tinguish between two surfaces differing in degree of roughness. Experiments such as this one show that performance after early brain
damage is task-dependent and that conclusions regarding the effects
of age at the time of brain damage are not necessarily generalizable
from one set of testing conditions to the next.

Status of Remaining Brain Areas

There has been increasing recognition of the fact that the results of
any brain-lesion study will depend not only on the locus of the
damage, but also on the functional status of remaining brain tissue
(Finger & Stein, 1982). In terms of accounting for variability across
studies, this notion has broad applicability and is pertinent when
attempting to understand the different types of effect that can follow
early brain damage. In particular, the status of the remaining brain can
help to explain why diffuse early brain damage, such as that resulting
from early undernutrition, can have such severe consequences. Under
these conditions, brain regions that might normally compensate for a
particular damaged area may also be severely compromised. In contrast, with focal lesions, such as those that characterize most laboratory animal studies on the effects of cortical ablations, other functionally related parts of the brain may still be capable of responding
at the high level of efficiency necessary to compensate for the damaged area.

The developmental status of spared parts of the brain should also
be considered here. On the basis of an extensive series of studies on
young monkeys with forebrain lesions, Goldman (1974) has suggested
that one structure might even be capable of taking over for another
and of undergoing some sort of anatomical reorganization if it is not
yet mature or committed to its own functions at the time a related or
neighboring area is damaged. Such a change in neuronal organization could be mediated by axons failing to retract at a particular time
(Goldman & Galkin, 1978; Land & Lund, 1979), by aberrant inputs
projecting to an area (Schneider & Jhavari, 1974), or even by more
subtle physiological changes, all of which would depend at least in
part upon the developmental status of the areas spared at the time of
injury.

Complete versus Subtotal Lesions
Made in Infancy

The clinical and experimental evidence indicates a growing list of factors that can influence behavior and recovery following brain damage sustained early in life. This is consistent with what is also known about recovery processes in adult organisms (for review see Finger & Stein, 1982) and suggests that hard and fast rules concerning recovery of function must be qualified by the circumstances particular to the case at hand. In two studies from this laboratory (Finger, Simons, & Posner, 1978; Simons & Finger, 1983), another potential interacting variable has been examined in relation to performance after brain damage early in life. This is the effect of lesion size, especially as it relates to the use of remaining spared fragments of target tissue.

Our interest in the effects of lesions sustained in infancy stemmed from a series of experiments investigating factors that could affect ridge versus smooth discrimination performance following somatosensory forebrain damage in adult rats. In these experiments, animals that were previously blinded by enucleation were tested in a T maze on a series of five ridge–smooth problems (milled aluminum plates) that were graded in difficulty. The animals were allowed to palpate the discriminanda (which formed the floors in the wings of the maze) at the choice point, and exploration could involve receptors on the face, paws, and so forth. The rats received five trials per day and progressed to more difficult ridge–smooth problems as an a priori criterion was met. Animals that did not master a problem in 40 to 60 days were removed from further testing. Food served as the reinforcement in these studies.

Intact animals readily mastered the entire battery in about 35 days. In contrast, adult-lesioned rats with large, one-stage bilateral lesions of sensory–motor cortex areas I or II (SmI, SmII) or both were typically unable to complete the tactile battery and consistently showed severe impairments in the acquisition of these learned behaviors (Finger, Cohen, & Alongi, 1972; Finger & Reyes, 1975). Nevertheless, it was observed that under certain circumstances rats with similar sensory–motor cortex lesions could perform these tactile discriminations almost as well as sham-lesioned animals. One factor improving performance was the production of the lesion in discrete steps (i.e., the serial-lesion effect; Finger, Marshak, Cohen, Scheff, Trace, & Niemand, 1971; see also Simons, Puretz, & Finger, 1975; Finger & Simons, 1976). Another important factor proved to be the length of the postoperative recovery period, at least for rats with lesions restricted to either SmI or SmII (Finger, Hart, & Jones, 1982).

In this context, an attempt was made to assess tactile performance following one-stage bilateral lesions of the sensory–motor cortex in newborn rats. It was expected that the infant-lesioned animals would be significantly less impaired than their adult-lesioned counterparts; that is, that a Kennard-like sparing effect would be observed. However, after much testing it became clear that such a difference between infant- and adult-lesioned animals only occurred when both lesion groups experienced subtotal lesions, and that rats in both age groups performed very poorly after experiencing complete or nearly complete destruction of SmI + II.

The rats with lesions placed in infancy came from two groups. In both cases, the rat pups were 24–48 hours old when they received either bilateral lesions intended to include all of SmI and SmII bilaterally or sham operations. The lesions were produced by gentle aspiration and were guided by evoked-potential maps made with slightly older rats. Enucleations were performed at 90 days of age, and 2 weeks later the animals began behavioral testing. After mastering all five tactile problems or after failing to learn a given discrimination within 60 days, the animals were removed from testing. Because some of the comparison groups from other studies were allowed only a 40-day period to learn each problem, all scores to be presented here are adjusted to show performance based on the 40-day cutoff. In the first infant study, the rats were immediately sacrificed for histological study.

The performance scores of the first group of rats (Group A) were found to be fairly good (see Figure 1). Although they took more days ($\bar{X} = 75$) to complete the series of problems than did sham-lesioned animals, they learned the tasks much more rapidly than did adult-lesioned animals that had received large bilateral lesions of SmI + II in previous studies in our laboratory (e.g., $\bar{X} = 180$). Although these findings at first seemed indicative of a Kennard effect, careful examination of the gross surface topology of the infant cortices and of changes in the thalamic ventrobasal complex suggested that the neonatal lesions did not completely damage the entire SmI area and that these animals thus sustained less SmI + II damage than previously tested adult-lesioned rats. Nevertheless, it was difficult to determine which regions and how much cortex were spared because mechanical adjustments occur after large expanses of neocortex are ablated early in life, including a filling of the lesion abcess by growing cortical tissue.

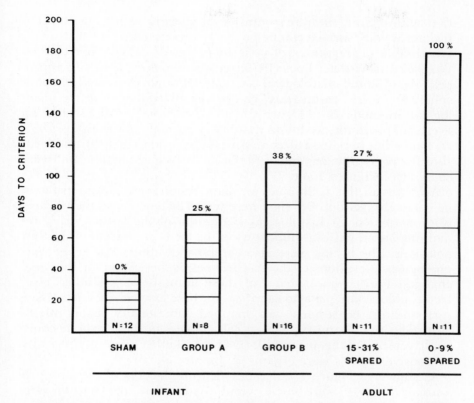

Figure 1. Performance scores of four groups of rats with sensory–motor cortex lesions and one group with sham operations on five successive tactile discriminations. Infant-lesioned animals sustained lesions (Groups A and B) or sham operations on the 2nd postnatal day, and adult-lesioned animals sustained lesions at 90 days of age that spared 15–31% or 0–9% of SmI in at least one hemisphere. Horizontal bars across columns indicate mean number of days to criterion on each tactile problem, and figures above the columns indicate the percentage of animals that failed to master the entire battery. The performance scores of the infant-lesioned rats were computed on the basis of a 40-day limit for mastering a given problem. Adult-lesioned animals were removed from testing if they failed to master a problem within 40 days. All animals that failed to meet this criterion were given conservative scores of 43 days for that problem and all remaining problems to which they fail to advance. (Graph based on data of Finger, Simons, and Posner, 1978, and Simons and Finger, 1983.)

In discussing this assessment problem with Thomas Woolsey, it was suggested that we use the barrels in Layer IV of the SmI as anatomical markers for a better understanding of what was being spared after the early lesions. Using rats, Welker (1976) had observed

that within SmI, the representation of specific regions of the contralateral body surface can be precisely correlated with consistently
identifiable aggregations of cells in Layer IV called "barrels" by
Woolsey and Van der Loos (1970; see also Woolsey, 1967). In appropriately oriented histological sections through the cortical hemisphere an entire "ratunculus" can be visualized using routine histological methods (see Figure 2[a]). With serial sections and an
overhead projector, we found that it was possible to reconstruct barrel fields that remained after an SmI lesion, and to identify and measure the particular regions of the body surface projection that were
spared (see Figures 2 and 3).

Armed with this technique, we made lesions in a second group of
newborn rats (Group B). They were tested as before and their brains
were processed for histological evaluation of the lesions using remaining barrel fields as indicators of the locus and extent of the SmI
ablations. The brains were also carefully examined for gross morphological alterations in the cerebral hemispheres and for thalamic
changes. Furthermore, many of these animals were studied electrophysiologically prior to sacrifice. In these experiments, the tissue
surrounding the lesions was mapped functionally using microelectrodes to determine whether cell clusters in these regions could
be driven by cutaneous stimulation and whether these peripherally
responsive regions were organized somatotopically.

As shown in Figure 1, the tactile-learning scores of the Group B
animals ($\bar{X} = 110$) were worse overall than those of the Group A rats.
Moreover, many of these animals displayed learning deficits as pronounced as those of adult-lesioned rats with large SmI + II lesions,
who typically scored about 175 days to criterion. Histological analyses revealed that the lesions of the Group B animals were larger than
those produced in the Group A animals. Nevertheless, close examination of the Group B brains showed that some of the lesions still failed
to include all of SmI bilaterally. Furthermore, a significant negative
correlation was found between lesion size and speed of learning; infant-lesioned rats with total or nearly total lesions (i.e., less than 10%
of SmI spared in the hemisphere with the smaller lesion) were severely impaired in learning the tactile discriminations, whereas rats
with less complete lesions (which typically spared 15–30% of SmI in
the oral and forepaw regions) were somewhat impaired relative to
control animals but were nevertheless able to complete all five tactile
problems within the alloted time (see Finger et al., 1978). Figure 2
includes representative histological sections of the cortex and
thalamus from an infant-lesioned animal that learned the tactile dis-

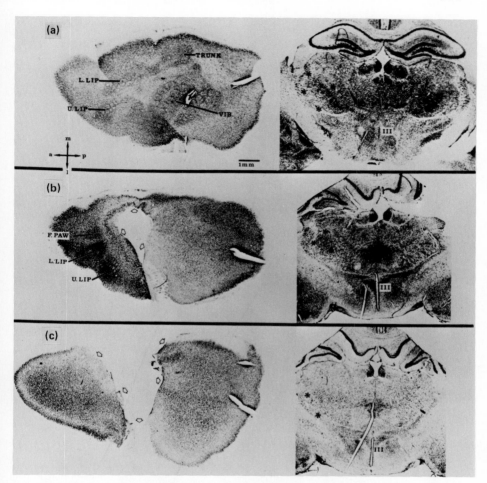

Figure 2. Photomicrographs showing left cortical hemispheres and thalami of (a) a control animal, (b) a fast learner (10B 5), and (c) an animal that failed to master even the easiest tactile discrimination. (a) Barrel fields can be visualized that correspond to the projections of the lower lip (L.LIP), upper lip (U.LIP), trunk, and mystacial vibrissae (VIB); the boundaries of the ventrobasal complex (on the left side) are marked with asterisks in the corresponding photomicrograph on the right. (b) The lesion in this rat (79% complete) spared some of the projections from the forepaw and the oral–facial regions. A much reduced ventrobasal complex can be seen in the corresponding left thalamus. (The right hemisphere of this animal sustained a complete SmI ablation). (c) The left cortical hemisphere and the thalamus of an animal with complete bilateral removal of SmI. Asterisks indicate the approximate position at which the ventrobasal complex normally would have developed. Arrows indicate the perimeters of the lesion cavities. (a) anterior; (p) posterior; (m) medial; (l) lateral; (III) third ventricle. (From Finger, Simons, & Posner, 1978.)

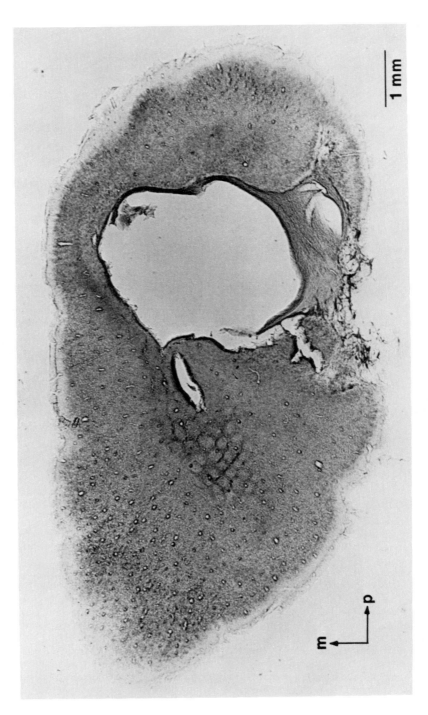

1 mm

p

m

criminations rapidly and from a rat that failed to master even the easiest discrimination. Note that in the former case (Figure 2[b]), barrels in the forepaw and facial regions are visible and the ventrobasal complex in the thalamus is not completely degenerated. In the latter case, barrels are not visible and the ventrobasal complex has virtually disappeared.

These findings implied that adult- and infant-lesioned animals may be equally impaired after sensory–motor cortex damage provided that the lesions are large and spare little or no SmI. To formally test this hypothesis we chose the 10 infant-lesioned rats with the largest lesions and compared their performance scores to two groups of adult-lesioned animals with comparably large lesions from previous studies in our laboratory (see Figure 1, 0–9% spared). One group was matched for recovery time after surgery and the other group was matched for age at time of testing. Three groups of sham-lesioned controls completed the experimental design. An analysis of variance on these data showed a highly significant lesion effect but no effect of age at time of surgery, indicating that all groups of animals with large lesions of SmI + II were severely impaired in tactile learning, regardless of the developmental age at which the lesions were produced (Finger, *et al.*, 1978).

Effect of Subtotal Lesions in Infancy and Adulthood

Although these findings failed to demonstrate recovery of function following nearly complete lesions of the sensory–motor cortex in infancy, they clearly suggested that the relatively good tactile learning observed in many of the infant-lesioned rats is mediated by spared

---

Figure 3. Photomicrograph of a 100-μm thick tangential section through the left hemisphere of an adult-lesioned rat (4G) that sustained an incomplete lesion of the SmI cortex. Barrels in Layer IV were observed only in the anterolateral aspects of the SmI cortex, and in this section, cellular aggregates corresponding to part of the representation of the upper lip are clearly visible. Serial reconstruction of remaining barrel fields revealed the lesion to be 76% complete, sparing portions of the representation of the upper and lower lip and, to a lesser extent, the forepaw. On the basis of lesion size and location this animal was matched to infant-lesioned animal 10B 5, histology from which is shown in Figure 2(b). The tangential orientation of the section in this figure is more lateral than that in Figure 2(b). (p) posterior; (m) medial. See also Figure 1 and Simons and Finger (1983).

fragments of the sensory–motor cortex. This was especially interesting inasmuch as data from earlier studies in our laboratory often suggested that spared fragments of cortical tissue may not be used in a very effective manner by adult-lesioned animals with one-stage, bilateral sensory–motor cortex lesions.

In order to look more carefully at the possibility that infant-lesioned animals with SmI + II lesions could be making more efficient use of spared fragments of target tissue than adult-lesioned animals, we (Simons & Finger, 1983) gave 30 adult-lesioned animals subtotal lesions that were made to closely match those of the infant-lesioned rats that had 13–28% of SmI remaining in at least one hemisphere. Following either a 1-month or 4-month recovery period, the animals were tested on the tactile discriminations. At the conclusion of behavioral testing, the animals were sacrificed and their brains were sectioned in a tangential plane so that remaining barrel fields could be visualized and the lesions reconstructed as before. The brains of these animals were then compared individually to those of the infant-lesioned rats. Because of the bilateral nature of the task, for each animal the hemisphere containing the most sparing was used for the comparisons. Matches were made, first on a qualitative basis in terms of which particular cytoarchitectonic zones could be visualized, for example, oral regions versus oral plus forepaw regions, and then on the basis of the lesion extent, measured quantitatively. Figure 3 shows the histology of the adult-lesioned animal (4G) that was matched to the infant-lesioned rat (10B-5) of Figure 2(b). Serial reconstructions showed that both animals had some sparing of regions representing the upper and lower lips and the forepaw.

Good matches were found for 11 of the infant-lesioned animals with incomplete lesions (see Figure 4). In every pair of animals, the SmI regions spared by the cortical lesions included at least a portion of the representation of the upper and lower lips, including the furry bucal pad within the mouth. Of these, 9 animals also had some sparing of the forepaw projections and in 5 cases there was some sparing of the vibrissae and dorsal head regions. The infant-lesioned group had an average of 21.6% of SmI spared (in the hemisphere with the smaller lesion), and the adult-lesioned group had an average of 22.3% of Sm1 spared; the difference between each pair did not exceed 4%.

In spite of the similarities in the lesions, the tactile-learning scores presented in Figure 4 show that the two groups of animals performed quite differently. As a group, the infant-lesioned rats required 63 days to complete the tactile battery, whereas the matched adult-lesioned animals needed 112 days. The sham-lesioned animals, by com-

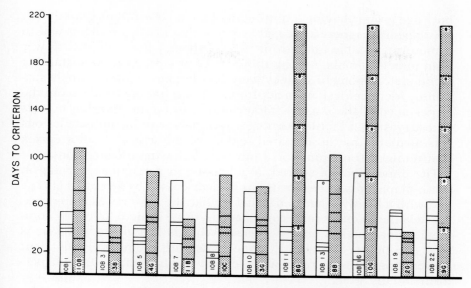

MATCHED LESIONS OF THE SENSORY-MOTOR CORTEX

Figure 4. Days to criterion (vertical bars) for each matched pair of infant- and adult-lesioned animals on five successive discriminations. Infant-lesioned rats (clear) had 13–28% of SmI remaining in at least one hemishpere; adult-lesioned rats (shaded) had 15–31% of SmI spared. Individual matches were made on the basis of lesion size and location. Circles signify that a discrimination was not learned within 40 days. Adult-lesioned animals in Group G had 120-day recovery periods; all other adult-lesioned rats had 35-day recovery periods. (After Simons & Finger, 1983).

parison, took 36 days. These data were subjected to statistical analyses, and overall the results were supportive of the hypothesis that infant-lesioned animals perform better than their adult counterparts when sizeable spared fragments of target tissue are left. That is, in contrast to what was observed after nearly complete lesions, evidence for a partial Kennard-like effect emerged when 15–30% of the SmI part of the system was spared.

Compensation or Reorganization?

The results of the aforementioned experiments show that tactile learning in infant- and adult-lesioned rats is severely impaired following large lesions of the sensory–motor cortex, but that animals in both age groups having a minimum of 15 to 30% of SmI spared in at least one hemisphere are capable of learning tactile problems within a more reasonable amount of time, although they are still slower than intact animals. Among these latter groups, animals sustaining incomplete lesions in infancy were less impaired than animals sustaining identical lesions in adulthood. These findings underscore the importance of the sensory–motor cortex in tactile learning by rats and suggest that tactile learning by animals with incomplete lesions was mediated by those spared regions of the sensory–motor cortex that retained some functional integrity following the ablations.

The importance of spared target tissue in perceptual learning in brain-damaged adult animals has been discussed by Frommer (1978), and with a highly organized structure like the sensory–motor cortex, the idea that behavioral recovery can be quite limited following complete lesions makes intuitive sense. What is less clear, however, is why the infant- and adult-lesioned rats with seemingly equivalent spared fragments of remaining sensory–motor cortex did not perform equally well.

One reason for this disparity might be that neurons in the remaining cortical areas of the two age groups have different functional response properties. In other words, it might be postulated that some sort of reorganization had taken place in the infant cortex but not in the adult cortex, perhaps as Kennard believed had occurred after motor cortex damage in her young monkeys. Nevertheless, all of the indices employed seemed to suggest that the spared fragments of the sensory–motor cortex continued to develop quite normally after the neonatal ablations. First, the SmI lesions did not appear to disrupt the continued development of the remaining cortical barrels that first become visible 4–5 days postnatally (see Killackey & Belford, 1979; Rice & Van der Loos, 1977). Second, the somatotopic organization and other receptive-field properties of the cells in the spared remnants of the SmI cortex were comparable to those seen in intact hemispheres. These units still showed short latency discharges, small receptive fields, and responses to stimulation of only those parts of the body that would normally project to these areas. And third, units in tissue outside the sensory–motor cortex continued to be unresponsive to cutaneous stimulation, just as in normal animals.

Although these relatively gross indices of central nervous system function are not sufficient to rule out some sort of reorganization at the cortical level, or even at some subcortical site, the data do suggest that the infant-lesioned animals were relying upon remaining, more or less normal tissue to guide behavior. This, in turn, would be consistent with a behavioral model that emphasizes only that the different age groups might not have been equally efficient in adapting effective compensatory strategies following brain damage.

This behaviorally oriented view also derives from a consideration of the nature of the tactile testing procedure and the topographical organization of the sensory cortex. In the discrimination tasks used here, the animals were not restricted to a particular receptor system for contacting the discriminanda. Thus the rats conceivably could have learned to use their forepaws or hindpaws, mystacial vibrissae, or perioral sinus hairs for making the discriminations. Each of these receptor systems is located on a different part of the body and each is represented in a separate region of the SmI cortex (Welker, 1976). Following an incomplete SmI lesion that may have spared a portion of only one or two of these projection zones, an advantage could have gone to those animals who were able to develop behavioral strategies that used these spared systems, even though performance may have been mediated by different cues or receptors than those normally chosen by intact animals in the particular situation. Thus, with the forepaw and hindpaw projections severely damaged by the cortical lesions, the younger animals may have learned in the course of development to rely on their facial hairs as the principal source of information in discriminating rough and smooth surfaces. Adult-lesioned animals, on the other hand, may have been slower in switching from one set of receptors to another, may have been less effective at devising strategies to use different receptors in unfamiliar settings, or may have persisted in using an inefficient component of the system as a result of previous learning experiences and well-established learning sets (Harlow, 1949).

Summary and Conclusions

Although the underlying basis of the present findings remains to be fully elucidated, the results of these experiments provide strong support for the contention that whether early brain damage results in a Kennard-like sparing effect or a performance just as poor as that seen in an adult-lesioned group depends on more than just age at the time of trauma. To the list of known variables that have the potential for affecting performance after a neonatal injury (e.g., lesion locus, task difficulty, length of posttraumatic recovery period) one can also cite degree of completeness of the lesion. In this case, there was some evidence for better tactile performance by infant-lesioned than adult-lesioned animals when the lesions spared 15–30% of the anterior part of SmI in both groups, but when only 0–10% of SmI remained, all animals performed poorly, regardless of age at the time of surgery.

If, as suggested here, the neonatal animals were simply making better use of spared fragments of target tissue that continued to develop normally, it might be expected that under the appropriate conditions even adult-lesioned subjects would be able to show that they too could use spared fragments of target tissue in an efficient manner. Lesions made in discrete stages (see Finger *et al.*, 1971), for example, might allow more effective use of remaining target tissue than lesions placed all at once, not only as a result of less neural shock, but because such subjects might already be learning new behavioral strategies that use spared tissue while the system is undergoing the slower dissolution. A differential ability to use spared fragments might also account for the better postoperative learning scores of adult animals raised under highly enriched environments, because these animals might have more opportunities than animals raised in more restrictive settings to learn that different receptors can be used effectively under certain circumstances (see Finger & Stein, 1982). In addition, very extensive but specific training (i.e., overtraining; Weese, Niemand, & Finger, 1973) may provide a greater advantage to subjects prior to incomplete lesions than prior to complete lesions for some of these same reasons.

Although it cannot be argued that all cases of good recovery following brain damage early or even later in life reflect a differential ability to use spared fragments of target tissue, an understanding of the effect of any potential interactive factor on performance in brain-damaged subjects can lead to a better understanding and appreciation of the variability that is often seen in experiments on laboratory animals, as well as in case studies involving human patients. It is in this context that variables such as spared fragments of target tissue deserve increased recognition and further study by those interested in the response to brain damage in subjects of any age.

Acknowledgments

The projects reported here were funded in part by NINCDS grant NS-11002 and by a Biomedical Research Support Grant (Division of Research Resources, NIH) to the second author.

References

Almli, C. R., Golden, G. T., & McMullen, N. T. (1976). Ontogeny of drinking behavior of preweanling rats with lateral preoptic damage. *Brain Research Bulletin, 1,* 437–442.

Beach, F. A. (1938). The neural basis of behavior: II. Relative effects of partial decortication in adulthood and infancy upon maternal behavior in the primiparous rat. *Journal of Genetic Psychology, 53,* 109–148.

Benjamin, R. M., & Thompson, R. F. (1959). Differential effects of cortical lesions in infant and adult cats on roughness discrimination. *Experimental Neurology, 1,* 305–321.

Finger, S., Cohen, M., & Alongi, R. (1972). The roles of somatosensory cortical areas 1 and 2 in tactile discrimination in the rat. *International Journal of Psychobiology, 2,* 93–102.

Finger, S., Hart, T., & Jones, E. (1982). Recovery time and sensorimotor cortex lesion effects. *Physiology and Behavior, 29,* 73–78.

Finger, S., Marshak, A., Cohen, M., Scheff, S., Trace, R., & Niemand, D. (1971). Effects of successive and simultaneous lesions of the somatosensory cortex on tactile discriminative ability in the rat. *Journal of Comparative and Physiological Psychology, 77,* 221–227.

Finger, S., & Reyes, R. (1975). Long-term deficits after somatosensory cortical lesions in rats. *Physiology and Behavior, 16,* 289–293.

Finger, S., & Simons, D. (1976). Effects of serial lesions of somatosensory cortex and further neodecortication on retention of a rough–smooth discrimination in rats. *Experimental Brain Research, 25,* 183–197.

Finger, S., Simons, D., & Posner, R. (1978). Anatomical, physiological and behavioral effects of neonatal sensorimotor cortex ablation in the rat. *Experimental Neurology, 60,* 347–373.

Finger, S., & Stein, D. G. (1982). *Brain damage and recovery: Research and clinical perspectives.* New York: Academic Press.

Frommer, G. P. (1978). Subtotal lesions: Implications for coding and recovery of function. In S. Finger (Ed.), *Recovery from brain damage: Research and theory* (pp. 217–280). New York: Plenum.

Goldman, P. (1974). An alternative to developmental plasticity: Heterology of CNS structures in infants and adults. In D. G. Stein, J. J. Rosen, & N. Butters (Eds.), *Plasticity and recovery of function in the central nersous system* (pp. 149–174). New York: Academic Press.

Goldman, P. S., & Galkin, T. W. (1978). Prenatal removal of frontal association cortex in fetal rhesus monkeys: Anatomical and functional consequences in postnatal life. *Brain Research, 152,* 451–485.

Guttman, E. (1942). Aphasia in children. *Brain, 65,* 205–219. Harlow, H. F. (1949). The formation of learning sets. *Psychological Review, 56,* 51–65.

Hécaen, H. (1979). Aphasias. In M. S. Gazzaniga (Ed.), *Handbook of behavioral neurobiology: Neuropsychology* (Vol 2. pp. 239–292). New York: Plenum.

Hicks, S. P., & D'Amato, C. J. (1970). Motor–sensory and visual behavior after hemispherectomy in newborn and mature rats. *Experimental Neurology, 29,* 416–438.

Hicks, S. P., & D'Amato, C. J. (1975). Motor–sensory cortex–corticospinal system and developing locomotion and placing in rats. *American Journal of Anatomy, 143,* 1–42.

Isaacson, R. L. (1975). The myth of recovery from early brain damage. In N. R. Ellis (Ed.), *Aberrant development in infancy* (pp. 1–25). Potomac, MD: Erlbaum.

Issacson, R. L., Nonneman, A. J., & Schmaltz, L. W. (1968). Behavioral and anatomical sequelae of damage to the infant limbic system. In R. L. Isaacson (Ed.), *The neuropsychology of development* (pp. 41–78). New York: Wiley.

Johnson, D. A. (1972). Developmental aspects of recovery of functions following septal lesions in the infant rat. *Journal of Comparative and Physiological Psychology, 78*, 331–348.

Johnson, D. A., & Almli, C. R. (1978). Age, brain damage, and performance. In S. Finger (Ed.), *Recovery from brain damage: Research and theory* (pp. 115–134). New York: Plenum.

Kennard, M. A. (1936). Age and other factors in motor recovery from precentral lesions in monkeys. *American Journal of Physiology, 115*, 138–146.

Kennard, M. A. (1938). Reorganization of motor function in the cerebral cortex of monkeys deprived of motor and premotor areas in infancy. *Journal of Neurophysiology, 1*, 477–497.

Kennard, M. A. (1940). Relation of age to motor impairment in man and sub-human primates. *Archives of Neurology and Psychiatry, 44*, 377–397.

Kennard, M. A. (1942). Cortical reorganization of motor function: Studies on a series of monkeys of various ages from infancy to maturity. *Archives of Neurology and Psychiatry, 48*, 227–240.

Killackey, H. P., & Belford, G. R. (1979). The formation of afferent patterns in the somatosensory cortex of the neonatal rat. *Journal of Comparative Neurology, 183*, 285–304.

Land, P. W., & Lund, R. D. (1979). Development of the rat's uncrossed retinotectal pathway and its relation to plasticity studies. *Science, 205*, 698–700.

Lenneberg, E. (1967). *Biological foundations of language.* kew York: Wiley.

Miller, E. A., Goldman, P. S., & Rosvold, H. E. (1973). Delayed recovery of function following orbital prefrontal lesions in infant monkeys. *Science, 182*, 304–306.

Milner, B. (1974). Sparing of language functions after early unilateral brain damage. In E. Eidelberg & D. G. Stein (Eds.), *Functional recovery after lesions of the nervous system. Neuroscience Research Program Bulletin, 12*, 213–216.

Murphy, E. H., & Stewart, D. L. (1974). Effects of neonatal and adult striate lesions on discrimination in the rabbit. *Experimental Neurology, 42*, 89–96.

Rice, F. L., & Van der Loos, H. (1977). Development of the barrels and barrel field in the somatosensory cortex of the mouse. *Journal of Comparative Neurology, 171*, 545–560.

Schneider, G. E., & Jhavari, S. R. (1974). Neuroanatomical correlates of spared or altered function after brain lesions in the newborn hamster. In D. G. Stein, J. J. Rosen, & N. Butters (Eds.), *Plasticity and recovery of function in the central nervous system* (pp. 65–110). New York: Academic Press.

Simons, D., & Finger, S. (1983). Neonatal vs. later sensorimotor cortex damage: The ability to use spared fragments of target tissue to guide tactile learning. *Physiological Psychology, 11*, 29–34.

Simons, D., Puretz, J., & Finger, S. (1975). Effects of serial lesions of somatosensory cortex and further neodecortication on tactile retention in rats. *Experimental Brain Research, 23*, 353–366.

Soltmann, O. (1876). Experimentelle Studien über die Functionen des Grosshirns der Neugeborenen. *Jahrbuck für Kinderheikunde, 9*, 106–148.

Teuber, H. L., & Rudel, R. G. (1962) Behavior after cerebral lesions in children and adults. *Developmental Medicine and Child Neurology, 4,* 3–20.

Thompson, C. I., Harlow, H. F., Blomquist, A. J., & Schiltz, K. A. (1971). Recovery of function following prefrontal lobe damage in rhesus monkeys. *Brain Research, 35,* 37–48.

Tsang, Y. C. (1937). Maze learning in rats hemidecorticated in infancy. *Journal of Comparative Psychology, 24,* 221–254.

Vulpian, A. (1866). *Lecons sur la Physiologie Generale et Comparee du Systeme Nerveux.* Paris: Bailliere.

Weese, G. S., Niemand, D., & Finger, S. (1973). Cortical lesions and somesthesis in rats: Effects of training and overtraining prior to surgery. *Experimental Brain Research, 16,* 542–550.

Welker, C. (1976). Receptive fields of barrels in the somatosensory neocortex of the rat. *Journal of Comparative Neurology, 66,* 173–190.

Winick, M. (1976). *Malnutrition and brain development.* New York: Oxford University Press.

Woolsey, T. A. (1967). Somatosensory, auditory and visual cortical areas of the mouse. *Johns Hopkins Medical Journal, 121,* 91–112.

Woolsey, T. A., & Van der Loos, H. (1970). The structural organization of layer IV in the somatosensory region (S1) of the mouse cerebral cortex: The description of a cortical field composed of discrete cytoarchitectonic units. *Brain Research, 17,* 205–242.

18

Early Brain Damage
and Early Environment

*Bruno Will
and Francoise Eclancher*

Introduction

Prenatal and neonatal brain damage produced by mechanically disrupting events (trauma, infarct, necrosis, surgical lesions) has often been reported to be followed by less severe outcome than similar brain damage in adults. The first experimental studies that showed this relationship between age and sparing or recovery[1] of function were conducted by Kennard in monkeys during the late 1930s and early 1940s (Kennard, 1942). Called the Kennard principle, this relationship was confirmed by several other studies (e.g., Bregman & Goldberger, 1982; Goldman & Galkin, 1978; Murphy, Mize, & Schecter, 1975; Nonneman & Corwin, 1981; Spear, 1979; Sutherland, Kolb, Whishaw, & Becker, 1982; Tees, 1975). The interpretation of the Kennard principle is generally based on the assumption that the infant brain displays greater plasticity than the adult brain.

However, a growing body of evidence suggests that the neonatal brain may well be more vulnerable than the adult brain (e.g., Brazier,

---

[1]Although sparing and recovery correspond to different biological processes, most studies we refer to do not allow an exact identification of the particular process underlying the reported effects. For greater convenience, when not otherwise stated, we use only the term *recovery* for either of these processes.

1975; Perry &Cowey, 1982; Prendergast & Stelzner, 1976). Such findings, as well as other considerations, led some authors, such as Isaacson (1975), Schneider (1979), and Teuber (1974), to question the Kennard principle. Olmstead and Villablanca (1979), for instance, who studied recovery of paw usage in cats and kittens that had sustained caudate nuclei or frontal cortical ablations, found that the quantitative changes observed were at best equivocal vis-à-vis the Kennard principle, whereas the qualitative features of both the neurology and behavior indicated similar defects for animals with early and late brain damage. No difference in recovery from early and late central nervous system (CNS) damage, even from a quantitative point of view, was found by many authors, such as Bland and Cooper (1969), Eclancher and Karli (1979b, 1981a), and Thompson (1981). Several groups even reported experimental data that definitely contradicted the Kennard principle either by showing that the effects of brain damage were not a monotonic function of age (Meisel, Lumia, & Sachs, 1982; Perry & Cowey, 1982) or by showing better recovery of function in animals damaged at juvenile or adult age than in those damaged as infants (Cowey, Henken, & Perry, 1982; Eclancher & Karli, 1979a, 1981b; Gramsbergen, 1982). Eclancher, Schmitt, and Karli (1975) have shown that interspecific aggressiveness is observed in 90 to 95% of the rats amygdalectomized at Day 7 postnatally, whereas the occurrence of muricide (35%) remains closer to control levels (10%) in those operated on in adulthood (90 days). Similarly, they have shown that a bilateral ventromedial hypothalamic (VMH) lesion performed on 90-day-old rats results in no increase in the probability of initiating mouse killing, whereas virtually identical lesions performed in 7-day-old rat pups induce a highly significant increase in that probability (Eclancher & Karli, 1981b; Eclancher & Schmitt, 1972). Gramsbergen (1982) has shown that locomotor behavior of rats that had sustained hemicerebellectomy on the 5th or 10th day remain more impaired than rats operated upon the 30th day of age. Finally, it should be emphasized that Passingham, Perry, and Wilkinson (1983) found results that provide no support for Kennard's conclusions (1942) although they replicated her experiments using virtually identical experimental conditions. Yet the criticism against the Kennard principle based on such data is not as recent as generally thought: On the basis of several clinical observations of dramatic sparing of function in adults, Hebb suggested, as early as 1949, that a lesion sustained by an adult brain may be followed by less severe deficits than a similar lesion sustained by an immature brain. His interpretation of such findings was based on the assumption that the ability to solve problems was less diminished in subjects with a rich pretraumatic or preoperative experience because the subjects could rely on a variety of preoperatively learned strategies, whereas more naive brain-damaged subjects would be forced to learn the alternative strategies for the first time in a postoperative situation.

Obviously, the Kennard principle remains open to question and its generality needs at least to be restricted. Some of the major factors that might explain the discrepancies found in the cited studies are now briefly considered. One of these factors, the pre- and postoperative environment, is analyzed more thoroughly in the following paragraphs.

The Study of the Age Factor: Some Methodological Problems

AGE CANNOT BE DISSOCIATED FROM SOME OTHER FACTORS

The study of the age factor raises several basic methodological questions. First, the age factor, like other factors such as sex, cannot be properly dissociated from other factors, simply because we cannot make a subject young or old at will. When an experimenter chooses to compare young and old subjects at a given moment, the subjects have clearly not been randomly assigned to either young or old treatment groups. Therefore, they may differ in numerous factors other than age. Conversely, when subjects born at the same time are randomly assigned to different age groups, they will necessarily be tested at different periods and, consequently, in testing conditions which are not, strictly speaking, identical.

BOTH BRAIN AND BEHAVIOR VARY THROUGHOUT THE LIFESPAN

When considering age–brain damage interaction, there are even more complicated problems. As clearly stated by Johnson and Almli (1978), neither brain nor behavior are homogeneous throughout an animal's lifespan. When the duration of the postoperative period is constant for all groups, as in most studies, young and old subjects will be tested at different ages, although the young subjects, "rarely have the advantage of the equivalent of a 'culture free' testing situation, as most testing procedures have been developed using normal intact adult animals" (Johnson & Almli, 1978, p. 131). It is also not clear whether young and old subjects show sensory, motor, or motivational equivalence for the behavioral tasks used. Various significant interactions between age and brain damage, concerning either CNS dimension or behavior, may therefore be observed (Finger, 1978a; Jeannerod & Hecaen, 1979; Stein, Rosen, & Butters, 1974; Van Hof & Mohn, 1981). It should be added—and we now stress this point and its implications—that experience (i.e., the interaction between an organism and its environment) also is not at all homogeneous throughout the lifespan.

Interactions between Environment, Lesion, and Age: Behavioral Studies

ENVIRONMENT–LESION INTERACTION

Experience and age are linked factors. Early- and late-damaged subjects differ by the numerous interactions they have with their environment. Even when the environment is maintained as constant as is possible, young and old subjects have differentially interacted with it, first because in most cases this interaction occurs either pre- or postoperatively, and second, because this interaction lasts for different periods when the animals are tested at the same age. These differences should not be underestimated, because it has become clear that the environment may play equally important roles in brain-damaged and intact subjects (e.g., Will, 1981). Both behavioral and brain measurements may be strongly affected by pre- and postoperative environments.[2] The environments most often used in experimental designs are the so-called standard, impoverished, and enriched conditions. As indicated by Rosenzweig, Bennett, and Diamond (1972b), in the standard laboratory colony there are usually three rats in a cage, in the impoverished environment a rat is kept alone in a cage, and in the enriched environment, 12 rats live together

[2]For the effects of interoperative experience on recovery of function, see, for instance, Greenough, Fass, and DeVoogd (1976a).

in a large cage furnished with a variety of objects that are changed daily.

An already large number of studies, particularly in rodents, provides evidence that the outcome of brain injury may be dependent largely on the social and physical environment in which the subject was living either before or after CNS injury.

PREOPERATIVE ENVIRONMENT

Several authors have organized their experimental design so that the preoperative experience and the postoperative behavioral task are specifically related. In these studies, better sparing or recovery of function has been reported following preoperative familiarization with some aspects of the postoperative testing situations (e.g., Levere & Morlock, 1973; Miller & Cooper, 1974; Singh, 1974), as well as following preoperative overtraining in the behavioral task used again in postoperative testing (e.g., Lukaszewska & Thompson, 1967; Weese, Neimand, & Finger, 1973). These results all indicate that the relationship between preoperative experience and postoperative behavioral expression may be quite specific. However, "this may reflect both the limited test selection and the experimental emphasis on primary sensory neocortex lesions" (Greenough, Fass, & DeVoogd, 1976a, p. 20).

In view of these results, it could be assumed that only specific preoperative experience can facilitate postoperative sparing or recovery of function. This assumption is not fully accurate, because several reports are indicative of rather generalized transoperative effects of a preoperative enriched or socially increased experience, at least in the case of limbic damage. In this case, however, as well as after neocortex damage, the effects of preoperative experience seem to depend on both the lesion locus and the behavioral task used (e.g., Donovick, Burright, & Swidler, 1973; Engellenner, Goodlett, Burright, & Donovick, 1982; Hugues, 1965; Lewis, 1975). For instance, Hugues (1965) reported that preoperative enriched experience diminished maze-learning deficits that were induced by lesions of the anterodorsal as well as the posteroventral parts of the hippocampus, whereas group housing had such an alleviating effect only on the deficits induced by posteroventral lesions. In another study (Donovick et al., 1973), preoperative rearing conditions have been shown to affect feeding and exploratory behaviors, but not performance in a spatial

354   BRUNO WILL AND FRANCOISE ECLANCHER

alternation task, of rats with septal lesions. Likewise, following large
hippocampal lesions, hyperreactivity of rats was affected by preoperative enrichment or isolation, whereas their learning performance was not altered (Lewis, 1975).

POSTOPERATIVE ENVIRONMENT

Postoperative enriched experience was also shown to attenuate
behavioral symptoms following brain damage. The earliest experimentation that presented an exclusive analysis of postoperative environmental effects was probably that of Schwartz (1964). He made
bilateral posterior cortical lesions in 1-day-old rats. These rats, as well
as sham-lesioned controls, were then reared for 90 days in either a
standard or an enriched environment before being tested in the Hebb–
Williams maze. Schwartz found that early enriched experience offset
the effects of the lesions so efficiently that rats with cortical lesions
from the enriched environment made fewer errors than intact rats
from the standard environment. The study by Schwartz had the merit
of being the first to indicate that significant functional recovery is
possible even after bilateral one-stage lesions, but with the limitation
of given environmental and age conditions.
    In collaboration with Rosenzweig and the Bennett group (at the
University of California, Berkeley), Will has replicated the experiment conducted by Schwartz. The results, like those of Schwartz,
indicated that even though brain-injured rats showed a deficit in
maze learning when compared to control rats, they nevertheless performed at a higher level when previously exposed to a complex environment. Furthermore, Will and his associates have shown that
this kind of environmental therapy remained efficient even when the
duration of differential experience was reduced from 90 to 7 days
(Will, Deluzarche, & Kelche, 1983), or to 2 hours per day during 1
month (Will, Sutter, & Offerlin, 1977b), as well as when it started
only several weeks after neonatal cortical lesions (Will, Rosenzweig,
& Bennett, 1976). It should be emphasized that the effects of cortical
or dorsal hippocampal lesions sustained at 30 days of age (Einon,
Morgan, & Will, 1980; Will, Rosenzweig, Bennett, Hebert, & Morimoto, 1977a) or at 120 days of age (Kelche & Will, 1978; Will &
Rosenzweig, 1976) can also be attenuated by an enriched postoperative experience. This environmentally induced attenuation of symptoms has been observed in several strains of rats, in both genders,

after neocortical as well as hippocampal lesions and for various learning and memory tasks.

Numerous other studies have shown that recovery of function can be significantly altered by postoperative environmental conditions following various types of brain insult. Facilitatory effects of complex social and physical experience have been reported after various kinds of surgically (*e.g.*, Cornwell & Overman, 1981; Eclancher & Karli, 1980, 1981a; Karli, Eclancher, Vergnes, Chaurand, & Schmitt, 1974) or chemically (*e.g.*, Diaz, Ellison, & Masuoka, 1978; Stricker & Zigmond, 1975) produced brain damage. It has also been shown that an enriched condition may compensate for the effects of malnutrition (*e.g.*, Frankova, 1974; Levitsky & Barnes, 1972), hyperthyroidism (*e.g.*, Sjöden, 1977; Sjöden & Lindqvist, 1978), hypothyroidism (*e.g.*, Davenport, 1976), or lead exposure during development (Petit & Alfano, 1978). Likewise, a beneficial effect of an enriched experience has been observed in rats genetically selected for their poor performance in a maze-learning task (Cooper & Zubek, 1958) as well as in "dwarf" mutant mice characterized by a primary deficiency of the anterior hypophysis and by deficits in various learning and memory tasks (Bouchon & Will, 1982a, 1982b, 1983).

Some studies have shown that either the social or the physical aspects of the housing conditions are sufficient for producing significant modifications in functional recovery. Eclancher and Karli (1980, 1981a, 1981b) have shown, for instance, that isolation or group rearing strongly affects the performance of adult rats in a two-way active avoidance task after neonatal amygdaloid, septal, or VMH lesions. In contrast, these postoperative rearing conditions were shown to exert no effect on the increase of mouse-killing behavior induced by these early lesions (Eclancher *et al.*, 1975, Eclancher & Karli, 1979a, 1979b, 1981b). Will and his associates have observed that the mere exposure of isolated rats to a set of different objects every day for 1 month is a powerful therapeutic tool for alleviating deficits induced by hippocampal lesions in maze learning and in neotic behavioral reactivity towards novelty (Will, Misslin, Deluzarche, & Kelche, in preparation).

In conclusion, a large number of reports indicate that preoperative as well as postoperative environments may strongly affect the outcome of brain damage. When impoverished and enriched conditions are compared, the difference between the effects of these treatments generally appears even larger among brain-damaged than among control animals (e.g., Davenport, 1976). It may be that brain-damaged animals profit more from an enriched experience (e.g., Will *et al.*, 1983) or are harmed more by an impoverished experience (e.g., Sara, King, & Lazarus, 1976) than are control animals just because they are more sensitive or reactive to the effects of environment (e.g., Bernstein & Moyer, 1970). However, another explanation of the interaction between brain condition and environment may be linked to the characteristics of the behavioral tasks used. In most of these tasks, the performance improvement of the brain-damaged animals is clearly less affected by a possible ceiling or floor effect than is the performance of controls.

ENVIRONMENT–AGE INTERACTION

A few studies have reported small or no behavioral effects of environmental conditions on brain-damaged as well as on intact populations. We here briefly mention some of the major interpretations of these findings that are indicative of an absence of environmental effects on functional recovery and we stress particularly one interpretation, based on the effects of the age factor.

Bland and Cooper (1969) were probably the first to report results indicative of the absence of environmental effects on functional recovery. They found that enriched experience was ineffective for improving the performance of rats in several visual-brightness and pattern-discrimination tasks when the rats had sustained visual cortex lesions as infants or adults. Similar results were reported by Cornwell and Overman (1981) in kittens. Likewise, dark- or light-rearing had no impact on pattern discrimination in rats that had sustained neonatal striate lesions (Tees, 1975), and enriched experience did not improve tactile discrimination after somatosensory cortex ablation in rats (Finger, 1978b).

All of these studies that failed to demonstrate any beneficial effects of environmental enrichment or sensory stimulation appear to concern specific sensory capabilities that are known to depend on rather limited regions of the brain. Therefore, as already stated by Greenough, Snow, and Fiala (1976b) as well as Finger (1978b), it appears that the impact of experience may depend on highly specific task variables (i.e., the extent to which skills acquired in the rearing environment can be carried over to the test situation).

However, task variables are certainly not the only factors that may account for the presence or absence of environmental effects. Several other factors may also interact with the environmental factor, such as species (Stuurman & Van Hof, 1980), sex (McConnell, Uylings, Swanson, & Verwer, 1981), lesion size (Will *et al.*, 1976; Eclancher & Karli, 1981b), and as shown in the following, lesion locus and age.

With regard to lesion locus, Eclancher and Karli (1979a, 1979b, 1981b) showed that amygdaloid, septal, and VMH neonatal lesions in rats provoke a significant increase in the probability of occurrence of mouse-killing behavior, irrespective of the postoperative rearing conditions (in groups or in isolation). Since the same behavioral measurement (elicitation of mouse killing) was affected by the same rearing conditions following lesions of other structures, such as olfactory bulbs (Karli *et al.*, 1974; Didiergeorges & Karli, 1966) or mediodorsal thalamus (Eclancher & Karli, 1981b), it cannot be argued that the absence of environmental effects following amygdaloid, septal, and VMH lesions is due to task specificity. A study by Will, Kelche, and Deluzarche (1981) provides another example of a situation in which such an argument cannot be used. They tested young rats that had sustained bilateral entorhinal cortex lesions on spontaneous alternation and a maze-learning task. They found that environmental enrichment improved performance only in sham-lesioned rats and that there was virtually no environmental effect in the rats with lesions. Because highly significant environmental effects were previously found using the same maze-learning task with rats of the same strain, sex, and age, but which had sustained lesions of the occipital cortex (Will *et al.*, 1977a), it has been suggested that the effects of postoperative environmental conditions are, in part at least, dependent on the lesion locus.

Finally, one more important factor that might modulate the environmental effects should be mentioned, namely, age. It is known that the effects of differential experience may vary as a function of age in intact as well as in brain-damaged animals (e.g., Rosenzweig & Bennett, 1977). Forgays and Read (1962), for instance, have reported that intact rats show the highest sensitivity to their environmental conditions immediately after weaning. Similarly, for brain-damaged animals, it has been reported that young animals may be more sensitive or reactive to the environmental conditions than those that have sustained brain damage when older (e.g., Goldman, 1976; Sjödén, 1977).

The same environmental conditions may be differentially perceived by young and adult subjects and may thus lead to different behavioral changes. For instance, Eclancher (in press) has observed that rearing rats in groups from weaning (25 days) until adult age (85 days) prevents the increase of the probability of occurrence of mouse-

killing behavior in the rats that have sustained olfactory bulb ablation at weaning. In contrast, these same rearing conditions do not
prevent the increase of the probability of occurrence of the same
behavior in rats that have sustained virtually the same ablation at
adult age (85 days). Thus, it can be assumed that the same environmental rearing, given at the same age and time, is not equally experienced by the rats operated on in infancy and those operated on at
adult age. Furthermore, in a study carried out in 1966, Didiergeorges
and Karli found that group rearing, contrary to isolation rearing,
prevents an increase of muricide in rats that have sustained olfactory
bulb ablation at adult age. It appears from the results of these studies
that the postoperative environment is more critical than the preoperative environment for the development of mouse-killing behavior following early as well as late olfactory bulb ablations. This age-
dependent sensitivity to the environment may, of course, be quite
critical for certain particular developmental periods, referred to as
critical or sensitive periods.

Although we have shown that there exists sufficient evidence that
demonstrates that, at least under certain circumstances, brain-
damaged subjects are also (and sometimes highly) responsive to their
environment, it is far less clear whether brain-damaged and intact
subjects are identically responsive to their environment and whether
differentially reared subjects are identically responsive to a given
brain injury.

Interactions between Environment, Lesion, and Age: Brain Measures

LESION–AGE INTERACTION

Brain damage in infants is followed by the degeneration of many
more neurons than in adults (e.g., Bleier, 1969; Perry & Cowey, 1982;
Prendergast & Stelzner, 1976) and often results in an overall shrink-
ing of brain size which has never been reported, to our knowledge,
after similar lesions sustained in adulthood. For instance, inflicting
cortical or limbic lesions within 10 days of birth has been reported to
reduce the growth of the cortical bulk in cats (Issacson, Nonneman, &
Schmaltz, 1968), rabbits (Nonneman, 1970), and rats (Will et al.,
1976). Such findings obviously should be correlated with functional
modifications that contradict the Kennard principle, unless the defi-

cits induced by early lesions would be more efficiently compensated for by whatever process underlies apparent recovery of function.

Although Kalil and Reh (1979) have stated that mammalian CNS axons severed early in life may regenerate into original terminal sites, even over a long distance and via a new anomalous pathway, the evidence seems to indicate that functional recovery after infant CNS injury may be alternatively explained. The infant CNS was shown to have a capacity greater than the adult CNS for preservation of projections that develop late and thereby escape the effects of direct damage (e.g., Bregman & Goldberger, 1982), for preservation of normally transient projections (e.g., Perry & Cowey, 1982), and for reorganization (e.g., Lund, Cunningham, & Lund, 1973; Lynch & Gall, 1979; Schneider, 1973). Furthermore, maturation and aging add restrictions not only to extent but also to latency and speed of at least some of the processes involved in reorganization (Gall & Lynch, 1978). Thus, infant or young brain-damaged subjects may show greater recovery of function than do adults by means of their greater capacity for neuronal preservation or reorganization. However, reorganization often appears to take the form of quite anomalous projections and connections (e.g., Crutcher, 1981; Kalil & Reh, 1979; Loy & Moore, 1977; Schneider, 1973, 1979). As shown, for instance, by Schneider (1979) as well as Smith, Steward, Cotman, and Lynch (1973), these new connections can be functionally maladaptive. The causal relationship between this anomalous neuronal reorganization and functional maladaptation was further demonstrated by an experiment in which Schneider (1979) partially corrected the observed dysfunction by sectioning the aberrant projections.

In summary, the brain that is injured in infancy is paradoxically characterized both by a larger susceptibility to neuronal death and by a larger potentiality for reorganization (larger plasticity) than the mature or senescent brain; this larger plasticity of the infant brain either may help overcome the deleterious effects of CNS injury or, on the contrary, may increase the lesion-induced symptoms.

ENVIRONMENT–LESION INTERACTION

What clouds the issue even more is the possibility of an interaction between abnormal cellular processes and environmental conditions. As previously shown, recovery of function may be quite different for animals reared in different environments. When there exists a genu-

ine biological interaction in recovery of function between brain condition and environment, this interaction may be explained in two
different ways, according to whether pre- or postoperative environment is considered. When the subjects have the opportunity to experience different environments before surgery, they obviously have
different brains at the time of surgery (e.g., Bennett, 1976; Greenough, 1976; Rothblat & Schwartz, 1978).

Transoperative survival of knowledge or capacity may, of course,
be dependent on the preoperative structural and functional characteristics of the injured brain. When differential experience is postoperatively given, functional recovery may also be dependent on several
structural and functional CNS characteristics that can be shown to
be modified by that experience. Although the evidence remains too
scarce to give us any clear indications of the mechanisms by which
postoperative experience could affect the outcome of brain injury, the
few published results are supportive of enrichment-dependent compensatory effects such as increase of cellular survival (Will et al.,
1977a), increase in metabolism (Will et al., 1977a), or increase in
synaptic connectivity (Kelche & Will, 1982) in areas adjacent to the
lesion. It has been suggested that these mechanisms might be trig-
gered by an initial glial trophic response to differential experience
(Will, 1981).

ENVIRONMENT–AGE INTERACTION

Several studies conducted on intact animals have shown that the
magnitude of the cerebral effects of differential experience varies
with age at the onset of the experience. For instance, Bennett (1976)
reported that, whatever the age at the onset of differential rearing
(25, 60, 185, or 290 days), the occipital cortex of rats enriched for 30
days was heavier than that of the rats impoverished for the same
period. However, the magnitude of this difference regularly decreased with age (9.6, 7.2, 6.0, and 4.8%, respectively). Likewise,
Greenough et al. (1976b) stated that dendritic branching in the occipital cortex was significantly affected by differential rearing (enriched versus impoverished) that started at weaning, whereas no
such effect was found when differential rearing started at 90 days,
even though in this case the controlled rearing lasted for three times
as long (90 days versus 30 days).

However, when considering other cerebral variables, such as the
activity of acetylcholinesterase (ACHE), cholinesterase (CHE), or cortical thickness (Rosenzweig, Bennett, & Diamond, 1972b) or RNA/

DNA (Bennett & Rosenzweig, unpublished; in: Rosenzweig & Bennett, 1977), it appears that the effects of differential experience seem relatively age-independent. Cortical weight as well as occipital ACHE and CHE activities were significantly modified by differential rearing (lasting 30, 60, or 90 days in enriched, standard, or impoverished conditions) even when this experience began at about 285 days (Riege, 1971). However, the enzyme activities were affected by the environmental conditions only when the rats had remained in those conditions for at least 90 days. The older the animals are when differentially reared, the longer must this rearing period be if it is to significantly affect their brain measurements.

Conclusion: The Kennard Principle Needs Qualification

Although numerous authors have reported data that confirm the Kennard principle, especially when the effects of cortical lesions were considered, there are too many experimental studies that fail to corroborate or even contradict that principle. Even though some discrepancies in results might be explained by methodological differences, it should be remembered that recovery of function following brain damage depends on many factors other than age (and developmental status of the system studied), such as lesion locus, species, and sex; but also, as was shown, it depends on the experience provided by the environment either pre- or post-CNS injury. This environmental factor is able to strongly modulate recovery in the direction of functional impairment (e.g., Sara *et al.*, 1976) or improvement (e.g., Will *et al.*, 1983) and thus, under certain circumstances, may be used as a therapeutic tool. The indirectly adaptive or maladaptive environmental effects often appear to be more pronounced in young than in adult animals, and it can thus be assumed that recovery of function in infants or juveniles can be either greater or more limited than in adults. For all these reasons, it could even be considered astonishing to find the Kennard principle so often restated.

Acknowledgments

This work was supported by CNRS grant ATP 6580085.40 to B. Will and by DRET Grant n° 80/424 to P. Karli. The authors are greatly indebted to P. Karli, V. H. Perry, and T. Leis for their critical reading of the manuscript and for their suggestions.

References

Bennett, E. L. (1976). Cerebral effects of differential experience and training. In M. R. Rosenzweig & Bennett E. L. (Eds.), *Neural mechanisms of learning and memory* (pp. 279–287). London: MIT Press.

Bernstein, H., & Moyer, K. E. (1970). Aggressive behavior in the rat: Effects of isolation and olfactory bulb lesions. *Brain Research, 20,* 75–84.

Bland, B. H., & Cooper, R. M. (1969). Posterior neodecortication in the rat: Age at operation and experience. *Journal of Comparative and Physiological Psychology, 69,* 345–354.

Bleier, R. (1969). Retrograde transsynaptic cellular degeneration in mammillary and ventral tegmental nuclei following limbic decortication in rabbits of various ages. *Brain Research, 15,* 365–393.

Bouchon, R., & Will, B. (1982a). Effets des conditions d'élevage après le sevrage sur les performances d'apprentissage des Souris "Dwarf." *Physiology and Behavior, 28,* 971–978.

Bouchon, R., & Will, B. (1982b). Effects of early enriched and restricted environments on the exploratory and locomotor activity of Dwarf mice. *Behavioral and Neural Biology, 35,* 174–186.

Bouchon, R., & Will, B. (1983). Effects of post-weaning environment and apparatus dimension on spontaneous alternation as a function of phenotype in "Dwarf" mice. *Physiology and Behavior, 30*(2), 213–219.

Brazier, M. A. B. (Ed.) (1975). *Growth and development of the brain: Nutritional, genetic, and environmental factors* (Vol. 1). International Brain Research Organization Monograph Series. New York: Academic Press.

Bregman, B. S., & Goldberger, M. E. (1982). Anatomical plasticity and sparing of function after spinal cord damage in neonatal cats. *Science, 217,* 553–555.

Cooper, R. M., & Zubek, J. P. (1958). Effects of enriched and restricted early environments on the learning ability of bright and dull rats. *Canadian Journal of Psychology, 12*(3), 159–164.

Cornwell, P., & Overman, W. (1981). Behavioral effects of early rearing conditions and neonatal lesions of the visual cortex in kittens. *Journal of Comparative and Physiological Psychology. 95*(6), 848–862.

Cowey, A., Henken, D. B., & Perry, V. H. (1982). Effects on visual acuity of neonatal or adult tectal ablation in rats. *Experimental Brain Research, 48,* 149–152.

Crutcher, K. A. (1981). Cholinergic denervation of rat neocortex results in sympathetic innervation. *Experimental Neurology, 74,* 324–329.

Davenport, J. W. (1976). Environmental therapy in hypothyroid and other disadvantaged animal populations. In R. N. Walsh & W. T. Greenough (Eds.), *Environments as therapy for brain dysfunction (pp. 71–114).* New York: Plenum.

Diaz, J., Ellison, G., & Masuoka, D. (1978). Stages of recovery from central norepinephrine lesions in enriched and improverished environments: A behavioral and biochemical study. *Experimental Brain Research, 31,* 117–130.

Didiergeorges, F., & Karli, P. Stimulations "sociales" et inhibition de l'agressivité interspécifique chez le rat privé de ses afférences olfactives. *Comptes Rendus des séances de la Société de Biologie, 1966, 160,* 2445–2447.

Donovick, P. J., Burright, R. G., & Swidler, M. A. (1973). Presurgical rearing environment alters exploration, fluid consumption, and learning of septal lesioned and control rats. *Physiology and Behavior, 11,* 543–553.

Eclancher, F. (1984). Early and adult olfactory bulbectomy: Role played by the environment in the initiation of mouse-killing behavior. *Aggressive Behavior.*

Eclancher, F., & Karli, P. (1979a). Effects of early amygdaloid lesions on the development of reactivity in the rat. *Physiology and Behavior, 22,* 1123–1134.

Eclancher, F., & Karli, P. (1979b). Septal damage in infant and adult rats: Effects on activity, emotionality and muricide. *Aggressive Behavior, 5,* 389–415.

Eclancher, F., & Karli, P. (1980). Effects of infant and adult amygdaloid lesions upon acquisition of two-way active avoidance by the adult rat: Influence of rearing conditions. *Physiology and Behavior, 24*(5), 887–893.

Eclancher, F., & Karli, P. (1981a). Influence of rearing conditions on the acquisition of the two-way active avoidance responses by rats septalectomized at an early age. *Behavioural Brain Research, 3,* 83–98.

Eclancher, F., & Karli, P. (1981b). Environmental influences on behavioural effects of early and late limbic and diencephalic lesions in the rat. In M. W. Van Hof & G. Mohn (Eds.), *Functional recovery from brain damage* (pp. 149–165). Amsterdam/New York/Oxford: Elsevier.

Eclancher, F., & Schmitt, P. (1972). Effets de lésions précoces de l'amygdale et de l'hypothalamus médian sur le développement du comportement d'agression interspécifique du rat. *Journal de Physiologie, 65,* 231.

Eclancher, F., Schmitt, P., & Karli, P. (1975). Effets de lésions précoces de l'amygdale sur le développement de l'aggressivité interspécifique du Rat. *Physiology and Behavior, 14,* 277–283.

Einon, D. F., Morgan, M. J., & Will, B. E. (1980). Effects of post-operative environment on recovery from dorsal hippocampal lesions in young rats: Tests of spatial memory and motor transfer. *Quarterly Journal of Experimental Psychology, 32,* 137–148.

Engellenner, W. J., Goodlett, C. R., Burright, R. G., & Donovick, P. J. (1982). Environmental enrichment and restriction: Effects on reactivity, exploration and maze learning in mice with septal lesions. *Physiology and Behavior, 29*(5), 885–893.

Finger, S. (Ed.) (1978a). *Recovery from brain damage. Research and theory* (pp. 1–423). London: Plenum.

Finger, S. (1978b). Environmental attenuation of brain-lesion symptoms. In S. Finger (Ed.), *Recovery from brain damage* (pp. 297–329). London: Plenum.

Forgays, D. G., & Read, J. M. (1962). Crucial periods for free-environmental experience in the rat. *Journal of Comparative and Physiological Psychology, 55*(5), 816–818.

Frankova, S. (1974). Interaction between early malnutrition and stimulation in animals. In J. Cravioto, L. Hambraeus, & B. Vahlquist (Eds.), *Early malnutrition and mental development, Symposia of the Swedish Nutritional Foundation* XII (pp. 202–209). Uppsala: Almqvist & Wiksell.

Gall, C., & Lynch, G. (1978). Rapid axon sprouting in the neonatal rat hippocampus. *Brain Research, 153,* 357–362.

Goldman, P. S. (1976). Maturation of the mammalian nervous system and the ontogeny of behavior. *Advances in the study of behavior, 7,* 1–90.

Goldman, P. S., & Galkin, T. W. (1978). Prenatal removal of frontal association cortex in the fetal rhesus monkey; anatomical and functional consequences in postnatal life. *Brain Research, 152,* 451–485.

Gramsbergen, A. (1982). The effects of cerebellar hemispherectomy in the young rat. I. Behavioural sequelae. *Behavioural Brain Research, 6,* 85–92.

Greenough, W. T. (1976). Enduring brain effects of differential experience and training. In M. R. Rosenzweig & E. L. Bennett (Eds.), *Neural mechanisms of learning and memory* (pp. 255–278). Cambridge, MA: M.I.T. Press.

Greenough, W. T., Fass, B., & DeVoogd, T. J. (1976a). The influence of experience on recovery following brain damage in rodents: Hypotheses based on developmental research. In R. N. Walsh & W. T. Greenough (Eds.), *Environments as therapy for brain dysfunction* (pp. 10–50). London: Plenum.

Greenough, W. T., Snow, F. M., & Fiala, B. A. (1976b). Environmental complexity versus isolation. A sensitive period for effects on cortical and hippocampal dendritic branching in rats? *Neuroscience Abstracts, 2*(1184), 824.

Hebb, D. O. (1949). *Organization of behavior.* New York: Wiley.

Hughes, K. R. (1965). Dorsal and ventral hippocampus lesions and maze learning: Influence of preoperative environment. *Canadian Journal of Psychology, 19*(4), 325–332.

Isaacson, R. L. (1975). The myth of recovery from early brain damage. In N. R. Ellis (Ed.), *Aberrant development in infancy.* Potomac: Erlbaum.

Isaacson, R. L., Nonneman, A. J., & Schmaltz, L. W. (1968). Behavioral and anatomical sequelae of damage to the infant limbic system. In R. L. Isaacson (Ed.), *The neuropsychology of development.* New York: Wiley.

Jeannerod, M., & Hecaen, H. (1979). *Adaptation et restauration des fonctions nerveuses* (pp. 1–392). Villeurbanne: Simep.

Johnson, D., & Almli, R. (1978). Age, brain damage, and performance. In S. Finger (Ed.), *Recovery from brain damage* (pp. 115–134). New York: Plenum.

Kalil, K., & Reh, T. (1979). Regrowth of severed axons in the neonatal central nervous system. Establishment of normal connections. *Science, 205,* 1158–1161.

Karli, P., Eclancher, F., Vergnes, M., Chaurand, J. P., & Schmitt, P. (1974). Emotional responsiveness and interspecific aggressiveness in the rat: Interactions between genetic and experiential determinants. In J. H. F. Van Abeelen (Ed.), *Genetics of behaviour* (pp. 291–319). Amsterdam: Elsevier.

Kelche, C. R., & Will, B. E. (1978). Effets de l'environnement sur la restauration fonctionnelle après lésions hippocampiques chez des rats adultes. *Physiology and Behavior, 21,* 935–941.

Kelche, C., & Will, B. (1982). Effects of postoperative environments following dorsal hippocampal lesions on dendritic branching and spines in rat occipital cortex. *Brain Research, 245,* 107–115.

Kennard, M. A. (1942). Cortical reorganization of motor function. *Archives of Neurology and Psychiatry, 48,* 227–240.

Levere, T. E., & Morlock, G. W. (1973). Nature of visual recovery following posterior neodecortication in the hooded rat. *Journal of Comparative and Physiological Psychology, 83,* 62–67.

Levitsky, D. A., & Barnes, R. H. (1972). Nutritional and environmental interactions in the behavioral development of the rat: Long-term effects. *Science, 176,* 68–71.

Lewis, M. E. (1975). *The influence of early experience on the effects of one and two-stage hippocampal lesions in male rats.* Unpublished Masters thesis, Clark University.

Loy, T., & Moore, R. Y. (1977). Anomalous innervation of the hippocampal formation by peripheral sympathetic axons following mechanical injury. *Experimental Neurology, 57*(2), 645–650.

Lukaszewska, I., & Thompson, R. (1967). Retention of an overtrained pattern discrimination following pretectal lesion in rats. *Psychonomic Science, 8,* 121–122.

Lund, R. D., Cunningham, T. J., & Lund, J. S. (1973). Modified optic projections after unilateral eye removal in young rats. *Brain Behavior and Evolution, 8,* 51–72.

Lynch, G., & Gall, C. (1979). Organization and reorganization in the central nervous system: Evolving concepts of brain plasticity. In F. Falkner & J. M. Tanner (Eds.), *Human Growth* (Vol. 3, pp. 125–144). New York: Plenum.

McConnell, P., Uylings, H. B. M., Swanson, H. H., & Verwer, R. W. H. (1981). Sex differences in effects of environmental stimulation on brain weight of previously undernourished rats. *Behavioural Brain Research, 3,* 411–415.

Meisel. R. L., Lumia, A. R., & Sachs, B. D. (1982). Disruption of copulatory behavior of male rats by olfactory bulbectomy at two, but not ten, days of age. *Experimental Neurology, 77,* 612–624.

Miller, L. G., & Cooper, R. M. (1974). Translucent occluders and the role of visual cortex in pattern vision. *Brain Research, 79,* 45–59.

Murphy, E. H., Mize, R. R., & Schecter, P. B. (1975). Visual discrimination following infant and adult ablation of cortical areas 17, 18, and 19 in the cat. *Experimental Neurology, 49,* 386–405.

Nonneman, A. J. (1970). *Anatomical and behavioral consequences of early brain damage in the rabbit.* Unpublished doctoral dissertation, University of Florida.

Nonneman, A. J., & Corwin, J. V. (1981). Differential effects of prefrontal cortex ablation in neonatal, juvenile, and young adult rats. *Journal of Comparative and Physiological Psychology, 95*(4), 588–602.

Olmstead, C. E., & Villablanca, J. R. (1979). Effects of caudate nuclei or frontal cortical ablations in cats and kittens: Paw usage. *Experimental Neurology, 63,* 559–572.

Passingham, R. E., Perry, V. H., & Wilkinson, F. (1983). The long-term effects of removal of sensorimotor cortex in infant and adult rhesus monkeys. *Brain.*

Perry, V. H., & Cowey, A. (1982). A sensitive period for ganglion cell degeneration and the formation of aberrant retinofugal connections following tectal lesions in rats. *Neuroscience, 7*(3), 583–594.

Petit, T., & Alfano, D. P. (1978). Differential experience following developmental lead exposure: Effects on brain and behavior. *Pharmacology Biochemistry and Behavior, 11,* 165–171.

Prendergast, J., & Stelzner, D. J. (1976). Changes in the magnocellular portion of the red nucleus following thoracic hemisection in the neonatal and adult rat. *Journal of Comparative Neurology, 166,* 163–172.

Riege, W. H. (1971). Environmental influences on brain and behavior of year-old rats. *Developmental Psychobiology, 4*(2), 157–167.

Rosenzweig, M. R., & Bennett, E. L. (1977). Effects of environmental enrichment or impoverishment on learning and on brain values in rodents. In A. Oliverio (Ed.), *Genetics, environment and intelligence* (pp. 163–196). Amsterdam: Elsevier.

Rosenzweig, M. R., Bennett, E. L., & Diamond, M. C. (1972a). Brain changes in response to experience. *Scientific American, 226,* 22–29.

Rosenzweig, M. R., Bennett, E. L., & Diamond, M. C. (1972b). Chemical and anatomical plasticity of the brain; replications and extensions, 1970. In J. Gaits (Ed.), *Macromolecules and behavior* (2nd ed., pp. 205–277). New York: Appleton-Century-Crofts.

Rothblat, L. A., & Schwartz, M. L. (1978). Altered early environment: Effects on the brain and visual behavior. In R. D. Walk & H. L. Pick (Eds.), *Perception and experience* (pp. 7–36). New York: Plenum.

Sara, V., King, T., & Lazarus, L. (1976). The influence of early nutrition and environmental rearing on brain growth and behaviour. *Experientia, 32,* 1538–1539.

Schneider, G. E. (1973). Early lesions of superior colliculus: Factors affecting the formation of abnormal retinal projections. *Brain Behavior and Evolution, 8,* 73–109.

Schneider, G. E. (1979). Is it really better to have your brain lesion early? A revision of the "Kennard principle." *Neuropsychologia, 17*, 557–583.

Schwartz, S. (1964). Effect of neonatal cortical lesions and early environmental factors on adult rat behavior. *Journal of Comparative and Physiological Psychology, 57*, 72–77.

Singh, D. (1974). Role of preoperative experience on reaction to quinine taste in hypothalamic hyperphagic rats. *Journal of Comparative and Physiological Psychology, 86*, 674–678.

Sjöden, P. O. (1977). *Behavioral disturbances induced by neonatal thyroid hormone stimulation in rats.* Unpublished doctoral dissertation, University of Uppsala.

Sjöden, P. O., & Lindqvist, M. (1978). Behavioral effects of neonatal thyroid hormones and differential postweaning rearing in rats. *Developmental Psychobiology, 11*(4), 371–383.

Smith, R. L., Steward, O., Cotman, C., & Lynch, G. (1973). Axon sprouting in the hippocampal formation and behavioral recovery following unilateral entorhinal cortex lesions. *Third Annual Meeting of the Society for Neuroscience*, San Diego.

Spear, P. D. (1979). Behavioral and neurophysiological consequences of visual cortex damage: Mechanisms of recovery. *Progress in Psychobiology and Physiological Psychology, 8*, 45–90.

Stein, D. G., Rosen, J. J., & Butters, N. (Eds.) (1974). *Plasticity and recovery of function in the central nervous system* (pp. 1–516). London: Academic Press.

Stricker, E. M., & Zigmond, M. J. (1975). Recovery of function following damage to central catecholamine-containing neurons: A neurochemical model for the lateral hypothalamic syndrome. In J. M. Sprague & A. N. Epstein (Eds.), *Progress in psychobiology and physiological psychology* (Vol. 6, pp. 121–188). New York: Academic Press.

Stuurman, P. M., & Van Hof, M. W. (1980). Pattern discrimination in rabbits kept in environments of different complexities after unilateral removal of the occipital cortex. *Behavioural Brain Research, 1*, 211–226.

Sutherland, R. J., Kolb, B., Whishaw, I. Q., & Becker, J. B. (1982). Cortical noradrenaline depletion eliminates sparing of spatial learning after neonatal frontal cortex damage in the rat. *Neuroscience Letters, 32*, 125–130.

Tees, R. C. (1975). The effects of neonatal striate lesions and visual experience on form discrimination in the rat. *Canadian Journal of Psychology, 29*(1), 66–85.

Teuber, H. L. (1974). Recovery of function after lesions of the central nervous system: History and prospects. In E. Eidelberg & D. G. Stein (Eds.), *Functional recovery after lesions of the nervous system. Neuroscience Research Program Bulletin, 12*, 197–211.

Thompson, C. I. (1981). Learning in rhesus monkeys after amygdalectomy in infancy or adulthood. *Behavioural Brain Research, 2*, 81–101.

Van Hof, M. W., & Mohn, G. Eds.) (1981). *Functional recovery from brain damage* (pp. 1–449). Amsterdam: Elsevier/North-Holland.

Weese, G. D., Neimand, D., & Finger, S. (1973). Cortical lesions and somesthesis in rats: Effects of training and overtraining prior to surgery. *Experimental Brain Research, 16*, 542–550.

Will, B. E. (1981). The influence of environment on recovery after brain damage in rodents. In M. W. Van Hof & G. Mohn (Eds.), *Functional recovery from brain damage* (pp. 167–188). Amsterdam: Elsevier.

Will, B., Deluzarche, F., & Kelche, C. (1983). Does post-operative environment attenuate or exacerbate symptoms which follow hippocampal lesions in rats? *Behavioural Brain Research*, 7, 125–132.

Will, B., Kelche, C., & Deluzarche, F. (1981). Effects of postoperative environment on functional recovery after entorhinal cortex lesions in the rat. *Behavioral and Neural Biology*, 1981, *33*, 303–316.

Will, B., Misslin, R., Deluzarche, F., & Kelche, C. (in preparation). The effects of postoperative physical environment on novelty seeking behavior and maze learning in rats with hippocampal lesions.

Will, B. E., & Rosenzweig, M. R. (1976). Effets de l'environnement sur la récupération fonctionnelle après lésions cérébrales chez des rats adultes. *Biology of Behaviour*, *1*, 5–16.

Will, B. E., Rosenzweig, M. R., & Bennett, E. L. (1976). Effects of differential environments on recovery from neonatal brain lesions, measured by problem-solving scores and brain dimensions. *Physiology and Behavior*, *16*, 603–611.

Will, B. E., Rosenzweig, M. R., Bennett, E. L., Hebert, M., & Morimoto, H. (1977a). Relatively brief environmental enrichment aids recovery of learning capacity and alters brain measures after postweaning brain lesions in rats. *Journal of Comparative and Physiological Psychology*, *91*, 33–50.

Will, B. E., Sutter, A. R., & Offerlin, M. R. (1977b). Effets de la métamphétamine et d'un environnement complexe sur la récupération comportementale après atteinte cérébrale. *Psychopharmacology*, *51*, 273–277.

Author Index

The numerals in italics indicate pages on which the complete references appear.

A

Adolph, E. F., 78, *92*
Adrien, J., 88, *92*
Aggarwal, N., 238, *250*
Agnati, L. F., 21, *33*
Ajmone-Marsan, C., 182, 196, *207*
Akers, R. M., 202, *207*
Akert, K., 141, 142, *151*, 212, *224*, *225*
Al Salti, M., 258, 261, *265*
Albert, D. J., 302, *306*
Alderson, L. M., 76, *92*
Alexander, G. E., 144, *151*
Alfano, D. P., 355, *365*
Alkana, R. L., 300, *311*
Allin, J. T., 80, *93*
Almli, C. R., 74, 78, 84, 88, *95*, *96*, 99,
    101, 101, 102, 104, 105, 106, 107,
    110, 111, 113, *114*, *115*, *116*, 140,
    152, 158, *175*, 328, 330, *345*, *346*,
    351, 352, *364*
Alongi, R., 333, *345*

Altman, J., 82, *93*, 120, 121, 122, 133,
    134, 157, *175*, 264, *267*
Amano, T., 315, *324*
Ambrosio, E., 315, *325*
Anand, B. K., 87, *93*
Anderson, W. J., 157, *175*
Angaut, P., 199, *206*
Antelman, S. M., 256, *265*
Arai, Y., 323, *324*
Ariel, M., 244, *248*
Arigbede, M. O., 241, *251*
Arimatsu, Y., 315, *324*
Armand, J., 195, *209*
Arnott, G., 205, *206*
Aron, C., 258, 261, *265*
Ary, M., 119, *135*, 244, *249*
Asano, T., 299, *310*
Asratian, E. A., 156, 164, *175*
Astic, L., 264, *265*
Austin, G. M., 205, *206*
Avery, D. L., 183, 186, *209*
Avissar, S., 315, *324*
Azuara, M. C., 315, *325*

Subject Index

A

Aberrant connections, 164, 175, 203–206, 238, 240, 243, 332, 359; *see also* Axonal sprouting
Acetylcholine, 88
Acetylcholinesterase, 360–361
ACTH, *see* Corticosteroids
Adrenalectomy, 299
Adrenal glands, 316
Aggression, 86, 212, 298, 350
Agonistic behavior, 298
Alcohol, 300
Alpha-methylparatyrosine, 27
Amphetamines, 26–30, 51, 81, 83, 213
Amygdala, 212–214, 264, 350, 355, 357
Androgen, 313–324
Angiotensin II, 279
Anomalous projections, *see* Aberrant connections
Aphagia, 28, 87, 104–114
Aphasia, 328
Apomorphine, 27, 30, 83
Arborization, 18, 23
Autoradiography, 189, 190, 195, 242
Avoidance behavior, 76, 297, 303, 355; *see also* Passive avoidance
Axonal proliferation, 24; *see also* Axonal sprouting
Axonal retraction, *see* Retraction of axons
Axonal sprouting, 18, 35, 43, 101, 114, 175, 180, 204–206, 263

B

Barrell organs, 335–342
Basal ganglia, 75–76
Body temperature, *see* Temperature regulation
Body weight, 106–108, 158, 160, 183, 259–285
Butaclamol, 27

C

Catecholamines, 19, 20, 244, 296
Caudate nucleus, 75, 140–151, 201–202, 350
Cell death, 9, 13, 359
Cerebellorubral connections, 37, 165, 167–168, 193, 198–199
Cerebellum, 35–37, 50, 55–57, 102, 131, 155–175, 189, 204, 350
Cerebral cortex,
 frontal, 17, 18, 23, 64, 118, 138–151, 201, 212–214, 223, 254, 264, 299, 303, 304, 350
 dorsomedial, 140–151
 dorsolateral, 140–151, 329
 motor, 54, 59, 67, 130, 189, 197, 211, 327, 328
 occipital, 23, 52–60, 67, 133, 215–222, 229–247, 303, 354, 356, 357, 360–361
 orbital, 140–151
 parietal, 28, 37, 40, 42, 55–58, 62, 67, 133, 212, 332–344, 356
 posterior, *see* occipital
 somatosensory, *see* parietal
 striate, *see* occipital
 sucal, 140–151
 visual, *see* occipital
Cerebral peduncle, 37
Cerebrorubral connections, 37
Cholinesterase, 360–361
Cholecystokinin, 83
Chromatin cells, 29–30
Chromatin body, 8